Emerging and Re-Emerging infectious Diseases

Editor

GERALD KAYINGO

PHYSICIAN ASSISTANT CLINICS

www.physicianassistant.theclinics.com

Consulting Editors
KIM ZUBER
JANE S. DAVIS

July 2023 • Volume 8 • Number 3

ELSEVIER

1600 John F. Kennedy Boulevard ● Suite 1800 ● Philadelphia, Pennsylvania, 19103-2899

http://www.theclinics.com

PHYSICIAN ASSISTANT CLINICS Volume 8, Number 3
July 2023 ISSN 2405-7991, ISBN-13: 978-0-323-93857-0

Editor: Taylor Hayes
Developmental Editor: Axell Ivan Jade Purificacion

Physician Assistant Clinics (ISSN: 2405–7991) is published quarterly by Elsevier Inc., 360 Park Avenue South, New York, NY 10010-1710. Months of issue are January, April, July, and October. Periodicals postage paid at New York, NY and additional mailing offices. Subscription prices are $150.00 per year (US individuals), $305.00 (US institutions), $100.00 (US students), $150.00 (Canadian individuals), $320.00 (Canadian institutions), $100.00 (Canadian students), $150.00 (international individuals), $320.00 (international institutions), and $100.00 (international students). Foreign air speed delivery is included in all *Clinics* subscription prices. All prices are subject to change without notice. POSTMASTER: Send address changes to *Physician Assistant Clinics*, Elsevier Periodicals Customer Service, 11830 Westline Industrial Drive, St. Louis, MO 63146. Customer Service Health Sciences Division, Subscription Customer Service, 3251 Riverport Lane, Maryland Heights, MO 63043. **Customer Service: 1-800-654-2452 (U.S. and Canada); 314-447-8871 (outside U.S. and Canada). Fax: 314-447-8029. E-mail: journalscustomerservice-usa@elsevier.com (for print support); journalsonlinesupport-usa@elsevier.com (for online support).**

Reprints. For copies of 100 or more, of articles in this publication, please contact the Commercial Reprints Department, Elsevier Inc., 360 Park Avenue South, New York, NY 10010-1710. Tel. 212-633-3874; Fax: 212-633-3820; E-mail: reprints@elsevier.com.

Physician Assistant Clinics is covered in *EMBASE/Excerpta Medica and ESCI.*

www.physicianassistant.theclinics.com. The CME program is available to subscribers for an additional annual fee of USD 149.00.

METHOD OF PARTICIPATION
In order to claim credit, participants must complete the following:
1. Complete enrolment as indicated above
2. Read the activity
3. Complete the CME Test and Evaluation. Participants must achieve a score of 70% on the test. All CME Tests and Evaluations must be completed online

CME INQUIRIES/SPECIAL NEEDS
For all CME inquiries or special needs, please contact elsevierCME@elsevier.com.

Contributors

CONSULTING EDITORS

KIM ZUBER, PAC, MS
American Academy of Nephrology PAs, St Petersburg, Florida, USA

JANE S. DAVIS, DNP
Division of Nephrology, The University of Alabama at Birmingham, Birmingham, Alabama, USA

EDITOR

GERALD KAYINGO, PhD, MBA, PA-C, DFAAPA
Assistant Dean, Executive Director and Professor, Physician Assistant Leadership and Learning Academy, Graduate School, University of Maryland, Baltimore, Baltimore, Maryland, USA

AUTHORS

JOSHUA ANDERSON, MS, PA-C
Crossroads Medical Associates, Ellicott City, Maryland, USA

GORDON H. BAE, MD
Department of Dermatology, Stanford University School of Medicine, Redwood City, California, USA

JUSTINA BENNETT, MPAS, PA-C
Department of PA Medicine, Frostburg State University, Hagerstown, Maryland, USA

VANESSA BESTER, EdD, PA-C
Associate Professor, Augsburg University PA Program, Minneapolis, Minnesota, USA

FREDERICK BROWNE, MD
Sacred Heart University PA Program, College of Health Professions, Sacred Heart University, Fairfield, Connecticut; Griffin Hospital, Derby, Connecticut, USA

JAMES F. CAWLEY, MPH, PA-C, DHL(hon)
Scholar in Residence, Visiting Professor, Physician Assistant Leadership and Learning Academy, University of Maryland, Baltimore, Baltimore, Maryland; Professor Emeritus of Prevention and Community Health, Milkin Institute School of Public Health, The George Washington University, Washington, D.C, USA

JENNIFER COMINI, MSPAS, PA-C
Assistant Professor, Charles R. Drew University of Medicine and Science Physician Assistant Program, Los Angeles, California, USA

NANCY HAMLER, DMSc, MPA, RDN, PA-C
Clinical Assistant Professor, Faculty Chair, Departments of MS Physician Assistant Science, and MS Clinical Nutrition, University of the Pacific School of Health Sciences, Sacramento, California, USA

SARA KADIU, PharmD
Partners Pharmacy, Marlborough, Massachusetts, USA

TEUTA KADIU, RN, MSL
UC Davis Betty Irene Moore School of Nursing, Sacramento, California, USA

GERALD KAYINGO, PhD, MBA, PA-C, DFAAPA
Assistant Dean, Executive Director and Professor, Physician Assistant Leadership and Learning Academy, Graduate School, University of Maryland, Baltimore, Baltimore, Maryland, USA

LUCY W. KIBE, DrPH, MS, MHS, PA-C
Program Director and Associate Professor, PA Program, Charles R. Drew University School of Medicine and Science, Los Angeles, California, USA

TRICIA LEPAGE, PA-C
Sacred Heart University PA Program, College of Health Professions, Sacred Heart University, Fairfield, Connecticut, USA

JEFFREY LIEN, PharmD
Walgreens, Mill Valley, California, USA

CLAIRE LIEPMANN, MD
Department of Infectious Diseases, Indiana University School of Medicine, Maywood, Illinois, USA

MARGARITA LOEZA, MD
Assistant Dean, Student Affairs and Admissions, Charles R. Drew University of Medicine and Science, Venice Family Clinic, Los Angeles, California, USA

BRENT LUU, PharmD, BCACP
Associate Clinical Professor, UC Davis Betty Irene Moore School of Nursing, Sacramento, California, USA

VIRGINIA MCCOY-HASS, DNP, MSN, RN, FNP-C, PA-C
UC Davis Betty Irene Moore School of Nursing, Sacramento, California, USA

ERIC C. NEMEC, PharmD, MEd, BCPS
Clinical Professor, Sacred Heart University PA Program, College of Health Professions, Sacred Heart University, Fairfield, Connecticut, USA

VICTORIA NGO, PhD
UC Davis Betty Irene Moore School of Nursing, Sacramento, California, USA

MOLLY O'NEILL, PA-C
Sacred Heart University PA Program, College of Health Professions, Sacred Heart University, Fairfield, Connecticut, USA

SAMUEL PAIK, PA-C
Assistant Professor, Charles Drew University PA Program, Los Angeles, California, USA

SUMATHI SANKARAN-WALTERS, PhD
University of California, Davis, Sacramento, California, USA

OLIVIA SAWH, MS, PA-C
Instructional Faculty and Stanford Educators4Care (E4C)-PA, Master of Science in PA Studies, Stanford School of Medicine, Stanford, California, USA

JENN STAUFFER, MHS, PA-C, AAHIVS
Clinical Assistant Professor, Oklahoma State University Center for Health Sciences Physician Assistant Program, Tulsa, Oklahoma, USA

GRETA VINES-DOUGLAS, MSHS, PA-C
Assistant Professor, Charles R. Drew University of Medicine and Science Physician Assistant Program, Los Angeles, California, USA

ANNE WALSH, MMSc, PA-C, DFAAPA
Clinical Associate Professor, Chapman University–MMS-PA Studies Program, Irvine, California, USA

CHELSEA WARE, MS, PA-C
Sacred Heart University, Fairfield, Connecticut, USA

SAMPATH WIJESINGHE, DhSc, AAHIVS, PA-C
Clinical Assistant Professor, Stanford School of Medicine–MSPA Education, Stanford, California, USA

HENRY YOON, MD
Clinical Associate Professor, Sacred Heart University, Fairfield, Connecticut; Department of Family Medicine, Stamford Hospital, Stamford, Connecticut, USA

PETER A. YOUNG, MPAS, PA-C
Department of Dermatology, The Permanente Medical Group, Sacramento, California; Department of Dermatology, Stanford School of Medicine, Redwood City, California, USA

OTIS ZEON, MD, MBS
Assistant Professor, Clinical Coordinator, PA Program, Charles R. Drew University School of Medicine and Science, Los Angeles, California, USA

Contents

> Infectious diseases have not been eradicated and continues to threaten humankind worldwide. Emerging infections are newly appeared in a population or have been known for some time but are rapidly increasing in incidence or geographic range. Reemerging diseases reappear after they have been on a significant decline. Most of these infections have a zoonotic origin, crossing from wildlife and domesticated animals to humans. Globalization, climate change, and other human factors are precipitating the rapid spread. Recent cases of Zika, Ebola, COVID-19, and Mpox underscore the need for continued vigilance. Pandemic preparedness will require global collaboration, advanced surveillance, rapid diagnostics, and vaccines.

> Antimicrobial resistance, a process by which germs invade antimicrobial agents, remains one of the most important challenges in health care today. Without appropriate coordinated actions, it is projected to cause the death of 10,000,000 people annually in addition to costing a global GDP of US $3.4 trillion dollars.

> Gonococcal and chlamydial infections are some of the most common communicable sexually acquired bacterial infections worldwide. Strains of gonococcus have developed resistance to several antimicrobials. This chapter discusses the epidemiology, risk factors, diagnosis, treatment, and prevention of gonococcal and sexually transmitted chlamydial infections in the United States.

> Fungal infections are prevalent worldwide and for most of the population are not life-threatening illnesses. Immunocompromised individuals, such as those with hematologic malignancies, solid-organ transplant recipients, and patients on tumor necrosis factor inhibitors among other high-risk conditions, have a significant threat of severe disease, mortality, or long-term

PHYSICIAN ASSISTANT CLINICS

SERIES OF RELATED INTEREST

Primary Care: Clinics in Office Practice
https://www.primarycare.theclinics.com/

THE CLINICS ARE AVAILABLE ONLINE!
Access your subscription at:
www.theclinics.com

Foreword

The Bugs Are Winning

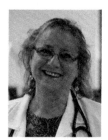 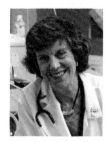

Kim Zuber, PAC, MS   Jane S. Davis, DNP
Consulting Editors

The renown Harvard sociobiologist E.O. Wilson once noted, "The variety of genes on the planet in viruses exceeds, or is likely to exceed, that in all of the rest of life combined." While we cannot review all the types of viruses, bacteria, fungi, and/or parasites, we do want to talk about emerging diseases. This issue of *Physician Assistant Clinics* highlights the new, the old, and the genetically modified emerging viruses, bacteria, and parasites.

As COVID-19 demonstrated, when there is a contest between viruses and organisms, the viruses and bacteria have been here and will always be here. Any temporary victory will be short-lived, and we will always lose in the end. While we may believe we can "cure" a disease state, the common cold has proven to us that managing is not eradicating. Viruses, with slight modifications, will survive in the population for many, many years.

Dr Kayingo has put together an impressive collection of authors and an especially scary collection of diseases. As you peruse this issue, it's fascinating to see how diseases that we once thought defeated (think smallpox and its resurgence in early 2000s) are appearing again. As we all know, the ability of a bacteria to adapt to our latest and greatest antibiotic is simply a patient away from a new, more-aggressive version of disease. We know, and at a gut level understand, that we are simply just surviving the newest onslaught. We will never truly win.

This issue highlights the ubiquity of the fight against bacteria, viruses, and parasites. Not only do we understand we will not truly win, but also we understand that we are fighting this battle throughout all areas of medicine: in the ICU, on the hospital floor, in the surgery suite, in the office, in the outpatient clinics, in the field, and in the classroom. As any parent can tell you, the most virulent infections seem to be the ones running through the elementary school.

As you enjoy (?) the update on what are expected to be the emerging disease states of the next 5 years, and we revisit those diseases that maintain the upper hand, we also

Physician Assist Clin 8 (2023) xv–xvi
https://doi.org/10.1016/j.cpha.2023.03.007
2405-7991/23/© 2023 Published by Elsevier Inc.

need to discuss vaccine hesitancy. With all our science, if we are not connecting with our patients, all of this is for naught. We know and have seen losses to infections, and we need to share what we have seen with the next generation of caregivers. We have generational amnesia; those of us who remember polio, smallpox, mumps, or measles are being lost, and with that, so too is the organizational knowledge of the toll of these diseases. While we look for and fight the newest derivatives of viruses and bacteria, let us not let our guard down and forget the successes we had. We cannot go back.

Kim Zuber, PAC, MS
American Academy of Nephrology Pas
131 31st Avenue North
St Petersburg, FL 33704, USA

Jane S. Davis, DNP
Division of Nephrology
University of Alabama at Birmingham
3605 Oakdale Road
Birmingham, AL 35223, USA

E-mail addresses:
zuberkim@yahoo.com (K. Zuber)
jsdavis@uabmc.edu (J.S. Davis)

Preface

Are You Ready for the Next Pandemic?

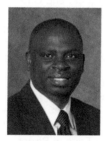

Gerald Kayingo, PhD, MBA, PA-C, DFAAPA
Editor

Despite advancements in vaccines and antimicrobial development, life-threatening pathogens continue to emerge and reemerge globally. With the increasing globalization, climate change, and human encroachment on nature, the next pandemic is more likely to appear in not so much of a distant future. Recent cases of Zika, Ebola, COVID-19, and Monkeypox underscore the need for continued vigilance. The global impact of these infectious diseases is staggering, and the threat to humankind, economic, and political stability is real. The COVID-19 pandemic has clearly illustrated the fragility of our health systems and the overall global inefficiency for pandemic preparedness. At both a global and a local level, interventions are urgently needed to develop rapid monitoring systems and coordinate resources for real-time surveillance, prevention, and eradication.

Clinicians have a responsibility to stay current on best practices, advance infection control, prescribe responsibly, and continually address the care disparities that are endemic to the field of infectious diseases. The goal of this issue is to equip health care practitioners with the knowledge on current trends and best practices in managing emerging and reemerging infectious diseases.

The article in this issue entitled "Emerging, Reemerging Infectious Diseases and Global Pandemic Preparedness" introduces the concepts of emerging and reemerging infections. It also discusses risk factors and provides an overview on global pandemic preparedness. This article is strategically followed by concepts on antimicrobial resistance by Zeon and Kibe. Following a systematic approach, the issue then covers significant examples of bacteria, viruses, spirochetes, parasites, and fungal pathogens. A unique feature of this issue is the inclusion of recent literature on bioterrorism, the intersection between emerging infections and addiction as well as recent understanding on antivaccination and vaccine hesitancy. Not all pathogens could be covered, but we

Physician Assist Clin 8 (2023) xvii–xviii
https://doi.org/10.1016/j.cpha.2023.03.006
2405-7991/23/© 2023 Published by Elsevier Inc.

hope that the general concepts and exemplars provided here will be applied to other emerging and reemerging infectious diseases worldwide.

Paik covers the concept of emerging infectious diseases and bioterrorism, identifying the major players, and provides perspectives on what health professionals can do to prepare for the inevitable. Wijesinghe and colleagues discuss how substance use disorders increase user's odds of contracting emerging infectious diseases, particularly HIV and hepatitis. Individuals may contract or transmit a viral infection when they inject drugs and share needles or other drug equipment. Cawley summarizes trends on the antivaccine movement and how it is rapidly growing in the era of social media. Cawley and Kidd's article makes a call for action for new approaches to mitigate the antivaccine movement, build trust between patients and providers, and dispel the myths and misinformation that erode public confidence in vaccines.

Gerald Kayingo, PhD, MBA, PA-C, DFAAPA
Physician Assistant Leadership and Learning Academy
Graduate School
University of Maryland, Baltimore
520 West Fayette Street, Suite #130
Baltimore, MD 21201, USA

E-mail address:
gkayingo@umaryland.edu

Emerging, Reemerging Infectious Diseases and Global Pandemic Preparedness

Gerald Kayingo, PhD, MBA, PA-C, DFAAPA

KEYWORDS

- Emerging • Reemerging • Infectious diseases • Global pandemics preparedness

KEY POINTS

- Despite advancements in vaccines and antimicrobial development, life-threatening pathogens continue to emerge and reemerge globally.
- Most emerging pathogens have zoonotic origins and spillover to humans. Globalization, climate change, and human encroachment into nature accelerate emergence and spread of infectious diseases.
- Microbial adaptation and breakdown of public health measures are also major drivers for emergence and reemergence of human pathogens.
- An integrated approach to global surveillance, vector control, early detection, drug and vaccine development, public hygiene and sanitation, public education, and health policy interventions will be essential.
- Pandemic preparedness plans should be developed at all levels to facilitate rapid responses, prevent spread, and reduce morbidity and mortality.

INTRODUCTION/HISTORY/DEFINITIONS/BACKGROUND

The past 100 years have been marked with astonishing progress in the knowledge of infectious disease, the invention of antibiotics, and breakthrough vaccines. Consequently, the mortality associated with infectious diseases has significantly been reduced particularly in the western world. Despite this remarkable progress, there remains a major global threat from emerging and reemerging infectious diseases.[1] As a definition, the World Health Organization (WHO) refers to an emerging infectious disease as one that has newly appeared in a population or that has been known for some time but is rapidly increasing in incidence or geographic range.[2] On the other hand, reemerging diseases are diseases that reappear after they have been on a significant decline. Examples of emerging infectious diseases include human immunodeficiency virus infection/acquired immunodeficiency syndrome (HIV/AIDS), coronaviruses, and

Physician Assistant Leadership and Learning Academy, Graduate School, University of Maryland, 520 West Fayette Street, Suite # 130, Baltimore, MD 21201, USA
E-mail address: gkayingo@umaryland.edu

Physician Assist Clin 8 (2023) 405–409
https://doi.org/10.1016/j.cpha.2023.02.001
2405-7991/23/© 2023 Elsevier Inc. All rights reserved.

ebolaviruses (**Table 1**) which have been some of the greatest challenges over the past 100 years (**Table 2**). Examples of reemerging infectious diseases include multidrug-resistant tuberculosis, drug-resistant malaria, and drug-resistant *Staphylococcus aureus*. There are six major types of infectious agents: viruses, bacteria, fungi, protozoa, helminths, and a new class, called prions. Most of these infections have a zoonotic origin,[3] crossing from wildlife and domesticated animals to humans (**Fig. 1**). Other key contributing factors include climate change, microbial adaptation, antimicrobial resistance, global travel, and migration. Similarly, weakened health services, population growth, and changing human susceptibility are all playing a key role in the reemergence of infectious diseases.[4] Micro and macro interventions are urgently needed to develop rapid monitoring systems, coordinate resources for surveillance, prevention, and eradication.

Global Pandemic Preparedness

Given the raising trends in risks factors, new pathogens are more likely to appear, and old ones are also likely to reappear in the future. Local, national, and global agencies must develop pandemic preparedness plans that can respond rapidly and halt the spread infection as well as the associated morbidity and mortality. Preparedness plans should be integrated and interdisciplinary with capacity to engage both domestic and international partners. Preparedness should leverage the rapidly growing

Table 1
Global examples of emerging and reemerging infectious diseases

Newly Emerging Diseases[8–10]	Region	Reemerging and Resurging Diseases	Region
Ebola hemorrhagic fever	Africa	Drug–resistant malaria	Africa, Asia, South America
HIV	Africa	Multi–drug tuberculosis,	Africa, Europe, Asia, North America
Marburg hemorrhagic fever	Africa	Yellow fever	Africa, South Africa
Lassa fever	Africa	Plague	Africa
SARS	Asia	Human mpox	Africa, North America
Escherichia coli O157:H7	Asia & North America	Rift Valley fever	Africa
H5N1 influenza	Asia	Cholera	Africa, Asia, South America
Hendra virus	Australia	Dengue	South America, North America
Cryptosporidiosis	North America	Lyme disease	North America
Hantavirus pulmonary disease	North America and South America	West Nile Virus	North America
COVID-19	Global	Vancomycin-resistant *S aureus*	North America, Asia
Whitewater Arroyo virus	North America	Measles	North America
MERS	Asia	Zika virus disease	Africa

Abbreviations: MERS, Middle East respiratory syndrome; SARS, Severe acute respiratory syndrome.

Table 2
Global examples of emerging and reemerging infectious disease

1899–1923 Sixth cholera pandemic Begins in India, spreads to Russia, Middle East and Africa	*1918–1920* 1918 flu (Influenza virus) Infects roughly one-third of population and kills 50 million	*1957–1958* Asian flu pandemic Begins in Singapore, spreads to China, Europe and North America	*1961–present* Cholera pandemic Begins in Indonesia, spreads to globally. Endemic in over 50 countries	*1968–1969* Hong Kong flu pandemic H3N2 strain emerges in Hong Kong, spreads globally
1981–present HIV/AIDS pandemic Originated in nonhuman primates in Central Africa and spread globally. Killed> 40 million	*2002–2003* SARS Begins in China and spreads globally. Origins likely form Civet cats	*2009–2010* H1N1 pandemic Also known as swine flu Begins in Mexico and Spreads to Northen America, affecting mostly young people	*2012* MERS New coronavirus Middle east respiratory syndrome. Likely form camels begins in Saudi Arabia	*2014* Polio Reemerges in Africa and Asia Young people mostly affected Widespread mistrust of vaccine
2014-2016 Ebola (West Africa) Begins in Guinea, Liberia, and Sierra Leone, spreads globally. First Ebola outbreak to reach epidemic proportions. Over 28,500 people infected and > 11,300 deaths. Bats suspected to be involved	*2015–2016* Zika Emerges in Brazil and spreads to the Americas. First discovered in Uganda in 1940s	*2018–2020* Ebola Reemerges in war-torn areas of Congo and spreads in regionally. Approximately 2300 deaths	*2019–present* COVID-19 Emerges from China's Hubei province, rapidly spreads globally per WHO, over 752,517,000 Confirmed cases and over 6,804,000 deaths by January 2023	*2022–present* Mpox First reported in United Kingdom rapidly spreads globally. Outside endemic areas, cases are primarily among men who have sex with men.

Sources for this table include references from[8–11]

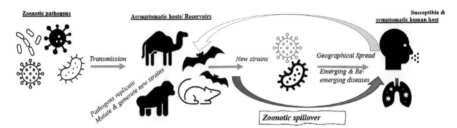

Fig. 1. Wild animals play a key role the in transmission, amplification, and spread of emerging and reemerging infectious diseases. (*Adapted from* Rahman M.T., et al.[3], Cupertino, M.C. et al.[12])

knowledge of infectious diseases, incorporate biomedical technologies, build a robust infrastructure, and improve coordination and communication.

At global level, the United Nations and the WHO describe preparedness as *"the ability (knowledge, capacities, and organizational systems) of governments, professional response organizations, communities, and individuals to anticipate, detect and respond effectively to, and recover from, the impact of likely, imminent or current health emergencies, hazards, events or conditions. It means putting in place mechanisms that will allow national authorities, multilateral organizations, and relief organizations to be aware of risks and deploy staff and resources quickly once a crisis strikes."*[5]

Subsequently, these international agencies have outline key elements that should constitute a global pandemic preparedness and response (PPR) architecture.[6] These include

- Surveillance, collaborative intelligence, and early warning
- Prioritized research and equitable access to countermeasures and essential supplies
- Public health and social measures and engaged resilient communities
- Lifesaving, safe, and scalable health interventions and resilient health systems
- PPR strategy, coordination, and emergency operation

In the United States, the Federal Emergency Management Agency encourages the use of an incident command system model in situation of large-scale disasters including pandemics. Such models can involve Hospital Incident Command System or a Joint Operations Center that can centralize communication and coordination to rapidly respond to a pandemic crisis.[7]

CLINICS CARE POINTS

- The threat of emerging infections and the reemergence of old ones are here to stay; Underlying risk factors such as globalization and climate change are just increasing.
- Heath care practitioners must keep up to date with epidemiological trends and management guidelines.
- Health care practitioners should be knowledgeable with federal and state policies regarding diseases and conditions that must be reported to authorities.
- It is imperative to practice effective infection control practices and standard precautions such as hand hygiene and use of personal protective equipment.
- Taking a good travel history is vital for early interventions.

- Individuals should be familiar of with incident command systems at their place of work to support rapid responses in case of a suspected infectious emergency.
- Clinicians should prescribe responsibly to minimize antimicrobial resistance.
- As discussed by Dr Anthony S Fauci,[1] the global impact of infectious diseases is staggering, and the threat to humankind is real. The COVID-19 pandemic has clearly illustrated the fragility of our health systems and the overall global inefficiency for pandemic preparedness. At a clinic level, there is a responsibility to improve capabilities, stay current on best practices, and continually address the care disparities that are often associated with emerging and reemerging infectious diseases.

DISCLOSURE

The author has nothing to disclose.

ACKNOWLEDGEMENT

Physician Assistant Leadership and Learning Academy, Graduate School, University of Maryland Baltimore.

REFERENCES

1. Fauci AS. It ain't over till it's over but it's never over - emerging and reemerging infectious diseases. N Engl J Med 2022;387(22):2009–11.
2. Morse SS. Factors in the emergence of infectious diseases. Emerg Infect Dis 1995;1(1):7–15.
3. Rahman MT, Sobur MA, Islam MS, et al. Zoonotic diseases: etiology, impact, and control. Microorganisms 2020;8(9):1405.
4. Baker RE, Mahmud AS, Miller IF, et al. Infectious disease in an era of global change. Nat Rev Microbiol 2022;20(4):193–205.
5. Gpmb A. World at risk: annual report on global preparedness for health emergencies. 2019 [Available at: https://reliefweb.int/sites/reliefweb.int/files/resources/GPMB_annualreport_2019.pdf.
6. Lal A, Abdalla SM, Chattu VK, et al. Pandemic preparedness and response: exploring the role of universal health coverage within the global health security architecture. Lancet Glob Health 2022;10(11):e1675–83.
7. Farcas A, Ko J, Chan J, et al. Use of incident command system for disaster preparedness: a model for an emergency department COVID-19 response. Disaster Med Public Health Prep 2021;15(3):e31–6.
8. Morens DM, Folkers GK, Fauci AS. The challenge of emerging and re-emerging infectious diseases. Nature 2004;430(6996):242–9 [published correction appears in Nature. 2010 Jan 7;463(7277):122].
9. Bhadoria P, Gupta G, Agarwal A. Viral pandemics in the past two decades: an overview. J Family Med Prim Care 2021;10(8):2745–50.
10. Centers for Disease control. Past pandemics. Available at: https://www.cdc.gov/flu/pandemic-resources/basics/past-pandemics.html.
11. Ndow G, Ambe JR, Tomori O. Emerging infectious diseases: a historical and scientific review. Socio-cultural Dimensions of Emerging Infectious Diseases in Africa 2019;31–40. https://doi.org/10.1007/978-3-030-17474-3_3.
12. Cupertino MC, Resende MB, Mayer NA, et al. Emerging and re-emerging human infectious diseases: a systematic review of the role of wild animals with a focus on public health impact. Asian Pac. J. Trop. Med 2020;13:99–106.

Antimicrobial Drug Resistance and Antimicrobial Resistant Threats

Otis Zeon, MD, MBS, Lucy W. Kibe, DrPH, MS, MHS, PA-C*

KEYWORDS

- Antimicrobial resistance (AMR) • Antimicrobial use (AMU) • Global impact
- Call to action • Crisis • Antimicrobial stewardship

KEY POINTS

- Antimicrobial resistance poses one of the serious global health crises of this century.
- Global coordinated efforts by key stakeholders are required in order to eradicate this crisis related to antimicrobial resistance.
- Antimicrobial stewardship, global education, and awareness programs are essential in the fight against antimicrobial resistance.
- Failure to fight against antimicrobial resistance has the potential to undo advancement made in disease eradication.

BACKGROUND

Antimicrobial resistance (AMR) poses one of the greatest threats to the advancement of modern medicine. Worldwide, an estimated 700,000 people die each year from AMR, and this number is expected to reach 10 million annually by 2050.[1] An estimated 2.8 M people experience AMR and 48,000 people die annually in the United States.[2] In India, 58,000 babies die each year because of transmission of a resistant bacterial infection.[3] In Europe, 25,000 people die each year specifically due to antibiotic resistance.[4] The World's Health Organization posits that AMR poses one of the serious global health crises of this century. The Britain's House of Lords on antimicrobial resistance, the European Union, the US Institute of Medicine on emerging infections, Center for Disease Control (CDC) of the Asian pacific, the CDC of Europe (ECDC), the WHO and World bank, are all on high alert due to the AMR global crisis.

There has been no better time in history, than now, to discuss the impact of AMR on health care and the global economy. During the last 3 decades, our understanding of

PA Program, Charles R. Drew University School of Medicine and Science, 1731 East 120th Street, Los Angeles, CA 90059, USA
* Corresponding author.
E-mail address: lucykibe@cdrewu.edu

Physician Assist Clin 8 (2023) 411–420
https://doi.org/10.1016/j.cpha.2023.03.001
2405-7991/23/© 2023 Elsevier Inc. All rights reserved.

microorganisms and their ability to adapt to their environment has improved tremendously. However, our response to this outcome has been lagging. For example, SARs-COV-1, a coronavirus known for its ability to mutate, has been studied for nearly 2 decades. Yet in 2019, a new variant, SARs-COV-2, what we now know as COVID-19 was able to invade the world and was declared a pandemic in 2020. This virus has mutated to various forms, for example, the Delta and Omicron variants. The mounting resistance of these variants has been compared with those of Ebola and Zika virus of recent years.

In addition to the more recent focus on viral infections, most AMR cases are secondary to bacterial infection. Penicillin-resistant *Staphylococcus aureus (PRSA)*, Methicillinresistant *Staphylococcus aureus (MRSA)*, Multidrug-resistant *Tuberculosis*, Infection secondary to *Clostridium difficile*, and Multidrug-resistant *Pseudomonas (MDRP)* are prominent bacteria that endanger the human species. Microbial resistance is a cause of concern because of 3 main reasons. First, we created this crisis by our various practices. For example, the agriculture industry accounts for 73% of antimicrobial use (AMU), which is one of the reasons for an alarming rate of resistance.[5] Second, we ignored the warning signs of microbial resistance for far too long. For example, health care has known about bacterial resistance to antibiotics for many decades, yet we continue with irresponsible prescribing practices. Finally, complexities of AMR have a negative economic impact and threaten progress made in health care.

IMPACT OF THE ANTIMICROBIAL RESISTANCE PROBLEM

To truly understand the magnitude of the problem, scientists and practitioners must measure and dissect its impact from a historical, population, health care, and economic burden perspective. Additionally, institutions and governing bodies must allocate both human capital and resources to conduct research about the pressing danger of AMR.

The World Bank posits that AMR economic impact could amount to 3.8% of the global GDP by 2050. At its current rate, AMR impact is expected to cause an annual shortfall of US$3.4 trillion in global GDP by 2030.[6] The loss of productivity from human resources, the impact on agriculture, livestock, manufacturing, and increase in health-care expenditure have all contributed to the AMR impact on the economy. Developing countries, minority, and disadvantaged populations are most vulnerable to these changes.

A "tragedy of the commons" is the term used by the World Bank when describing AMR. This phenomenon happens when individuals privately use communal resources in a manner to only benefit themselves. An effective antimicrobial stewardship in this case being the "commons" resource. The tragedy then would be how individual countries, institutions, and organizations are privatizing their antimicrobial stewardship programs while the rest of the world is inflicted by this crisis.

In the health-care setting, AMR cases leading to higher hospital stay has 2 main impacts. First, it increases the risk for hospital-acquired infection, and second, it increases the cost associated with the consumption of hospital resources during the stay. In Europe, patients are spending an additional 2.5 million days per year with an estimated cost of 1.5 billion euros each year attributed to antibiotics resistance alone.[4] In developing countries, AMR problems can be attributed to individual self-prescription, limited education, lack of enforceable standardized practice, and massive imports of fraudulent manufactured antimicrobials. In developed nations, the failure to practice a cohesive antimicrobial stewardship, prolonged hospital stay, and under production of antimicrobials are among the many causes of AMR. To prevent a future tragedy, it is imperative that the world take notice of AMR and that resources are allocated toward solving this global crisis.

CALL TO ACTION AGAINST ANTIMICROBIAL RESISTANCE

Because of the complex nature of AMR, solutions need to be multipronged and multi-disciplinary. The universal term "antimicrobial stewardship" is used to refer to a set of coordinated actions that promote the responsible use of antimicrobials by all stake-holders including health-care providers, health-care systems, health insurance com-panies, pharmaceutical companies, policy makers, educators, researchers, and the public. The CDC action plan for antimicrobial stewardship includes strategies for accelerating drug development, preventing the spread of resistant infections, devel-oping better diagnostic tools, improving data collection and surveillance, educating stakeholders, and improving global coordination for antibiotic resistance concerns. Resources on how to implement these strategies are outlined on the CDC website, for example, how to develop an antimicrobial stewardship program in large hospitals, small and critical access hospitals, outpatient settings, and resource limited settings.

At the provider level, it is necessary to practice actions that promote quality patient care while observing antimicrobial stewardship. Recommended actions include the use of universal precautions to prevent microbial transmission between patients, judi-cious and accurate prescription of antibiotics, awareness of local resistance patterns, use of diagnostic tools to guide prescriptive decisions, and patient education on sani-tation practices and appropriate antibiotic use.

MECHANISM OF ANTIMICROBIAL RESISTANCE ON A CELLULAR LEVEL

The objective of all living things is to propagate their genetic material to their progeny and to ensure survival of their species. Both macro and microorganisms alike, ensure survival by performing basic tasks: consumption of energy, responding to stimuli, maintaining a stable environment, reproduction, organizing, and adapting to their envi-ronment. Most microorganisms prefer an organic source to which they can form a symbiotic relationship; many of these organisms live with a plant, animal, or human host and do not cause disease. However, when there is a breakdown of host defense, an opportunistic organism will cause an infection. If resistant to antibiotics, this be-comes problematic, for example, *S aureus*, which is commonly found on the skin of people, can cause a life-threatening skin infection known as *MRSA*. Germs cause dis-ease and are capable of directly evading their host's protective barriers. By virtue of their nature, they simply want to invade their host, replicate, and spread.

To fight against microorganisms, scientists created antimicrobial agents. The objec-tive of these agents is either to stop the growth (*static*) or to kill microbes completely (*cidal*). Due to their genetic makeup, the more exposure an organism has with an agent, the better it can evade its static or cidal effects. Organisms use plasmids, which are circles of DNA that can move from 1 cell to another. They use transposon, a tiny piece of DNA that can join another cell's chromosome to be replicated. A phage is a vehicle tasked with infecting new microorganisms with genetic material. Germs can also change their surface coating, their genetic behavior, adapt to harsh environ-ments to resist antimicrobials.

Genetic drift is the most impressive way a microbial can invade antimicrobial agents. Genetic drift can be likened to a game of chess. Germs have genetic elements that are like the pawns on a chessboard. These elements mostly increase the total gene content and are used to either protect essential gene elements or be sacrificed in times of nutrient scarcity or toxic stress (when an antimicrobial is introduced). Plasmid, transposons, or phases in this analogy would be likened to the queen of a chessboard. When the queen can transport the most essential gene (the king of the board) to a new living host, it becomes a checkmate for the germs. In short, the different tactics used by the genetic elements to change their total genetic content and evade antimicrobials is the process of genetic drift and the critical mechanism used by germ for mounting resistance.

AMR in higher pathogens such as fungi, parasites, and viruses are a mechanism in which microorganisms evolved to become resistant to the drugs and treatments used to kill them. This can occur through genetic mutations, horizontal gene transfer, and the overuse or misuse of antimicrobials such as antifungal, antiviral, and antiparasitic agents. In horizontal gene transfer, the organism transfers its genetic material without the need of reproduction. They use conjugation, transduction, and transformation. Conjugation as mentioned previously involves a direct cell-to-cell contact, often facilitated by plasmids, which carried the AMR. Transduction involves the use of bacteriophage (a type of virus that infects bacterial) and transformation involves the update of naked DNA from the environment by a bacterium into a cell.

MECHANISM OF ANTIMICROBIAL RESISTANCE ON A COMMUNITY LEVEL

Germs can spread from person to person, animal to person, and surface to person. The spreading of germs maximizes its survivability and contributes to its overall resistance. The negative habits of people and industry alike increase the survivability of germs and directly contribute to its overall resistance. For example, when a sick person visits social events, they directly participate in the survivability of the germ, increasing its biomass ultimately fueling resistance.

Inappropriate use of antimicrobial agents to treat infected persons within a community can also result in resistance. The more people that get exposed to a given microorganism, the higher the likelihood that said organism gets exposure to a given antimicrobial agent. Excessive exposure of a specific agent may very well trigger the genetic drift phenomenon leading to resistance.

An essential part of being human is having the ability to eliminate waste and means of disposing of said waste. In the developing world, human feces are frequently disposed of directly into water sources such as rivers and lakes, whereas in developed nations, these waste goes through the sewer system and directly to water treatment plants. The result of waste elimination by humans is the high level of active antimicrobials agent's ingredients that end up in water sources.

In pharmacology (the study of drugs and their effect on living systems), there is a concept called bioavailability. This concept describes the available quantity of a given agent within a living system, which can have an effect. When an agent is taken orally, a portion of it gets destroyed by the digestive system, another portion gets absorbed into the bloodstream and leads to the desired outcome and a large quantity gets eliminated in the digestive tract. This eliminated portion, which still contains active antimicrobial properties, makes its way through the sewer system to water sources and treatment plants. These active ingredients may be ingested by humans and animals through their survival in water sources and agriculture. This process is one of the leading causes of AMR globally.

TIMELINE AND HISTORY OF ANTIMICROBIAL RESISTANCE

The discovery of penicillin in 1928 served as a critical and monumental turning point in health care. Less than 10 years later, the discovery of sulfonamides coupled with the clinical application of penicillin completely changed the way scientists thought about the nature of microorganisms and associated diseases. The next 2 decades were marked by applications and discovery of multiple types of antimicrobial agents, specifically antibiotics. By the 1960s health care experienced an increase of *PRSA*.[7] *MRSA* was very problematic in the 1960s as well, and subsequently, scientists developed vancomycin, nalidixic, cephalosporins to fight against the various AMR of the times.[4] By the early 1980s, the development of carbapenem and monobactam were completed to fight against Extended-Spectrum Beta-Lactamase (ESBL)-producing gram-negative bacilli. In the midtwentieth century, the focus of scientists was the development and discovery of antimicrobial agents, although acknowledgment of AMR was given.[7]

By the end of the twentieth century, it seems that scientists had slowed down their efforts on researching and development of new antimicrobial agents. One of the arguments made was that scientists had confidence in the agents that already existed in the market and that resources were diverted elsewhere. This decision added to the increase of AMR. *MRSA*, *PRSA*, and *MDRP*, continued to rampage the health-care sector and were now part of a list of germs known as the "superbugs."

TIMELINE OF GLOBAL EFFORT TO ANTIMICROBIAL RESISTANCE

Coordinated global efforts have been made by various institutions and organizations during the last 2 decades to fight against AMR. Although the timeline, resources, and methods are different for each entity tasked with this matter, the objectives have essentially been the same: collecting data regarding AMR cases, making these data available to scientists and researchers, making sense of these data, developing and deploying policies, awareness, funding, and other incentive programs.

WHO held its first conference on antibiotics and antibiotic resistance in 1959. In attendance were the likes of Selman Waksman and Lawrence Garrod. Dispute over definition of AMR, coupled with optimism and confidence in the pharmaceuticals industry, halted the discussions of microbial resistance.[8] The Prudent Use of Antibiotics (APUA) was founded in 1981 by Stuart B. Levy in response to the AMR crisis. The APUA mission was to formulate a uniform regulation process, which involved labeling, prescription, sales, and resistance tracking of antibiotics.[8]

The "Global Strategy for Containment of Antimicrobial Resistance" was formed in 1990. The United States increased its resource allocation to combat AMR by the creation of the National Antimicrobial Resistance Monitoring System (NARMS) in 1996. Three federal bodies combined resources to the creation of this system. The CDC, Food and Drug Administration, and the United States Department of Agriculture (NARMS, 2022). Other organizations were formed are as follows: European Antimicrobial Resistance Surveillance System (subsequently European Antimicrobial Resistance Surveillance System [EARS]-Net) in 1998, United Nations Environment Assembly's Interagency Coordination Group on AMR, The Food and Agriculture Organization, the World Organization for Animal Health (OIE), the ECDC, European Medicine Agency, and the World Bank.

COMMON MICROORGANISM CAUSING RESISTANCE

The WHO proposes more than 3 dozen antimicrobial agents that are subjected to resistance based on the organism they target.[9] More than 30 of these agents belong to the antibacterial class of agents. Antiviral drugs with strong focus on (HIV-AIDS), agents against malaria infection, and top antifungal agents such as fluconazole, amphotericin B, and voriconazole are top priority agents.

The 7 key bacteria that pose a great threat and are classified as the "superbugs" are as follows:

- *MRSA*
- Vancomycin-resistant *Enterococcus*

- ESBL-producing *Enterobacteriaceae* (extended-spectrum β-lactamases)
- Multidrug-resistant *Pseudomonas aeruginosa*
- Multidrug-resistant *Acinetobacter*
- Carbapenem-resistant *Enterobacteriaceae*
- Antibiotic-resistant *Escherichia coli* (H30-Rx strain)

Multidrug resistant *tuberculosis* is also an area of major concern. *TB* according to the CDC infected about 1.7 billion people in 2018 accounting for about 23% of the world's population.[10] *Mycobacterium tuberculosis (TB)*, a difficult bacterium to kill, has a strong correlation with the increase of HIV-AIDS during the last 2 decades. TB also, a highly contagious bacterial infection has a high case fatality rate within the immunocompromised population. Isoniazid and rifampin are the 2 most important anti-TB agents subjected to resistance by the *TB* organisms.

Not mentioned on the list of superbugs is *C difficile (C diff)*. This gram-positive bacterium is a common cause of colitis, an inflammatory process of the large intestine, which causes chronic diarrhea.[11] *C difficile* colitis or pseudomembranous colitis diarrheal illness is a great example of practices in health care, which contributes to AMR. For example, the overuse of second-generation and third-generation cephalosporins, fluoroquinolones, ampicillin/amoxicillin, and clindamycin has been shown to cause *C diff* infection. *C diff* is part of an AMR class of bugs, which are highly contagious and at its worst can cause a toxic enlargement of the colon, a highly fatal outcome.

The WHO is also concerned about the drug-resistant HIV (HIVDR) especially with the nonnucleoside reverse-transcriptase.[12] As mentioned, HIV, a viral infection that compromises the immune system has a high case fatality rate and is strongly correlated with TB, the *world's superbug*. HIVDR also increases the rate of opportunistic infections with bugs such as *Streptococcus pneumoniae*, common cause of pneumonia, *Pneumocystis carinii* pneumonia, *candidiasis*, *cryptococcosis*, invasive cancers, to name a few.

AMR poses a serious threat to the management and control of malaria around the world. The malaria epidemic affects many Asian and African nations and has a high mortality and morbidity rate. Artemisinin-based combination therapies (ACTs) is the first-line treatment of uncomplicated malaria caused by *Plasmodium falciparum*. However, this highly effective therapy is now facing AMR in countries such as Cambodia, Lao People's Democratic Republic, Myanmar, Thailand, and Viet Nam and Sub-Saharan Africa (WHO: Antimicrobial resistance, 2021).

Among the microorganisms causing problems, AMR relating to fungal infection, might be extremely alarming. The available antimicrobial agents for fungal infections are highly toxic, expensive, and usually require multiple cycles of treatment. Because most fungal infections, such as candidiasis, are opportunistic, it is highly probable that AMR to antifungal could exacerbate treatment progress regarding both primary and secondary causes of infections. The result of antifungal resistance is a high human and economic cost, health-care burden, and high mortality rate.

ANTIMICROBIAL RESISTANCE THREAT AND IMPACT ON HEALTH CARE

Antimicrobials are prescribed by a variety of prescribing providers in multiple health-care settings, including outpatient and inpatient. Providers specialized in the field of infectious disease are usually consulted when a patient requires a more specialized diagnostic formulation and care plan. Practitioners will typically place a patient on an antimicrobial agent while awaiting support from an infectious disease specialist. This practice of automatic prescription of broad-spectrum antimicrobial agents increases the risk of AMR.

Clinical Pearl 1

- *Question 1: How has the automatic use of broad-spectrum antimicrobials affected the AMR crisis?*
- *Thought Exercise 1: Before a broad-spectrum agent is used, it would be prudent to devise a quick, real-time diagnostic safeguard, or a decision-making tool to determine if the broad spectrum antimicrobial is needed in the immediate term.*

The CDC, in its attempts to help reduce AMR cases, has continued to provide specific guidelines on the AMU as well as guidelines on treatment recommendations for various forms of infections. When an infection enters the bloodstream and causes a massive systemic reaction and shutdown, this is called sepsis, resulting in septic shock. Sepsis has a high mortality rate and is usually a clinical concern for patients who have had a prolonged uncontrollable infection, those with long hospital stay, or those in critical condition. One of the concerns of the CDC is that AMR to a patient may increase the risk of sepsis, which has a high mortality rate and serves as an example of AMR direct impact in the hospital setting.[13] At the same time, the CDC encourages clinicians to treat patients' infections effectively without fear of an AMR taking place. The evidence-based practice of treating a chronic infection regardless of AMR is clear; however, the paradox remains, that excessive AMU is correlated with resistance.

Clinical Pearl 2

- *Question 2: How has the use of antimicrobial, especially antibiotics been able to add to the resistance of bugs commonly known to cause sepsis?*
- *Thought Exercise 2: Close attention must be given to the drastic shift from gram-negative to gram-positive as common organisms known to cause nosocomial infections leading to sepsis. It must be clear that, when an infection is persistent, aggressive treatment with antimicrobials is paramount regardless of the AMR risk; however, the paradox must be recognized.*

Infection control is an essential part of a comprehensive care delivery in many disciplines of health care. For example, when providing chemotherapy treatment of patients with cancer, it is standard practice to prescribe prophylaxis antimicrobial to prevent an infection from occurring or to be aggressive with AMU when an infection ensues. Nosocomial, community inquires and or opportunistic infections are a major cause of high mortality in cancer and immunocompromised patients. Other cases that require AMU are surgical operation, solid organ transplants, treatment of HIV/AIDS and other immunocompromised conditions, and artificial device implants to name a few. The key point is, in order to have a firm grasp on AMR in health care, we must take a comprehensive audit of AMU in all essential and nonessential use cases.

Clinical Pearl 3

- *Question 3: The use of antimicrobials in other health-care disciplines is essential; however, are there checks and balances for AMU within these various disciplines and use cases?*
- *Thought Exercise 3: Practitioners should often consult with infectious disease specialists when formulating care plans for patients receiving other forms of treatment, which may increase the risk for infection. Staying away from excessive use of broad-spectrum antimicrobials and focusing on highly effective organisms and specific agents to optimum their infection control protocols is essential.*

ANTIMICROBIAL RESISTANCE CRISIS AND TAKING ACCOUNTABILITY

The pathway to defeating the AMR crisis requires scientists, governments, industries, institutions, policy makers, and individuals around the world to take personal responsibility for its occurrence. For more than half a century, scientists and institutions have been made aware of microbials resistance and the need to take actions. For the most part, this matter has not been given the resources and attention, and its threat levels have been perceived to be low. Fortunately, the recent action plans and attention by major institutions such as the WHO, World Bank, CDC to name a few has shown the need to increase the threat level of AMR.

Much like the start of the midtwentieth century, industries such as pharmaceuticals, health care, agriculture and food, need to divert their attention, resources, and human capital to working on the AMR crisis. Pharmaceutical industries need to do more research and development on new agents, especially those agents known to treat high-risk organisms. The market needs to provide more incentive for the creation of antimicrobials that are designed to combat resistance. Regulatory and governmental institutions need a more efficient approval process regarding R&D for these antimicrobials' agents.

Individuals and practitioners can participate in the fight against resistance by increasing their knowledge base. Public knowledge is usually lacking when it comes to understanding the differences between microorganisms, the type of infection they cause, and how to treat them. For example, in nations without prescription guidelines, people often buy and use antibiotics for viral illness. In the fight against resistance, a strong antimicrobial prescription stewardship program coupled with public education is necessary.

CALL TO ACTION FOR THE ANTIMICROBIAL RESISTANCE CRISIS

The global-call-to-action (GCTA) for the AMR crisis requires that the problem be declared a global crisis. This call-to-action needs to be globally accepted and acted on by required institutions and organizations around the world. The WHO has provided 2 "Global Action plans," the World Bank has also provided research and action plans, and so has many other institutions. A unified effort by key stakeholder would optimize the use of current resources and human capital needed to combat this problem.

The AMR challenge requires both public and private sectors. For example, pharmaceuticals R&D, manufacturing, and after market surveillance is a very cost-intensive process. Funds and human resources should be made available by global financial institutions to fund both public and private organizations working on AMR. Companies should be rewarded or penalized for the effort regarding the fight against this crisis. For example, in developing nations, where regulations and enforcement are minimal, there is an unusually high influx of artificial drugs into pharmacies and drug stores. The self-prescription of fake antimicrobial drugs by people further exacerbates the resistance crisis. Companies manufacturing such drugs should be penalized while their product is removed from the market.

Finally, the GCTA AMR plan is not likely to be effective without a coordinated educational and knowledge base campaign.[14] Practicing clinicians and individuals need to be educated on the importance of antimicrobial stewardship as well as the threat it imposes. Making this matter a topic of conversation, by teaching this in schools and community events. Rewarding clinicians who provide patient education on the subject matter, placing marketing campaigns in various media and setting required standards regarding AMU. The primary goal regarding education would be achieved, once the idea of microbial resistance becomes a topic of conversation in everyday life.

Furthermore, every practitioner should, especially primary care clinicians such as physicians assistants/associates should have a standing protocol on the prescription of antimicrobial. They should get in the habit of asking questions about their use of antimicrobial, the setting in where it is appropriate and if their use of a given agent would add or detract from the increase of antimicrobial drug resistance.

Clinical Pearl 4

- *Question 4: How can clinicians effectively prescribe antimicrobials at the point of care without adding to the antimicrobial resistance crisis?*
- *Thought Exercise 4: Practitioners could limit the automatic prescription of broad-spectrum antibiotics until a definitive diagnosis is made. In nonemergent clinical cases involving the top microbials, a short window period of waiting for results is probable.*

Clinical Pearl 5

- *Question 5: On a macroscale, how can an entire country practice antimicrobial stewardship and join the fight against AMR?*
- *Thought Exercise 5: Nation states have the power to create enforceable policies and guidelines regarding AMU. They also have autonomy to create incentive and disincentive programs for practitioners, private and public organizations involved in the fight against resistance.*

CLINICS CARE POINTS

- Use antibiotics judiciously: Only prescribe antibiotics when they are truly needed, and choose the most appropriate antibiotic based on the type of infection and the susceptibility of the organism.

- Follow infection control measures: Implement standard precautions, such as hand hygiene and personal protective equipment, to prevent the spread of resistant organisms.

- Monitor antibiotic use and resistance: Collect data on antibiotic use and resistance patterns in your facility or community, and use this information to guide antibiotic prescribing practices.

- Consider antibiotic stewardship programs: Implement programs that promote the appropriate use of antibiotics and help to reduce unnecessary antibiotic use.

- Educate patients and families: Provide education on the appropriate use of antibiotics and the importance of infection prevention measures, such as vaccination and hand hygiene.

- Practice antimicrobial susceptibility testing: Test the susceptibility of organisms to antimicrobial agents, especially in cases of recurrent or persistent infections.

- Use combination therapy judiciously: Consider combination therapy for severe infections caused by multidrug-resistant organisms, but only when it is supported by evidence and appropriate.

- Consider the source control: Treat the source of the infection, such as draining abscesses or removing foreign bodies, in addition to using antimicrobial therapy.

- Follow-up patients: Monitor patients closely after initiation of antibiotic therapy to ensure that their infection is responding appropriately and to assess for adverse effects.

- Advocate for antimicrobial resistance awareness: Participate in advocacy efforts to raise awareness of antimicrobial resistance and the importance of appropriate antibiotic use and infection prevention measures.

DISCLOSURE

The authors have nothing to disclose.

REFERENCES

1. Shankar Pr. Book review: Tackling drug-resistant infections globally. Arch Pharm Pract 2016;7(3):110.
2. Prevention USC for DC and. Antibiotic Resistance Threats in the United States, 2019, *AR Threats Report*, 2019. Available at: https://www.cdc.gov/drugresistance/pdf/threats-report/2019-ar-threats-report-508.pdf. Accessed December, 2019.
3. CDC Global Health - Infographics. Antibiotic Resistance The Global Threat, Accessed 21 September, 2022. 2020. Available at: https://www.cdc.gov/globalhealth/infographics/antibiotic-resistance/antibiotic_resistance_global_threat.htm.
4. Prestinaci F, Pezzotti P, Pantosti A. Antimicrobial resistance: a global multifaceted phenomenon. Pathog Glob Health 2015;109(7):309–18.
5. McKernan C, Benson T, Farrell S, et al. Antimicrobial use in agriculture: critical review of the factors influencing behaviour. JAC-Antimicrobial Resistance 2021; 3(4). https://doi.org/10.1093/jacamr/dlab178.
6. Jonas. Drug-resistant infections : a threat to our economic future (Vol. 2) : final report. World Bank. Accessed September 21, 2022. 2017. Available at: https://documents.worldbank.org/en/publication/documents-reports/documentdetail/323311493396993758/final-report.
7. Saga T, Yamaguchi K. History of antimicrobial agents and resistant bacteria. JMAJ 2009;52(2):102–8.
8. Podolsky SH. The evolving response to antibiotic resistance (1945–2018). Palgrave Communications 2018;4(1):1–8.
9. World Health Orginization. WHO global priority pathogens list of antibiotic-resistant bacteria. Combat AMR. 2021. Accessed 21, September 2022. Available at: https://www.combatamr.org.au/news-events/who-global-priority-pathogens-list-of-antibiotic-resistant-bacteria.
10. CDC. Global Health - Newsroom. Tuberculosis, 2020. Accessed 21 September, 2022. Available at: https://www.cdc.gov/globalhealth/newsroom/topics/tb/index.html.
11. CDC. Most cases of C. diff occur while taking antibiotics or soon after. Centers for Disease Control and Prevention, Accessed 21 September, 2022. 2022. Available at: https://www.cdc.gov/cdiff/index.html
12. World Health Organization: WHO. Antimicrobial resistance. World Health Organization: WHO. 2021. Available at: https://www.who.int/news-room/fact-sheets/detail/antimicrobial-resistance. Accessed 21 September, 2022.
13. CDC. How Do healthcare professionals diagnose and treat sepsis? centers for disease control and prevention, Accessed 21 September, 2022. 2022. Available at: https://www.cdc.gov/sepsis/diagnosis/index.html.
14. CDC. The biggest antibiotic-resistant threats in the U.S. Centers for Disease Control and Prevention. Accessed 21 September, 2022. 2022. Available at: http://www.cdc.gov/DrugResistance/Biggest-Threats.html.

Gonococcal and Chlamydia Infections

Joshua Anderson, MS, PA-C[a],*, Sumathi Sankaran-Walters, PhD[b]

KEYWORDS

- Gonococcal infections • Chlamydia • Lymphogranuloma venereum • Urethritis
- Vaginitis

KEY POINTS

- Gonorrhea is among the most commonly reported infectious diseases in the United States.
- Infection rates have been increasing in the past years, especially in the 15 to 24 age group.
- Significant racial disparities exist in gonococcal infection rates.
- Gonococci strains that are resistant to penicillin, tetracycline, cephalosporins, and ciprofloxacin have been observed.
- Chlamydia infections are one of the leading causes of infertility in women in the United States.

GONOCOCCAL EPIDEMIOLOGY

In the United States, *Neisseria gonorrhea* is one of the most commonly reported bacterial communicable diseases. Many of these infections are asymptomatic, thus statistics only capture a fraction of the true disease incidence. Overall rates of infection declined after the mid-1970s, reaching an all-time low of 98.1 cases per 100,000 persons in 2009, but there was a subsequent increase in gonococcal infection rates, with 179.1 cases per 100,000 persons reported in 2018. According to the Centers for Disease Control and Prevention (CDC), in 2018 about 1.6 million new gonococcal infections occurred in the United States, with more than half of these infections occurring in young people aged 15 to 24 years.[1]

Transmission and Risk Factors

Transmission of *N gonorrhea* occurs during sexual activity including oral, anal, or vaginal sex. It can also be vertically transmitted from an infected mother to her

[a] Crossroads Medical Associates, 4801 Dorsey Hall Drive Suite 201, Ellicott City, MD 21043, USA;
[b] University Of California Davis, Betty Irene Moore Hall, 2570 48th Street, Sacramento, CA 95817, USA
* Corresponding author.
E-mail address: janderson995@gmail.com

Physician Assist Clin 8 (2023) 421–431
https://doi.org/10.1016/j.cpha.2023.02.005
2405-7991/23/© 2023 Elsevier Inc. All rights reserved.

baby during childbirth. The incubation period is typically 2 to 10 days. Factors that increase the risk of contracting gonorrhea include a recent new sexual partner, multiple sexual partners, being unmarried, young age, being of an underrepresented ethnic population, low educational and socioeconomic levels, substance abuse, or having history of previous gonorrhea.[2] Major racial and ethnic disparities exist in disease prevalence. Gonococcal infection rates are particularly high in specific populations, with the highest reported rates seen among adolescents and young adults, African Americans, and persons living in the southeastern United States.[3]

Signs and Symptoms

Key point: infections are often asymptomatic.
Urethritis:
Males: typical symptoms include dysuria and a serous or milky penile discharge. This discharge can turn purulent in a matter of days.
Females: typical symptoms include dysuria, and urinary frequency/urgency.
Cervicitis and vaginitis: typical symptoms include vaginal discharge, vaginal bleeding not associated with menstruation, pelvic pain, lower abdominal pain, dyspareunia, and inflammation of Bartholin glands.
Proctitis: most cases are asymptomatic. When symptoms occur, they can include tenesmus, anorectal pain, rectal fullness, constipation, anorectal bleeding, and mucopurulent anal discharge. This type of infection is common in men who have sex with men (MSM). It can also occur in women with existing genital infections in the absence of sexual contact through spread from the genital tract.
Pharyngitis: the pharynx is an atypical site of primary infection. "90% of infections are asymptomatic."[4] Infected patients may experience sore throat, odynophagia, and/or cervical lymphadenopathy.
Conjunctivitis: typical symptoms include conjunctival inflammation/swelling, mucopurulent discharge, eyelid edema, globe tenderness, and preauricular lymphadenopathy. This is common in babies born via vaginal birth to infected mothers.

Laboratory Testing

The importance of laboratory testing for gonococcal infections cannot be understated. A specific diagnosis of *N gonorrhoeae* can help to reduce complications, reinfections, and transmission.

Types of Tests

Nucleic acid amplification testing (NAAT) is the primary test of choice for microbiologic diagnosis of *N gonorrhoeae* infection[5] with excellent sensitivity and specificity. The sensitivity is typically superior to culture.[1] This type of testing can be run from urethral, endocervical, vaginal, rectal, or oropharyngeal swabs, as well as first-catch AM urine in men.[6]

Bacterial culture
This is an important diagnostic tool, especially when antibiotic resistance is suspected.[2] A culture requires an endocervical swab for women or a urethral swab for men. Cultures can also be used for detecting rectal, oropharyngeal, or conjunctival gonococcal infections. If there is a suspected or documented treatment failure, clinicians should perform both culture and antimicrobial susceptibility testing.[1]

Gram stain (microscopy)
Because of the high specificity (>99%), Gram stains of urethral discharge or secretions that demonstrate polymorphonuclear leukocytes with intracellular gram-negative

diplococci can confirm infection with *N gonorrhoeae* among symptomatic men. However, because of lower sensitivity (>95%), a negative Gram stain cannot rule out infection among asymptomatic men. Infection detection by using Gram stain of endocervical, pharyngeal, and rectal specimens is also insensitive and is not recommended.[1]

Rapid tests
There are several point-of-care tests available and can be useful, as NAAT results are not typically available the same day.

Antigen detection
Recently an enzyme immunoassay was developed to detect gonococcal antigens. This assay can be performed from cervical swabs or urine specimens but is not widely used because its positive predictive value is only acceptable in populations with a high prevalence of infection.[5]

Screening asymptomatic individuals
The USPSTF recommends screening annually for all sexually active women younger than 25 years and those aged 25 years or older who have a new sex partner, more than one sex partner, a sex partner with concurrent partners, or a sex partner who has a sexually transmitted infection (STI).[1] The USPSTF also recommends routine screening in people who have previously tested positive for gonorrhea or have multiple sexual partners. Because of increased risk individuals who use condoms inconsistently, provide sexual favors for money, or have sex while under the influence of alcohol or drugs should also be tested routinely.[7–9]

Additional testing
Commonly infection with *N gonorrhea* is accompanied by infection with *Chlamydia trachomatis*. Thus when a diagnostic test for *N gonorrhoeae* is performed, testing for coinfections, specifically *C trachomatis*, should also be performed.[5]

Men with Urogenital Symptoms

NAAT of the first-catch urine is the diagnostic test of choice. A urethral swab is also an acceptable specimen for NAAT. Extragenital infections are also common. Screening with oral and rectal swabs should be collected in high-risk individuals. Self-collected pharyngeal and rectal swabs can also be used.5 Urethral swab collection can be used to establish a microscopic diagnosis of *N gonorrhoeae*. The presence of polymorphonuclear leukocytes with intracellular gram-negative diplococci on Gram stain confirm the diagnosis.

Women with Urogenital Symptoms

The preferred diagnostic test is NAAT of either a self- or clinician-collected vaginal swab. An endocervical swab can also be used if a pelvic examination is being performed. Urine and liquid Pap smear medium can also be used for NAAT.[5] If NAAT methods are unavailable, culture, antigen detection, and genetic probe methods can be used instead.[5] Point-of-care testing can also be performed.

Patients with Extragenital Symptoms

Extragenital symptoms are relatively a rare presentation. Thus, sexually active individuals with symptoms and signs of proctitis, even in the absence of self-reported anal sexual exposure, should undergo diagnostic testing for *N gonorrhoeae*. In women with proctitis a thorough history needs to be taken in addition to testing for *N gonorrhoeae.* Patients who present with symptoms of pharyngitis with a history of unprotected oral sex should also be tested.[5] In patients, especially babies with symptoms of gonococcal conjunctivitis, microbiological diagnosis can be made by Gram stain and/or culture of conjunctival discharge.[5]

Differential Diagnosis

The symptoms of vaginal discharge in women and urethral discharge in men need to be differentiated from other STIs. Nongonococcal urethritis, cervicitis, and vaginitis due to *C trachomatis*, *Gardnerella vaginalis*, *Trichomonas*, and *Candida* have similar symptoms in women. Gonococcal infections can progress to result in pelvic inflammatory disease (PID).

Reactive arthritis (urethritis, conjunctivitis, arthritis) may mimic systemic infection with *N gonorrhoeae* or coexist with it.[6]

Treatment Overview

N gonorrhoeae has developed decreasing susceptibility to commonly used therapies; therefore, treatment options have changed over time.[5] Strains of gonococci that are resistant to penicillin, tetracycline, cephalosporins, and ciprofloxacin have been observed in greater frequency.[6] Cephalosporin treatment failures should be reported to the CDC. Empiric treatment can be provided to patients who have a known exposure to gonorrhea within 1 to 2 weeks. Treatment of gonorrhea is often combined with the treatment of chlamydia and will be covered at the end of this section.

Prevention

It is important to note that prior infection with *N gonorrhoeae* does not lead to immunity. Abstinence is a very effective method of prevention, however, not always practical. Education on safe sex practices, such as using protection or having sex with one partner who is not infected, is helpful to reduce gonococcal infections; this is a reportable communicable disease. The department of public health follows up with partner notification and referral of contacts for treatment. These actions can help lead to expedited treatment of partners. Mechanical prophylaxis using condoms reduces the risk of infection. Chemical prophylaxis, postexposure prophylaxis with effective drugs taken within 24 hours of exposure, can stave off an infection.[6]

Complications and Long-Term Sequelae

Males: epididymitis, inflammation of the periurethral glands. Prostatitis and urethral structures can occur with chronic infection. Penile edema, penile lymphangitis, and periurethral abscess can occur because of inflammation-associated scarring. Gonococcal infections are also associated with increased risk for prostate cancer.[10]

Females: the most common sequelae include salpingitis and scarring of fallopian tubes, resulting in hydrosalpinx. The most significant complication is PID (which can lead to infertility) as well as ectopic pregnancy and chronic pelvic pain.

Disseminated gonococcal infection (DGI): this occurs through the spread of the gonococci from the primary site via the bloodstream.

Gonococcal arthritis-dermatitis syndrome (triad: rash, tenosynovitis, and arthralgias): rash is typically maculopapular to pustular or hemorrhagic. Tenosynovitis typically occurs in the hands, wrists, feet, and ankles.[6] DGI must be differentiated from disseminated *Neisseria meningitidis* infection.

Suppurative arthritis: can occur in one or more joints as occurs with *N meningitidis* infection and must be differentiated.

Conjunctivitis: can occur through direct inoculation of the gonococci into the conjunctive, typically by autoinoculation of an individual with a genital infection or exposure in the birth canal. Purulent conjunctivitis may rapidly progress to panophthalmitis, resulting in loss of vision in the affected eye.[6]

Perihepatitis (Fitz-Hugh-Curtis syndrome): inflammation of Glisson capsule surrounding the liver can occur from extensions in the peritoneal cavity. This typically occurs in women and is associated commonly with *C trachomatis* infection.

Complications of Pregnancy

Urogenital gonococcal infections have been associated with chorioamnionitis, premature rupture of membranes, preterm birth, low-birth-weight or small for gestational age infants, and spontaneous abortions. Infants born to infected mothers may have neonatal conjunctivitis (ophthalmia neonatorum), pharyngitis, arthritis, and gonococcemia, and sepsis.[5]

Endocarditis and meningitis are rare complications while more common with *N meningitidis*.

CHLAMYDIA

C trachomatis is a sexually transmitted, gram-negative intracellular bacteria that causes infection worldwide. Infections can be asymptomatic, which can lead to quick disease transmission and chronic infections. Chlamydia infections are one of the leading causes of infertility in women in the United States.[6]

Epidemiology

In the United States, it is a commonly reported bacterial infection and cause of urethritis in men and cervicitis in women. In 2018, 1,758,668 chlamydial infections were reported to the CDC. With an incidence of 539.9 cases per 100,000 people, the rate of infection among women is about twice that among men, likely due to the fact that women are more likely to be screened while being asymptomatic.[11]

Transmission and Risk Factors

This is a sexually transmitted disease with a critical feature in that immunity to infection is not long-lived. Thus reinfection or persistent infection is common.[12,13] The incubation period of symptomatic disease ranges from 5 to 14 days following infection. This infection occurs commonly with *N gonorrhoeae*.

Race, ethnicity, economic disadvantage, and geographic region all play a role in the likelihood of contracting chlamydia. In 2018, the reported incidence among black individuals was almost 6 times that of white individuals. In 2015, it was estimated that American Indian or Alaska Native persons had an incidence of chlamydia 3.8 times higher than the rate among white persons in the United States.[12] Individuals younger than 25 years tend to have the highest prevalence of chlamydia. Other risk factors include new sexual partners or more than one sex partner in the prior 3 months, history of previous *C trachomatis* infection, inconsistent use of condoms, and MSM.

Signs and Symptoms

Women: most women are asymptomatic. When symptoms occur, the cervix is the most commonly infected anatomic site. Some women have an infection of the urethra. Left untreated, pelvic inflammatory disease may develop.

Cervicitis: nonspecific symptoms may include a change in vaginal discharge, intermenstrual vaginal bleeding, and postcoital bleeding. Physical examination findings include mucopurulent endocervical discharge, easily induced endocervical bleeding, or edematous ectopy.

Urethritis: symptoms may include urinary frequency, urgency, and dysuria.

Pelvic inflammatory disease: when symptoms of PID are present, abdominal and pelvic pain are the most common. Signs of PID include cervical motion tenderness, as well as uterine or adnexal tenderness. Systemic symptoms such as fever painful intercourse are also common.

Perihepatitis (Fitz-Hugh-Curtis syndrome): as mentioned previously this is an inflammation of the liver capsule and adjacent peritoneal surfaces associated with right-upper quadrant pain.

Complications of pregnancy: there is a risk of future ectopic pregnancy following chlamydia-associated PID. As seen with *N gonorrhoeae*, when a chlamydial infection occurs during pregnancy there can be an increased risk for premature rupture of the membranes, preterm delivery, and low-birth-weight infants (UTD).

Proctitis: can occur in both men and women. When symptoms occur, they can include tenesmus, anorectal pain, rectal fullness, constipation, anorectal bleeding, and mucopurulent discharge.

Men

Urethritis—Most males are asymptomatic. When symptoms are present, they typically include mucoid or watery urethral discharge which is often clear. Symptoms may also include dysuria.

Epididymitis—This is associated with unilateral testicular pain, tenderness, hydrocele, and palpable swelling of the epididymis. Scrotal ultrasound is helpful when concerned for epididymitis.

Other presentations include prostatitis and proctitis. Systemic symptoms such as fever and malaise may also occur. Anoscopic findings are nonspecific but may include mucosal friability, internal lesions, masses or polyps, and mucopurulent exudate.

Clinical Syndromes Occurring in Both Men and Women

Similar to *N gonorrhoeae*, patients may present with conjunctivitis or pharyngitis or genital lymphogranuloma venereum (discussed in later sections).

Reactive arthritis/reactive arthritis triad: reactive arthritis can occur following an STI and the classic triad includes arthritis, conjunctivitis or uveitis, and urethritis or cervicitis. *C trachomatis* seems to be the most common inciting pathogen for sexually acquired reactive arthritis.

Prevalence in Pregnancy

The risk of acquiring *C trachomatis* in an infant born vaginally to a woman with chlamydial cervicitis is approximately about 50%. The most frequent clinical manifestation of *C trachomatis* infection in the newborn is conjunctivitis. The incubation period for this type of conjunctivitis is 5 to 14 days after delivery. Pneumonia due to *C trachomatis* can also occur in infants between 4 and 12 weeks. Symptoms may include cough and nasal congestion and afebrile/minimal fever.

Laboratory Tests

NAAT: this is the diagnostic method of choice. Same-day results are not typically available.

Note: microscopy is not useful for the diagnosis of chlamydia. Because of superior sensitivity and specificity and wide availability, NAAT is the diagnostic technique of choice.

Women: *vaginal swab* can be self-collected and is the specimen of choice Endocervical swab can be collected by a provider and used as well.

First-catch urine: might detect 10% fewer infections compared with vaginal or endocervical swabs.

Men: first-catch urine is the specimen of choice. Urethral swab is an alternative site. Rectal swab and/or conjunctival swabs can also be used if they are the sites of infection.

Culture: these methods are typically reserved for research and reference laboratories due to expense and technical expertise required.

Antigen detection tests are performed from endocervical or urethral swabs. The sensitivity of this method is 80% to 95% when compared with culture.

Genetic probes are also performed from endocervical or urethral swabs. The sensitivity of this assay is approximately 80% when compared with culture.

Rapid tests: point-of-care testing is sometimes used in resource-limited regions. These tests offer same-day test results. Sensitivity 96%, specificity 99%, positive predictive value 91%, and negative predictive value 100% for *C trachomatis*.

Who to test?

Symptomatic and at-risk asymptomatic patients. Routine screening with NAAT should be offered to sexually active patients at high risk of infection and complications of chlamydia. Also, patients with documented gonococcal infection should also undergo testing for chlamydia. Patients who have been treated for chlamydia should be rescreened about 3 months after treatment due to high rates of reinfection. Patients who have had exposure to chlamydia within the past 1 to 2 weeks should be treated empirically.

Differential Diagnosis

Urethritis: differential diagnoses include low-colony count urinary tract infection (eg, infection caused by *Staphylococcus saprophyticus*) and urethritis due to other STIs, such as *N gonorrhoeae*, *Trichomonas vaginalis*, *Mycoplasma genitalium*, or *herpes simplex* virus.

Proctitis: differential diagnoses include *N gonorrhoeae*, herpes simplex virus, and *Treponema pallidum* infection.

Prevention

Prior infection does not lead to immunity. Abstinence is a very effective method of prevention; however, it is not always practical. Education on safe sex practices such as condom usage is a way to prevent infection.

Chemical prophylaxis— postexposure prophylaxis: effective drugs taken within 24 hours of exposure can stave off an infection.

Newborn prevention: maternal screening is recommended.

Screening: routine screening for chlamydial infection is recommended for all pregnant women younger than 25 years and women aged 25 years or older with risk factors for STI.

Potential Complications

Men: epididymitis, inflammation of the periurethral glands. Prostatitis and urethral structures can occur with chronic infection. Penile edema, penile lymphangitis, periurethral abscess.

Women: salpingitis, scarring of fallopian tubes; pelvic inflammatory disease (which can lead to infertility); ectopic pregnancy; and chronic pelvic pain.

TREATMENT OF *C TRACHOMATIS* AND *N GONORRHOEAE*

In general, *N gonorrhoeae* and *C trachomatis* are treated together.

Newborn Treatment

Conjunctivitis—for *N gonorrhoeae* ceftriaxone 1 g intramuscularly (IM) as a single dose.

Initial treatment of chlamydial conjunctivitis should be based on a positive diagnostic test with the preferred regimen of erythromycin, 50 mg/kg, PO in 4 divided doses x 14 days

Alternative: azithromycin, 20 mg/kg, given once daily PO x 3 days.

For neonatal pneumonia the initial treatment is empiric with the same protocol as discussed earlier until diagnostic test results come available.

Adult Treatment

C trachomatis is generally highly susceptible to tetracyclines, macrolides, and fluoroquinolones We often see resistance with penicillins. Sulfonamides and cephalosporins have limited activity. A comprehensive treatment approach includes antibiotic treatment of the infection as well as evaluation and treatment of other STIs, counseling on medication adherence and sexual activity, follow-up testing, and management of sex partners.

CERVICITIS AND URETHRITIS

For *N gonorrhoeae* ceftriaxone, 500 mg, IM (if < 150 kg) OR ceftriaxone, 1000 mg, IM (if > 150 kg) as a single dose is preferred.

In a case where cephalosporins are the only option, cefixime, 800 mg, PO x 1 can be used, but retesting to ensure successful treatment within 1 week is recommended in this case. For patients with urogenital or anorectal gonococcal infection who have severe cephalosporin allergies gentamicin, 240 mg, IM or gemifloxacin, 320 mg, PO x 1 plus azithromycin, 2 g, PO x 1 as a single dose can be used.

For *C trachomatis* doxycycline is the preferred antibiotic agent and is typically given as 100 mg BID x 7 days. Alternatively, single-dose azithromycin, 1 g, PO is preferred for pregnant individuals. It can be used in patients who are unlikely to complete a 7-day course of doxycycline. Additional alternative agents include levofloxacin, 500 mg, one PO QD x 7 days OR ofloxacin, 300 mg, one BID x 7 days. Fluoroquinolones can be more costly and also lead to potentially severe adverse effects.

Sulfonamides and cephalosporins should not be considered due to limited activity.

To avoid reinfection from both infectious agents, patients should be instructed to abstain from sexual intercourse until they and their sex partners have been completely treated (ie, after completion of a 7-day regimen or for 7 days after a single-dose regimen) and any symptoms have resolved.

Retesting after treatment: this is done on all patients with documented chlamydial infection 3 months after treatment.

Test of cure: it can be used to assess whether the administered antibiotic regimen eradicated the pathogen. Not required in all cases given a high rate of cure with appropriate treatment. It can be done in pregnant individuals, those with persistent symptoms, or those patients for whom you are concerned about nonadherence to the regimen.

PELVIC INFLAMMATORY DISEASE

Hospitalized patients are also treated for both infectious agents.

Ceftriaxone, 1 g, intravenously every 24 hours plus doxycycline, 100 mg, orally or intravenously every 12 hours plus metronidazole, 500 mg, orally or intravenously every 12 hours.

OR

Cefoxitin, 2 g, intravenously every 6 hours plus doxycycline, 100 mg, orally or intravenously every 12 hours.

OR

Cefotetan, 2 g, intravenously every 12 hours plus doxycycline, 100 mg, orally or intravenously every 12 hours.

Outpatient: mild-to-moderate PID.

A single intramuscular dose of a long-acting cephalosporin—ceftriaxone, 500 mg, IM (if < 150 kg) OR ceftriaxone, 1000 mg, IM (if > 150 kg) plus doxycycline, 100 mg, orally twice daily for 14 days plus metronidazole, 500 mg, orally twice daily for 14 days.

LYMPHOGRANULOMA VENEREUM

Lymphogranuloma venereum is both an acute and chronic STI caused by *C trachomatis* types L1 to L3 and is acquired through intercourse or through contact with contaminated exudate from active lesions. The incubation period is 5 to 21 days.

Signs/symptoms: lymphadenopathy, proctitis with rectal stricture in women or MSM. After the genital lesion disappears, the infection spreads to the lymph channels and lymph nodes of the genital and rectal areas. Inapparent infections and latent disease are unfortunately common.[6]

Men: initial vesicular or ulcerative lesion on the external genitalia is evanescent and often goes unnoticed. Inguinal buboes appear 1 to 4 weeks after exposure, often occurring bilaterally. They often fuse, soften, and break down into multiple draining sinuses, which can cause extensive scarring.[6]

Women: genital lymph drainage occurs at the perirectal glands. Early anorectal manifestations are proctitis with feelings of tenesmus and bloody purulent discharge. Late manifestations are chronic inflammation of the rectal and perirectal tissues, which can lead to rectal strictures as well as rectovaginal and perianal fistulas and can be mistaken for inflammatory bowel disease.[6]

LABORATORY FINDINGS

Serology: complement fixation test may be positive—titers greater than 1:64. Cross-reactivity with other chlamydiae can occur. High titers usually indicate active disease but may also represent remote infection.[6] NAAT for *C trachomatis* can be performed.

DIFFERENTIAL DIAGNOSIS

Early lymphogranuloma venereum lesions must be differentiated from the lesions of syphilis, genital herpes, and chancroid. Lymph node involvement should be differentiated from tularemia, tuberculosis, plague, neoplasm, or pyogenic infection. Rectal stricture must be distinguished from neoplasm and inflammatory bowel disease.[6]

TREATMENT
Urethritis and Cervicitis

C. trachomatis is a common cause of nongonococcal urethritis and cervicitis. In other cases, *Ureaplasma urealyticum* or *M genitalium* can be grown as the possible etiologic

agent. Coinfection with gonococci and chlamydiae is common.[6] Treatment is the same as listed earlier: doxycycline, 100 mg, BID x 21 days.
Alternative regimen: azithromycin 1 g orally once weekly for 3 weeks.

CLINICS CARE POINTS

- Take a complete sexual and travel history. It is essential in the diagnosis and treatment of *N gonorrhea* and *C trachomatis*.
- Be aware that many patients are asymptomatic and that reinfection is very common.
- When treating a patient for STI, investigate if there is an underlaying antimicrobial resistance
- In general *N gonorrhoeae* and *C trachomatis* are treated together.
- Educate patients about screening, prevention, and treatments of STIs.

DISCLOSURE

The authors have nothing to disclose.

REFERENCES

1. Centers for Disease Control and Prevention. 2022. Gonorrhea – CDC Detailed Fact Sheet. Available at: https://www.cdc.gov/std/gonorrhea/stdfact-gonorrhea-detailed.htm#ref1. Accessed April 24, 2022.
2. Price GA, Bash MC. Epidemiology and pathogenesis of Neisseria gonorrhoeae infection. In: Marrazzo J, editors. UpToDate. Waltham (MA): UpToDate. Available at: www.uptodate.com. Accessed April 29, 2022.
3. CDC. Sexually Transmitted Disease Surveillance, 2019. Atlanta, GA: Department of Health and Human Services; 2021.
4. Bernadette Z, Cantor MD, Amy G, et al. "Review: Screening for Gonorrhea and Chlamydia: A Systematic Review for the U.S. Prevententive Services Task Force". Ann Intern Med 2014;161(12):884–94. CiteSeerX.
5. Ghanem KG. Clinical manifestations and diagnosis of Neisseria gonorrhoeae infection in adults and adolescents. In: Marrazzo J. UpToDate. Waltham (MA): UpToDate. Available at: www.uptodate.com. Accessed April 29, 2022.
6. Papadakis MA, McPhee SJ, Rabow MW, et al, editors. Current medical diagnosis & treatment 2022. McGraw Hill; 2022. Available at: https://accessmedicine. mhmedical.com/content.aspx?bookid=3081&sectionid=258579240. Available at: Accessed June 1, 2022.
7. Smith L, Angarone MP. "Sexually Transmitted Infections". Urol Clin 2015;42(4): 507–18. CiteSeerX.
8. Workowski KA, Bachmann LH, Chan PA, et al. Sexually Transmitted Infections Treatment Guidelines, 2021. MMWR Recomm Rep (Morb Mortal Wkly Rep) 2021;70:1.
9. Seña AC, Cohen MS. Treatment of uncomplicated Neisseria gonorrhoeae infections. In: Marrazzo J. UpToDate. Waltham (MA): UpToDate. Available at: www. uptodate.com. Accessed April 29, 2022.
10. Saverio C, Sara G, Maria D, et al. "Sexually transmitted infections and prostate cancer risk: A systematic review and meta-analysis". Cancer Epidemiology 2014;38(4):329–38.
11. Centers for Disease Control and Prevention. Sexually transmitted disease Surveillance, 2018. Atlanta (GA): US Department of Health and Human Services; 2019.

Available at: https://www.cdc.gov/std/stats18/default.htm. Accessed on April 29, 2022.

12. Hsu K, Epidemiology of Chlamydia trachomatis infections. In: Marrazzo J. UpToDate. Waltham (MA): UpToDate. Available at: www.uptodate.com. Accessed April 29, 2022.

13. Hamill M. Lymphogranuloma venereum. In: Marrazzo J, editor. UpToDate. Waltham (MA): UpToDate. Available at: www.uptodate.com. Accessed June 28, 2022.

Concerning Features of Emerging Fungal Infections

Justina Bennett, MPAS, PA-C

KEYWORDS

- *Candida auris* • Coccidioidomycosis • *Cryptococcus gattii* • Histoplasmosis
- Pneumocystis pneumonia • Immunocompromised • Travel history
- HIV-negative persons

KEY POINTS

- Emerging fungal infections such as resistant *Candida auris* in health care facilities pose a significant risk for horizontal transmission and a high mortality rate for immunocompromised individuals.
- Knowledge of the changing demographic distribution of *Coccidioides* species along with an accurate travel history and a high degree of clinical suspicion is key in making a timely diagnosis of coccidioidomycosis.
- Recognizing nontraditional risk factors for *Cryptococcus gattii* infection including age greater than 50, chronic lung disease, smoking, and the more temperate demographic distribution of this new species.
- Educating high-risk patients to recognize recreational and occupational exposures that put them at risk for contracting histoplasmosis.
- Having a high index of suspicion for pneumocystis pneumonia in immunocompromised human immunodeficiency virus (HIV)-negative patients to make a timely diagnosis and improve outcomes.

INTRODUCTION TO EMERGING FUNGAL INFECTIONS

Many factors are at play in the changing landscape of fungal infections. According to a 2013 National Health Interview Survey, 3% of the population is immunosuppressed and this number is expected to grow due to improved lifespans and new indications for immunosuppressive therapies.[1] The pool of immunocompromised individuals has grown significantly with the use of monoclonal antibodies and small-molecule inhibitors for B-cell malignancies.[2] Additionally, we can more specifically identify genetic and phenotypic differences among known fungal pathogens and long-term antifungal and antibiotic use has led to an "altered global microbiome" and the emergence of drug-resistant fungal infections.[2]

Department of PA Medicine, Frostburg State University, 24 N. Walnut Street, Hagerstown, MD 21740, USA
E-mail addresses: Justina.Olsen@hotmail.com; jabennett@frostburg.edu

Physician Assist Clin 8 (2023) 433–452
https://doi.org/10.1016/j.cpha.2023.02.002
2405-7991/23/© 2023 Elsevier Inc. All rights reserved.

Candida Auris

Background

Candida auris is emerging primarily in hospital and long-term care facilities and is of significant concern due to its resistance to many antifungal medications. It was first identified in 2009 in a 70-year-old woman from Japan with ear drainage due to an ear canal infection.[3] From that time, *C auris* has been found in more than 30 countries worldwide including the United States of America in 2015.[4] It is typically associated with outbreaks in hospital facilities. Twenty-one states in the United States reported cases of *C auris* from 1/1/21 to 12/31/21 up from only four states in 2013 to 2016.[5] In some countries where *C auris* has been present for a decade, it is the leading cause of candidemia and is the most common *Candida* species in some settings.[4] Due to the highly specific laboratory testing needed to correctly identify *C auris,* it is likely that there is a greater spread than what is identified.[5]

PREVALENCE/INCIDENCE

Candidemia is the most common clinical manifestation of *C auris*. There is an in-hospital global crude mortality rate of 30% to 60%, up to 72% with candidemia cases.[6–8] A recent systematic review of nearly 5000 cases of *C auris* from 33 countries indicated a more specific overall crude mortality rate of 39%.[9] Risk factors for exposure are shown below (**Box 1**).

The high rate of mortality may be multifactorial including easy transmissibility in hospital settings, misidentification in the laboratories leading to delayed diagnosis, and multidrug resistance.[7,11] With the COVID-19 pandemic, there have been reports of spread in COVID-19 units. This may have been related to limitations in infection control and changes in cleaning and disinfection processes. For instance, early in the COVID-19 pandemic, there were personal protective equipment (PPE) limitations and protective wear was being used, reused, and used longer than recommended. Additionally screening for other pathogens such as *C auris* may have become secondary during the COVID-19 pandemic.[12]

C auris has been shown to live outside the human host on environmental surfaces such as plastics and medical devices for long periods.[13] A study by Welsh and colleagues[13] determined that *C auris* can live up to 2 weeks on surfaces in culture and remain metabolically active for up to 4 weeks. Patients and health care providers who are colonized with *C auris* can spread it asymptomatically.[9] *C auris* can be found on gloves, bedding, clothes, and medical devices that have been in contact with colonized or infected individuals.[9] A biofilm, which is drug-resistant, can form on indwelling catheters and medical devices serving as a venue for infection similar to what is seen with other *Candida* species.[8,13–15] Another significant risk is mechanical ventilation likely due to the presence and persistence of *C auris* on ventilation equipment as well as the risk factors

---

Box 1
Risk factors for candidemia due to *Candida auris*[10]

- Receiving care at a facility where *C auris* has been identified
- Prolonged hospital stays
- Immunocompromised patients including those with coronavirus disease (COVID-19)
- Central venous catheters or other invasive catheters or drains
- Recent broad-spectrum antibiotic or antifungal use

present in populations requiring mechanical ventilation.[16] It is unclear if climate change or other environmental factors are working to contribute to the spread of *C auris*.[17]

SIGNS/SYMPTOMS

Most patients with *C auris* are asymptomatic[9] and identified only by skin colonization testing.[18] Immunocompetent individuals often will not experience any symptoms when *C auris* is identified on the skin, in the respiratory tract, or in the urine,[18] however, they may be transmitting it to others.[9] *C auris* manifestations can be mild ranging from superficial and mucosal infections to severe causing disseminated disease (intra-abdominal infections, meningitis, myocarditis, osteomyelitis, surgical and nonsurgical wound infections) and bloodstream infections.[4,8,19] The clinical presentation of *C auris* is like candidemia from other species. It can vary from a minimal fever to a sepsis syndrome that is difficult to distinguish from severe bacterial etiologies making lab testing essential.[20]

EVALUATION

C auris infections share the same risk profile and clinical presentation as other *Candida* species, such as *Candida albicans* and *Candida glabrata*. Differentiating factors can be seen in the lab workup although the diagnostic workup to identify *C auris* is challenging due to multiple inconsistencies the species displays when cultured (**Table 1**). It is often misidentified as other species of *Candida* [21] and highly specialized lab equipment is needed.

TREATMENT

The current Centers for Disease Control (CDC) recommendation is that treatment of *C auris* only be implemented for clinically evident disease when isolated from a sterile specimen such as blood or cerebral spinal fluid.[23] Treatment is not recommended when *C auris* is found in non-invasive sites such as the respiratory tract, urine, or skin.[18,23] When *C auris* is identified in these non-invasive sites and patients do not manifest clinical disease, the appropriate infection control measures (**Box 2**) should be put in place to reduce invasive infections and prevent spread (**Box 3**) to others as spread in hospital settings is likely.[18,23]

Even with successful treatment of the disease, the patient may remain colonized with *C auris* long-term.[18] There is no specific literature documenting how long a patient may be colonized, but this could put them at risk for future infection as well as ongoing transmission to others.[23] There is no current recommended treatment to 'decolonize' patients.

The most concerning issue with *C auris* is that it is showing itself to be resistant to multiple antifungal medications. In some instances to all three classes of antifungals available (azoles, polyenes, and echinocandins).[24] Lockhart, and colleagues[24] (2017) noted almost half (44.29%) of *C auris* isolates from various studies were resistant to azole antifungals such as fluconazole. They also cite that 15.46% of *C auris* isolates are resistant to amphotericin B.[8,18] Echinocandin drugs such as Anidulafungin, Caspofungin, or Micafungin typically have been used first-line to treat *C auris* infections.[23] Up until recently, most strands of *C auris* have been susceptible to echinocandins although there is evidence of emerging resistance.[18,23] A combination of antifungal medications may be used.[23] Patients should be monitored to ensure clinical improvement with treatment and follow-up cultures with susceptibility testing should be repeated.[23] In the case of triple resistance to all antifungals (azoles, polyenes, and echinocandins), two new drug classes are in clinical trials. The *Fungerp* antifungal agent is also known as SCY-078

Table 1
Candida species diagnostic workup

Diagnostic Test	Pitfalls

Culture (from various specimen sites, sterile [blood] and nonsterile [skin for purpose of screening for colonization])[18]
• Chromogenic agar differentiates between *C auris* and *C haemulonii* because of growth characteristics[10]
  ○ *C auris* grows at elevated temperature (40 degree Celsius)[13,21]
  ○ *C auris* grows at increased salinity (10%wt/vol)[13]
	Characteristics[21]
	• Color—white, pink, red, or purple
	  ○ Inconsistent
	• Budding yeast rarely forming pseudohyphae
	  ○ Inconsistent
	• Does not form germ tubes
	• Some strains of *C auris* aggregate while others do not

Sequencing D1–D2 region of 28s rDNA to identify *C auris* (Gold Standard)[7,21]
• Diagnostic devices—MALDI-TOF
  ○ Differentiates *C auris* from other *Candida* species by their protein profile[7,21]
	• Many commercially available biochemical-based tests misidentify *C auris* as other phylogenetically related species[21,22]
	  ○ Vitek2 and API Auxacolor commonly misidentify *C auris* as *C famata, C haemulonii,* or *Rhodotorula glutinis*[7,21]
	• Not all reference databases included in MALDI-TOF devices allow for detection of *C. auris* species as it compares spectra and relies on input from previous isolates which are at times entered incorrectly[7,10,21]
	  ○ Differentiation between geographic strain is variable[10]

PCR assay specific to *C auris* using cultured colonies (in development) • Will allow rapid detection and proper identification of *C auris* species—useful in outbreak scenario[10]	• Need confirmation of sensitivity of these assays for different natural groups of *C auris*[10]

Abbreviations: MALDI-TOF, matrix-assisted laser desorption/ionization time-of-flight; PCR, polymerase chain reaction.

and is currently undergoing Phase III Clinical Trials.[8] APX001 is also proving to be effective against resistant *C auris* and is in the clinical development phase.[8]

SUMMARY

C auris is an important emerging fungal pathogen as it spreads easily within hospitals and long-term care facilities. If specific strains of *C auris* are found to be resistant to

Box 2
Infection control measures[16]

• Use of Standard Precautions and Contact Precautions

• Housing the patient in a private room

• Daily and terminal cleaning of the patient's room with a disinfectant that is active against *Clostridium difficile* spores

• Notification of receiving health care facilities when a patient with *C auris* colonization or infection is transferred

Note: Infection control measures are the same for colonized patients and those with evidence of active infection.[23]

Box 3
Prevention of *Candida auris* spread

- Screening for colonization with axilla/groin swab for high-risk patients and in facilities with known *C auris* presence[18]
- Specific attention to room cleaning
  - Products specific for *C auris* contain sodium hypochlorite-based disinfectant[16]
  - Correct product for the correct amount of time
  - Products with quarternary ammonia compounds are not effective in eliminating *C auris* despite their effectiveness against *C albicans*[23]
- Specific attention to device cleaning and care
  - Thoroughness in standards of infection control regarding device insertion and care
  - Routine re-evaluation of catheter, tubing, or device to determine if still warranted[23]
- Routine re-evaluation of antibiotic and antifungal use with timely discontinuation when appropriate[23]
- Infectious disease consultation[23]

multiple antifungal medications mortality rates are high. Diagnostic testing is challenging due to the misidentification of *C auris* as other *Candida* species. Culture characteristics can be inconsistent and even highly specific testing utilizing biochemical sequencing can be inaccurate. A low-cost method to get around the identification problems of commercial phenotypic assays is the use of chromogenic agar which can display specific features unique to *C auris* growth at elevated temperatures and salinity.[10] A guiding principle is if there is an increase in unidentified *Candida* species on culture in a hospital or long-term care facility *C auris* should be suspected.[21]

COCCIDIOIDOMYCOSIS
Background

Coccidioides species are diathermal dimorphic fungal species that are found endemically in the soil of the Western hemisphere.[25] It was first discovered in Argentina and then in California and is found primarily in the southwestern United States.[25] Even though it is considered endemic, it is distributed sparsely throughout the soil which has made it difficult to track.[25] Typically, it is found during arid weather after a period of rainfall.[25]

PREVALENCE/INCIDENCE

Table 2 discusses transmission and incubation. *Coccidioides* is considered infectious but not contagious.[25] Those most at risk are persons who live in or travel to endemic areas. Even short 1-day trips if exposed to *Coccidioides* can result in infection.[25] Approximately 60% of patients will be asymptomatic if they become infected, 40% of patients will develop primary disease affecting the pulmonary system, and less than 1% of cases will become disseminated.[25] Those at risk for disseminated disease include the elderly, solid-organ transplant recipients, HIV/AIDS patients, and those on tumor necrosis alpha antagonist therapies. Disseminated disease, particularly affecting the meninges without treatment, is often fatal.[25]

Coccidioides has been isolated in southwestern parts of the United States along the border of Mexico,[26] Arizona's Sonoran Desert including metropolitan areas of Phoenix and Tucson as well as California's southern San Joaquin Valley.[26] *Coccidioides* has also been found in Nevada, New Mexico, and Texas. Recently, new cases have occurred in Utah and south-central Washington.[26] Clinicians practicing in areas of the country where coccidioidomycosis is not endemic should be aware of their

Table 2
Comparison of fungal infections

	Coccidioidomycosis	Cryptococcus	Histoplasmosis
Location	• Historically: Southwest US ("Valley Fever") • Recently: Washington, Utah, Central/South America[26]	• Historically: Tropical/subtropical ○ Australia • Recently: Pacific Northwest[28,29]	• Ohio/Mississippi River Valleys[30] • Globally
Transmission	• Spore inhalation from disturbed soil (middens)[25,26] • Rare fomite-transmission[26]	• Spore inhalation from soil, plant debris, some trees[31]	• Microconidia inhaled from soil contaminated with bird/bat droppings[32,33] • High-risk exposures—spelunking, chicken coops, demolition/renovation old buildings[30,33]
Incubation	• 2 days to several weeks[25]	• 6 weeks to 35 months, most commonly 2 to 11 months[29]	• 3–17 days[33]

Presentation	• Pulmonary disease (40%)[25]
	  ○ Fever, cough, pleuritic pain
	• Disseminated disease (<1%)[25]
	  ○ Lymph
	  ○ Hematogenous—meningitis (most serious)
		• Pulmonary disease
		  ○ Cough, shortness of breath, chest pain, hemoptysis, pulmonary nodules[29,31]
		• CNS disease—meningoencephalitis
		  ○ Headache, ± nausea/vomiting, neck stiffness[29]
			• Pulmonary disease
			  ○ Fever, fatigue, cough, headache, chest pain, pulmonary nodules[33]
			  ○ Persistent pulmonary disease[34]
			• Disseminated[34]

Diagnostic workup	• Positive IgM/IgG immunodiffusion—diagnostic[25]
	• Culture—infection precautions needed in lab[25,27]
	• CBC w/differential—eosinophilia[25]
		• Imaging specific to presentation[29]
		  ○ CXR—CT chest—cryptococcomas
		  ○ CT/MRI brain—cryptococcomas, hydrocephalus
		• Culture—definitive diagnosis—turns culture medium blue on CGB agar[35]
		  ○ Specimen of concern—ie, LP for CNS disease[29,35]
			• Fungal culture[32]
			• Antigen and antibody testing via EIA[32,33]

Differential diagnoses	• Pulmonary[25]
	  ○ Community-acquired pneumonia d/t bacteria, viruses (COVID-19), fungus (blastomycosis, histoplasmosis)
	• Disseminated[25]
	  ○ Hematogenous—bacterial, viral, fungal etiologies of sepsis
	  ○ Meningitis—bacterial, viral, fungal etiologies
		• Pulmonary[29]
		  ○ Community-acquired pneumonia d/t bacteria, viruses, fungus
		• CNS[29]
		  ○ Meningoencephalitis d/t bacterial, viral, fungal etiologies
			• Pulmonary—acute
			  ○ Coccidioidomycosis, Blastomycosis, Community-acquired pneumonia due to bacteria, viral (including COVID-19) etiologies[36]
			• Pulmonary—chronic
			  ○ Tuberculosis, non-tuberculosis mycoplasma infections, blastomycosis, coccidioidomycosis, paracoccidioidomycosis, sporotrichosis, and sarcoidosis.[34]

Key points	• Know demographic locations *Coccidioides* found and obtain accurate travel history • Suspect in immunocompromised patients	• Travel history imperative but difficult to diagnose due to long incubation period[29] • Suspect in immunocompetent and immunocompromised patients[31]	• Occupational/recreational history of those living in or traveling to endemic areas, particularly if immunocompromised[30,33]

patients' travel history and patients who live in various parts of the country during different times of the year.[25]

SIGNS/SYMPTOMS

Primary pulmonary coccidioidomycosis causes fever, cough, and pleuritic pain.[25] If not appropriately identified and treated, it can become persistent or chronic.[25] This occurs most commonly in patients with other existing lung diseases. These patients may experience prolonged fever, cough, and weight loss.[25] Physical exam findings are very similar to other causes of community-acquired pneumonia.[25] In less than 1% of cases, coccidioidomycosis can become disseminated as either lymphatic or hematogenous.[25] Lymphatic disseminated disease manifests primarily as pericarditis or supraclavicular lymphadenitis and is less common than hematogenous.[25] Hematogenous coccidioidomycosis is classified by the body area it affects and can be found virtually anywhere with meningitis being the most serious of all the disseminated infections[25] (see **Table 2**).

EVALUATION

Table 2 displays the diagnostic workup. It is important to note that a culture-based diagnosis is definitive although it is imperative to notify the lab of potential cocci as they will need to take protocols to prevent inhalation of the spores while the culture is growing.[25,27] New lateral flow assays can detect total antibodies to *Coccidioides* in 30 minutes but are not widely used yet.[26] Non-specific findings include eosinophilia in the serum.[25]

DIFFERENTIAL DIAGNOSES

Primary pulmonary coccidioidomycosis is commonly mistaken for community-acquired pneumonia–bacterial or viral including COVID-19.[25] It can be differentiated from other types of pneumonia, bacterial or viral, by its prolonged and protracted clinical course and lack of improvement with antibiotics.[25] There will be non-specific lab findings. It is key to inquire about a detailed travel/leisure history if the patient is presenting outside areas known to be endemic to *Coccidioides*.[25] Disseminated coccidioidomycosis would present in various body systems like other fungal or bacterial or viral etiologies causing disease.[25]

TREATMENT

Treatment recommendations are still evolving, and progress has been slow but despite the work of many in areas of endemicity, none of the treatment recommendations are based on high-level evidence (**Table 3**).[37]

A live attenuated vaccine is being tested in dogs and may be effective in humans, the hope being that this would reduce the morbidity and mortality associated with severe disease presentations of coccidioidomycosis.[26] Regarding nonpharmacological interventions, there have been no proven methods to reduce the risk in endemic areas other than avoiding direct contact with uncultivated soil or soils containing visible dust.[38] Prevention strategies are challenging to create as there is no evidence of a reliable approach to determine if *Coccidioides* species are present in the soil. There is also variation between individuals, exposure dose, and immune status, and the development of symptoms.[26] The data we do have from outbreaks, typically from occupational situations (ie, construction sites), suggest that certain environmental modifications can be implemented to aid in reducing exposure. Wetting of the soil

Table 3
Approach to treatment of Coccidioidomycosis

	Pharmacological Treatment	Nonpharmacological Treatment
• Primary pulmonary disease ○ Mild to moderate	• Antifungal therapy may improve symptom intensity or duration in mild disease—more study needed[26]	• Will resolve without treatment[25]
• Primary pulmonary disease ○ Severe	• Triazole antifungal—fluconazole, itraconazole • Amphotericin B[25]	
• Disseminated disease ○ Meningitis	• Triazole antifungal—lifelong therapy, high-risk of relapse when medication stopped[25]	
• Disseminated disease ○ Complicated, ie, hydrocephalus	• Shunting, specialty care[25]	
• Transplant recipients	• Recent/active infection at time of transplant treat with antifungals for 6 months to 1 year[38] • No formal recommendations[38]	• Screen donors, if possible, to reduce incidences of donor transmitted infection[38]
• Persons living with HIV ○ No prophylactic antifungal recommendations for those living in endemic regions[38]	Starting high-risk medication such as tumor necrosis alpha antagonist with history of active coccidioidomycosis or positive serology treat triazole with antifungal[38]	

before disruption, PPE for workers including N95 respirators or higher when working in areas that are endemic, and not incarcerating high-risk populations such as Black and Filipino populations in areas where coccidioidomycosis is endemic.[26]

SUMMARY

Coccidioides is reportable in 26 states and the District of Columbia and has been nationally notifiable since 1995.[25] From a legislative standpoint, there should be a push for standardized reporting among states, particularly those known to be endemic for coccidioidomycosis. This would allow for better identification of disease presence and investigation of environmental factors that could affect coccidioidomycosis cases including climate change, disruption of land with increased population levels for housing, and urbanization.[26] It would give insight into population factors including elderly residents who are more likely immunocompromised and more susceptible to clinically evident disease.[26]

Cryptococcus

Background
Historically *Cryptococcus neoformans* rarely caused disease in humans. It became known as an opportunistic infection causing the AIDS-defining illness, cryptococcal meningitis, in the 1980s.[2,39] Another species of *Cryptococcus* gaining recognition as causing disease in humans is *Cryptococcus gattii*. Classically in tropical and subtropical areas (notably Australia), it has spread to new temperate climate zones outside these areas.[28,29] From scientific data, we know that *C gattii* has been in the United States, specifically California, since the 1960s[40] but in 1999, it was discovered in large case clusters in the Pacific Northwest on Vancouver Island in British Columbia and soon after in Oregon and Washington.[29,41] Additionally, it has been discovered in the Southeast United States.[42] *C gatti* is found in soil, plant debris, and on some trees and is inhaled leading to infection in humans.[31]

PREVALENCE/INCIDENCE

With the advent of antiretroviral therapy (ART), more intense virological monitoring and second-line options for ART in instances of resistance the incidence of cryptococcal meningitis due to *Cryptococcus neoformans* has decreased significantly in developed nations such as the United States.[39] Prevalence in developing nations without access to ART remains high.[39] *C gatti* gained attention in recent years as it appears to cause disease in immunocompetent patients as well as the immunosuppressed with its risk factors being more ill-defined (**Box 4**).[31] Cryptococcal infections appear to be rare in children regardless of HIV status.[31] Mortality rates are less clear in *C gattii* than in *Cryptococcus neoformans* although neurological disease carries a higher mortality rate across various genotypes and geographic locations.[29]

SIGNS/SYMPTOMS

As the incubation period can be variable, it is imperative that a specific travel history is obtained when patients present with suspicious disease manifestations in an area not considered endemic.[29] **Table 2** details pulmonary and central nervous system (CNS) manifestations of the disease. Immunocompetent patients can be asymptomatic or have pulmonary manifestations.[29,31] Less often sites such as the brain, skin, and bone can be affected in immunocompetent hosts.[31] Neurological disease presents with headache with or without vomiting and neck stiffness.[29] Molecular variations of

Box 4
Risk factors for *Cryptococcus gattii*[28,29,31]
• HIV infection
• Malignancy (hematologic malignancies)
• Solid-organ transplant recipients
• Patients receiving immunosuppressive medications including corticosteroids
• Age > 50[a]
• Chronic lung disease[a]
• Smoking[a]
[a]Specific to *Cryptococcus gattii*.

C gattii are thought to affect how the disease symptomatically manifests with the North American outbreak involving the pulmonary system to a greater extent than diseases seen in other areas of the world.[29] Neurological complications of *C gattii* include increased intracranial pressure, hydrocephalus, cranial nerve palsies, seizures, ataxia, focal long tract signs with ocular complications being significantly high compared to *C neoformans* with loss of visual acuity and blindness.[29]

EVALUATION

Table 2 details the diagnostic workup including imaging specific to the presentation. Pulmonary symptoms warrant chest imaging which most commonly shows nodules known as cryptococcomas.[29] Less commonly, lung infiltrates will be seen, alone or along with cryptococcomas.[29] Neurological imaging to assess for brain involvement includes computed tomography (CT) and MRI imaging. Cryptococcomas leading to obstructive hydrocephalus, or abnormal foci of reduced attenuation, contrast enhancement, edema, and mass lesions resembling abscesses may be seen.[29] Routine lumbar puncture of patients with suspected *Cryptococcus* is recommended.[29]

In terms of laboratory testing, *Cryptococcus* can be cultured from the appropriate clinical specimen (cerebrospinal fluid [CSF], lung tissue, sputum samples, and blood), this is essential for definitive diagnosis.[29] It will grow on canavanine-glycine-bromthymol (CGB) agar. *C. gattii* will turn culture medium blue differentiating it from *C neoformans,* which leaves the medium unaffected, a yellow-green color.[29,35] Cryptococcal antigen can be obtained via testing the serum or CSF although caution should be used as it may not reliably differentiate between *C neoformans* and *C gattii*.[29] Specimens should be sent for histopathological evaluation.[29] Nucleic acid tests are available to detect *Cryptococcus* and may be useful if there is a discrepancy with *Cryptococcus* seen in tissue pathology but not grown on culture but they are rarely needed to confirm diagnosis.[29]

TREATMENT

There are no antifungal drug trials to guide guidelines for *C gattii* infections but data from recent studies suggest that treatment should be guided by the affected site. Studies surrounding the outbreaks in the Pacific Northwest in Canada and the United States suggest that recommendations for antifungals should acknowledge the genotype of the *C gattii* strain whereas other data have not confirmed the benefit of testing antimicrobial susceptibility, but it may be beneficial in patients failing to respond to current antifungal treatment.[29] Treatment guidelines regarding induction and maintenance therapy are detailed in **Table 4**. Severe complications such as hydrocephalus and raised intracranial pressure should be addressed immediately.[29] Immune reconstitution inflammatory syndrome should not be confused with treatment failure but is instead a complication of cryptococcal infection when symptoms or imaging features show inflammation that worsened or occurred after clinical and/or microbiological response to anticryptococcal therapy and cultures were negative.[29] Surgical excision of single large cryptococcomas if they are accessible has been performed if they are intruding on local structures.[29]

Histoplasmosis

Background
Based on data from the 1940s/1950s, *Histoplasma capsulatum*, known as histoplasmosis, is considered the most prevalent endemic mycosis in North America.[32] It is difficult to establish if this is still true as histoplasmosis is only reportable in 13 states and not nationally reportable.[30] Geographic locations where histoplasmosis is endemic were established by performing nationwide skin testing to evaluate histoplasmin sensitivity in young adults during the 1940s/1950s.[30,34] Although this type of testing is no longer performed, the results showed the highest percentages of positive reactions in the areas surrounding the Ohio and Mississippi River valleys—approximately 60% to 90%.[30] Histoplasma grows well in the soil, particularly if infused with bird or bat droppings, so it is likely found outside of the defined endemic areas in small clusters.[30] Humans inhale airborne microconidia with disease severity depending on the amount of inoculum exposure.[32,33]

PREVALENCE/INCIDENCE

Histoplasmosis is not spread from human to human or from animal to human, rarely it is spread from an infected organ to a transplant recipient.[33] Most infections are sporadic but at times, there will be reports of outbreaks.[30] Exposure occurs after a disturbance of soil contaminated with bird or bat droppings.[30,33] Risk factors are detailed in **Box 5**. Immunocompetent patients may harbor the organism and have reactivation of infection in the future should they become immunocompromised.[30] Some data suggest that mortality is estimated to be 5% in children and 8% in adults.[32] Other sources state that fatality associated with acute disease is approximately 1% although this may be an underestimate as that was 1% of patients admitted to the hospital not taking into account those who were not admitted.[30] For patients with HIV who develop disseminated histoplasmosis mortality remains high.[33] Histoplasmosis is found nationwide as is evidenced by data showing it in each census region.[36] Histoplasmosis can also occur outside of the United States, thus, making a travel history imperative.[30]

Table 4 Approach to treatment of *Cryptococcus*		
	Induction Therapy	**Maintenance Therapy**
Pulmonary—moderate disease[29]	• Amphotericin B+ 5-flucytosine • 2 weeks duration	• Azole, specifically fluconazole • 12 months total therapy (induction + maintenance) duration
CNS disease[29]	• Amphotericin B+ 5-flucytosine • 6 weeks duration	• Same medication • 18–24 months duration

---

Box 5
Risk factors for histoplasmosis[30,32,33]

- Immunocompromising conditions
  - People living with HIV/AIDs
  - Organ transplant recipients
  - Immunosuppressive therapies including corticosteroids, TNF inhibitors
- Infants and individuals > 55 years of age
- High-risk activities
  - Spelunking
  - Chicken coop care
  - Demolition/renovation of buildings

TNF, tumor necrosis factor.

SIGNS/SYMPTOMS

Histoplasmosis may not cause symptoms in immunocompetent individuals but can cause acute pulmonary disease presenting with fever, fatigue, and cough (see **Table 2**).[33] The incubation period ranges from 3 to 17 days after inhalation of spores.[33] The severity of the infection will depend on the patient's immune status, the inoculum size as well as other factors.[30] Headache and chest pain can also be present and enlarged lymph nodes are a predominant finding associated with histoplasmosis.[30,36] Symptoms can persist for weeks or months and will be unresponsive to antibiotic therapy as they are fungal in etiology.[30] Long-term sequelae include pericarditis, broncholithiasis, pulmonary nodules, mediastinal granuloma, or mediastinal fibrosis.[34] Typically, these occur in patients who develop chronic, progressive disease or disseminated disease which can last for months.[34]

ASSESSMENT

The gold standard in the diagnostic workup of histoplasmosis is a fungal culture although this is time-consuming and often delays the diagnosis.[32] For more rapid assessment in patients presenting with severe pulmonary disease or with disseminated disease antigen and antibody testing can be used. EIA-based quantitative assays are becoming popular for antigen testing in the urine and serum and complement fixation and gel diffusion are the predominant methods for antibody testing.[32,33] The recommendation is to use antigen testing (serum or urine) in patients presenting with severe pulmonary disease or disseminated disease when the rapid diagnosis is essential for treatment and positive outcomes.[32] Antigen levels correlate with the severity of the illness and severity of exposure.[30,32,34] Cross-reactivity with other endemic fungal etiologies is the failure of antigen and antibody testing as well as the fact that antibodies can take up to 6 weeks to develop after exposure, testing can take 2 to 6 weeks, and patients who are immunocompromised may have a blunted immune response and lower antibody levels overall.[30,32,33] Combining antigen and antibody testing may increase diagnostic yield.[32] PCR testing for histoplasmosis is still experimental but is promising.[33]

DIFFERENTIAL DIAGNOSIS

The differential diagnoses of acute pulmonary histoplasmosis and chronic pulmonary histoplasmosis are included in **Table 2**.

TREATMENT

Treatment of mild to moderate histoplasmosis is itraconazole, and depending on the degree of illness, it may be continued for up to 6 months.[33,34] Itraconazole has fewer side effects than previously used high-dose ketoconazole.[34] Fluconazole has been found to be less effective and remains a second-line agent.[34] Severe pulmonary disease and disseminated infections are initially treated with amphotericin B and then switched to itraconazole upon improvement.[34] Antigen levels can be used to gauge response to antifungal therapy because antigen levels decline with improvement and rise with relapse.[32]

SUMMARY

A careful history of occupational and recreational exposures to known etiologies can help point the diagnosis to histoplasmosis as well as identifying if others around the patient doing similar activities have been affected.[34] Reactivation of previous illness when becoming immunosuppressed is an increasingly likely scenario in today's world where organ transplantation is more successful, people are living longer with HIV, and more people are exposed to immunosuppressive medications for various conditions. For those who are at risk of developing severe disease, the immunocompromised, health care providers should recommend avoidance of high-risk activities and educate patients as to what those activities are—disturbing the soil where there could be bird or bat droppings by digging, chopping wood, cleaning chicken coops which have become increasingly common in recent years, exploring caves, and cleaning/demolishing/renovating old buildings.[33]

Pneumocystis

Background

For many years, *Pneumocystis carinii* was thought to cause pneumocystis pneumonia (PCP). Later, scientists determined it was *Pneumocystis jirovecci* but chose not to change the name PCP to PJP.[43] *P jirovecci* is spread from person to person through aerosolized particles.[44] Asymptomatic people can carry the disease and transmit it to others.[45] It was thought that childhood exposure could reactivate in adults who become immunocompromised, but scientists believe it is more likely a new exposure from an asymptomatic immunocompetent person.[44,45] No environmental reservoir has been identified, *P jirovecci* is human-specific.[44] PCP was relatively rare before the HIV/AIDS epidemic[1] and was mainly seen in malnourished children with significant immunodeficiencies and adults who were immunosuppressed usually due to chemotherapy for malignancy.[46] During the AIDS epidemic cases of PCP, pneumonia rose significantly and became known as an AIDS-defining illness.[1] The consensus for PCP prophylaxis with Trimethoprim/sulfamethoxazole (TMP-SMX) for patients living with HIV has been the standard of practice for years when a patient's CD4 count is less than 200.[1] Prophylaxis and ART for HIV/AIDS patients contributed to PCP incidence decreasing significantly.[1] However, *P jirovecci* is a global pathogen.[46] There is a misconception that after the AIDS epidemic improved, PCP was a relatively rare disease and that is not the case.[46]

PREVALENCE/INCIDENCE

PCP is an emerging problem among populations that are HIV-negative.[46] Currently, the most at-risk populations are those who have immunosuppressive conditions that are not HIV. Risk factors for HIV-negative patients are listed in **Box 6**. Clinicians need increased

> **Box 6**
> **Risk factors for pneumocystis pneumonia in HIV-negative patients[1,46]**
>
> - Malignancy (hematologic malignancy)
> - Solid-organ transplant recipients
> - Chronic lung disease
> - Autoimmune disease
> - Primary immunodeficiency syndromes
> - Use of immunosuppressive medications including high-dose corticosteroids for prolonged courses
> - Male sex
> - Older age at presentation, mean age 58, when compared with patients living with HIV

awareness of the non-HIV risk factors associated with PCP and the lack of prophylactic measures in place for these populations.[46] There is no national surveillance of PCP.[45] Regardless of epidemiological risk factors and clinical presentation, patients who are HIV-negative presenting with PCP have a higher in-hospital mortality rate, with some studies suggesting up to 38%.[46] This is likely multifactorial due to delayed diagnosis and the start of treatment because of lack of suspicion secondary to their HIV-negative status, the presence of underlying conditions that make them more likely to suffer worse outcomes than those who are HIV-positive or secondary to a greater pulmonary inflammatory response to pneumonia depending on the underlying disease process.[46]

SIGNS/SYMPTOMS

Pneumocystis primarily affects the lungs and rarely causes disseminated disease.[44] Some cases of the disseminated disease have been reported in patients with advanced HIV infections.[44] Patients typically present with fever, chills, cough, fatigue, chest pain, and shortness of breath.[47] In HIV-positive patients, there is classically a subacute onset of progressive dyspnea, nonproductive or minimally productive cough, a low-grade fever, and malaise.[44] In HIV-negative immunocompromised individuals, there is more of an acute presentation of significant dyspnea, fever, and chills.[44] The dyspnea may be severe requiring mechanical ventilation with respiratory failure in these patients carrying a mortality rate of up to 40%.[44] Physical exam findings can range from an unremarkable lung exam to diffuse auscultatory crackles.[44] Extrapulmonary manifestations are rare but can include retinitis, thyroiditis, bone lesions, and pneumocystis of the brain, liver, spleen, or kidney.[44] These are rare complications and tend to occur in patients with a significant immunocompromised state such as advanced AIDS or who have been on prophylaxis (suggesting positive HIV status or hematologic malignancy) with aerosolized pentamidine.[44]

EVALUATION

The diagnostic workup includes a sputum sample collected from patient expectoration versus bronchoalveolar lavage or lung biopsy and is examined microscopically.[45] *Pneumocystis* cannot be cultured; the gold standard is microscopic visualization of the organism.[44] PCR testing for *Pneumocystis* DNA can be used in various types of samples and a blood test for beta-D-glucan, which is part of the cell wall in fungi, can help diagnose PCP.[45] Chest x-ray can be normal or have non-specific findings such as infiltrates, often bilateral and symmetrical.[44] On chest CT, the most common finding is bilateral ground-glass opacities.[44]

TREATMENT

The most important tool to differentiate PCP from other etiologies of pneumonia is a high index of clinical suspicion.[44] In Spain, there are now widely accepted recommendations for chemoprophylaxis of PCP in patients with hematologic malignancies, which has led to a decrease in the incidence of the disease in this population.[46] The study by Periera-Diaz suggests a relatively new risk group, those with chronic lung disease, are the second most likely risk group of HIV-negative persons to be affected by PCP.[46] Many studies suggest that patients with chronic lung diseases such as chronic obstructive pulmonary disease (COPD), cystic fibrosis, and interstitial lung disease are more likely to be colonized with *P jirovecci*.[46] Even though this may make those with chronic lung disease a reservoir for *Pneumocystis* infection, there are no specific guidelines for chemoprophylaxis in this specific population.[46] This may lead to a delayed diagnosis, worse outcomes, and higher costs for these patients and the medical system as a whole.[1] Future research needs to focus on earlier identification of PCP in HIV-negative patients, further characterize risk factors for diseases other than HIV, and data-driven guidelines for chemoprophylaxis in certain at-risk groups to reduce the incidence and mortality of PCP as we have done in the HIV population.[1,44,46]

SUMMARY

The main unifying thread among emerging fungal diseases is that immunosuppressed patients, those living with HIV but also those immunosuppressed for other reasons, is the main population affected by significant fungal infections. When seeing immunocompromised patients for illness, particularly pulmonary symptoms, we must keep fungal etiologies in our differential diagnoses. A detailed travel, occupational and recreational history is imperative. Atypical findings accompanying pulmonary diseases such as arthralgias, erythema nodosum, hyperhidrosis, and solitary pulmonary nodules are associated more so with fungal etiologies such as coccidioidomycosis and histoplasmosis.[36] Fever was a less predominant feature in fungal pulmonary diseases when compared with influenza causing community-acquired pneumonia.[36] When atypical findings such as these are evident, the clinician should be thinking of fungal etiologies. Laboratory testing with fungal culture or antigen combined with antibody testing is ultimately needed to confirm the exact diagnosis, but as clinicians, we need to maintain a high degree of suspicion for fungal etiologies of pulmonary disease and severe disseminated disease presentation, particularly in high-risk populations.[30,32]

CLINICS CARE POINTS

- Infection control measures are imperative to protect those most vulnerable to candidemia due to *C auris* including standard and contact precautions, private rooming, daily and terminal cleaning with a disinfectant active against *Clostridium difficile* spores, and notification to receiving facilities when a patient colonized or infected with *C auris* is transferred.[16]

- Despite inconsistencies in many of the diagnostic tests for *C auris*, a low-cost option is the use of chromogenic agar which can display features unique to *C auris*—growth at elevated temperatures and salinity.[10]

- The differential diagnoses for primary pulmonary coccidioidomycosis include community-acquired pneumonia due to other causes but coccidioidomycosis is differentiated by its prolonged and protracted clinical course and lack of improvement with antibiotics.[25]
- A focused travel/leisure history and knowledge of areas endemic to *Coccidioides* are imperative to making the diagnosis.[25]
- Primary pulmonary disease due to *Coccidioides* that is classified as mild to moderate will often improve without treatment although more studies are needed to determine if antifungal therapy may improve symptom intensity or duration.[25,26]
- Risk factors specific to *C gattii* include not only immunocompromising conditions but also nontraditional risk factors including age > 50, chronic lung disease, and smoking.[28,29,31]
- *Cryptococcus* can be cultured and will grow on CGB agar. *C gattii* will turn culture medium to blue differentiating it from *C neoformans*, which leaves the medium a yellow-green color.[29,35]
- Use antigen testing in patients presenting with severe pulmonary disease or disseminated disease for expedient diagnosis of histoplasmosis. Antibody testing can follow although it can take up to 6 weeks to develop antibodies after exposure.[30,32,33]
- Antigen levels can be used to gauge response to antifungal therapy as they decline with improvement and rise with relapse of histoplasmosis.[32]
- Patient education regarding high-risk activities (spelunking, chicken coop care, demolition, and renovation of buildings) for histoplasmosis exposure should be clearly delineated for those that are immunocompromised as this can be an unrecognized threat.[30,32,33]
- *Pneumocystis* pneumonia in HIV-negative immunocompromised patients presents with an *acute* presentation of significant dyspnea, fever, and chills in opposition to HIV-positive patients who have a more *subacute* onset of progressive dyspnea, nonproductive or minimally productive cough, low-grade fever, and malaise.[44]
- Future research is warranted to determine chemoprophylactic recommendations regarding the high-risk HIV-negative immunocompromised population.[1,44,46]

DISCLOSURE

I have no conflicts of interest.

REFERENCES

1. Gold JAW, Jackson BR, Benedict K. Possible Diagnostic Delays and Missed Prevention Opportunities in Pneumocystis Pneumonia Patients Without HIV: Analysis of Commercial Insurance Claims Data-United States, 2011-2015. Open Forum Infectious Diseases 2020;1:5–6. https://doi.org/10.1093/ofid/ofaa255.
2. Friedman DZP, Schwartz IS. Emerging fungal infections: new patients, new patterns, and new pathogens. Journal of Fungi 2019;5(3). https://doi.org/10.3390/jof5030067.
3. Satoh K, Makimura K, Hasumi Y, et al. Candida auris sp. nov., a novel ascomycetous yeast isolated from the external ear canal of an inpatient in a Japanese hospital. Microbiol Immunol 2009;53(1):41–4.
4. Tsay Sv, Mu Y, Williams S, et al. Burden of Candidemia in the United States, 2017. Clin Infect Dis 2020;71(9):E449–53.
5. Tracking Candida auris. Centers for Disease Control and Prevention. 2022. Available at: https://cdc.gov/fungal/candida-auris/tracking-c-auris.html. Accessed March 26, 2022.

6. Chakrabarti A, Sood P, Rudramurthy SM, et al. Incidence, characteristics and outcome of ICU-acquired candidemia in India. Intensive Care Med 2015;41(2): 285–95.

7. Calvo B, Melo ASA, Perozo-Mena A, et al. First report of candida auris in america: clinical and microbiological aspects of 18 episodes of candidemia. J Infect 2016; 73(4):369–74.

8. Bandara N, Samaranayake L. Emerging and future strategies in the management of recalcitrant Candida auris. Med Mycol 2022;60:8.

9. Proctor D.M., Dangana T., Joseph Sexton D., et al., Integrated genomic, epidemiologic investigation of Candida auris skin colonization in a skilled nursing facility, *Nature Medicine*, 27, 2021, 1401, 1407-1408. https://doi.org/10.1038/s41591-021-01383-w

10. Jeffery-Smith A, Taori SK, Schelenz S, et al. Candida auris: a review of the literature. Clin Microbiol Rev 2018;31(1). https://doi.org/10.1128/CMR.00029-17.

11. Arendrup MC, Patterson TF. Multidrug-resistant candida: Epidemiology, molecular mechanisms, and treatment. JID (J Infect Dis) 2017;216:S445–51.

12. Prestel C., Anderson E., Forsberg K., et al., MMWR, Candida auris Outbreak in a COVID-19 Specialty Care Unit — Florida, July–August 2020. *Morbidity and Mortality Weekly Report*, 70(2), 2021, 56-57. https://doi.org/10.15585/mmwr.mm6619a7

13. Welsh RM, Bentz ML, Shams A, et al. Survival, persistence, and isolation of the emerging multidrug-resistant pathogenic yeast Candida auris on a plastic health care surface. J Clin Microbiol 2017;55(10):2996–3005.

14. Sherry L, Ramage G, Kean R, et al. Biofilm-Forming Capability of Highly Virulent, Multidrug-Resistant Candida auris. Emerg Infect Dis 2017;23(2). https://doi.org/ 10.3201/eid2302.161320. Available at: www.cdc.gov/eid.

15. Larkin E, Hager C, Chandra J, et al. The Emerging Pathogen Candida auris: Growth Phenotype, Virulence Factors, Activity of Antifungals, and Effect of SCY-078, a Novel Glucan Synthesis Inhibitor, on Growth Morphology and Biofilm Formation. Antimicrobial Agents and Chemotherapy 2017;61(5):1–9. https://doi. org/10.1128/AAC.02396-16.

16. Tsay S, Welsh RM, Adams EH, et al. Notes from the Field: Ongoing Transmission of *Candida auris* in Health Care Facilities — United States, June 2016–May 2017. MMWR Morbidity and Mortality Weekly Report 2017;66(19):514–5.

17. Casadevall A. and Kontoyiannis D.P., On the Emergence of Candida auris: Climate Change, Azoles, Swamps, and Birds, mBio, 10 (4), e01397-19 https:// doi.org/10.1128/mBio.01397-19.

18. Karmarkar EN, O'Donnell K, Prestel C, et al. Rapid assessment and containment of candida auris transmission in postacute care settings-orange county, california, 2019. Ann Intern Med 2021;174(11):1554–62.

19. Kullberg BJ, Arendrup MC. Invasive candidiasis. N Engl J Med 2015;373(15): 1445–56. Campion EW.

20. Kauffman CA. Clinical manifestations and diagnosis of candidemia and invasive candidiasis in adults. UpToDate. 2022. Available at: https://www-uptodate-com. proxy-fs.researchport.umd.edu/contents/clinical-manifestations-and-diagnosis-of-candidemia-and-invasive-candidiasis-in-adults?search=clinical%20manifestations %20and%20diagnosis%20of%20candidemia%20and%20invasive%20candidiasis %20in%20adults&source=search_result&selectedTitle=1~150&usage_type= default&display_rank=1. Accessed April 30, 2022.

21. Identification of Candida auris. Centers for Disease Control and Prevention. 2020. Available at: https://www.cdc.gov/fungal/candida-auris/identification.html. Accessed April 30, 2022.
22. Borman A.M., Szekely A. and Johnson E.M., Comparative Pathogenicity of United Kingdom Isolates of the Emerging Pathogen Candida auris and Other Key Pathogenic Candida Species, mSphere, 1 (4), e00189-16 https://doi.org/10.1128/mSphere.00189-16.
23. Treatment and Management of Infections and Colonization. Centers for Disease Control and Prevention. 2021. Available at: https://www.cdc.gov/fungal/candida-auris/c-auris-treatment.html. Accessed March 26, 2022.
24. Lockhart SR, Etienne KA, Vallabhaneni S, et al. Clinical infectious diseases simultaneous emergence of multidrug-resistant candida auris on 3 continents confirmed by whole-genome sequencing and epidemiological analyses. Clin Infect Dis 2017;64(2):134–74.
25. Johnson RH, Sharma R, Kuran R, et al. Coccidioidomycosis: a review. J Investig Med 2021;69(2):316–23.
26. Redfield R.R., Bunnell R., Ellis B., et al., Surveillance for Coccidioidomycosis - United States, 2011-2017. *Morbidity and mortality weekly report*, 68(7), 2019, 1-2, 4-6.
27. Gastélum-Cano JM, Dautt-Castro M, García-Galaz A, et al. The clinical laboratory evolution in coccidioidomycosis detection: future perspectives. J Med Mycol 2021;31(3):101159.
28. Datta K, Bartlett KH, Baer R, et al. Spread of cryptococcus gattii into pacific northwast region of the United States. Emerg Infect Dis 2009;15(8). https://doi.org/10.3201/eid1508.081384.
29. Chen SCA, Meyer W, Sorrell TC. Cryptococcus gattii infections. Clin Microbiol Rev 2014;27(4):980–1024.
30. Benedict K, Mody RK. Epidemiology of histoplasmosis outbreaks, United States, 1938-2013. Emerg Infect Dis 2016;22(3):370–8.
31. MacDougall L, Fyfe M, Romney M, et al. Risk factors for cryptococcus gattii infection, British Columbia, Canada. Emerg Infect Dis 2011;17(2). https://doi.org/10.3201/eid1702.101020.
32. Hage C.A., Carmona E.M., Epelbaum O., et al., Microbiological Laboratory Testing in the Diagnosis of Fungal Infections in Pulmonary and Critical Care Practice An Official American Thoracic Society Clinical Practice Guideline, *Am J Respir Crit Care Med*, 200(5), 2019, 543-544. https://doi.org/10.1164/rccm.v200erratum8
33. Information for Healthcare Professionals about Histoplasmosis. Centers for Disease Control and Prevention. 2021. Available at: https://www.cdc.gov/fungal/diseases/histoplasmosis/health-professionals.html. Accessed May 6, 2022.
34. Kauffman CA. Histoplasmosis: a clinical and laboratory update. Clin Microbiol Rev 2007;20(1):115–32.
35. Diagnosis and testing for C. gattii infection. Centers for Disease Control and Prevention. 2020. Available at: https://www.cdc.gov/fungal/diseases/cryptococcosis-gattii/diagnosis.html. Accessed May 6, 2022.
36. Benedict K, Kobayashi M, Garg S, et al. Symptoms in blastomycosis, coccidioidomycosis, and histoplasmosis versus other respiratory illnesses in commercially insured adult outpatients-United States, 2016-2017. Clin Infect Dis 2021;73(11):e4336–44.
37. Deresinski S, Mirels LF. Coccidioidomycosis: what a long strange trip it's been. Med Mycol 2019;57:S3–15.

38. Ampel N., Coccidioidomycosis, In: Loscalzo J., Fauci A., Kasper D., et al., *Harrison's principles of internal medicine 21ed*, 2022, McGraw Hill. https://accessmedicine-mhmedical-com.proxy-fs.researchport.umd.edu/content.aspx?bookid=3095&sectionid=263965934.

39. Rajasingham R., Smith R.M., Park B.J., et al., Global burden of disease of HIV-associated cryptococcal meningitis: an updated analysis, *Lancet Infect Dis*, 17(8), 2017, 874- 881. https://doi.org/10.1016/S1473-3099(17)30243-8.

40. About C. gattii. Centers for Disease Control and Prevention. 2020. Available at: https://www.cdc.gov/fungal/diseases/cryptococcosis-gattii/definition.html. Accessed May 6, 2022.

41. Frieden T.R., Harold Jaffe D.W., Stephens J.W., et al., Emergence of *Cryptococcus gattii* - Pacific Northwest, 2004-2010, *Morbidity and Mortality Weekly Report*, 59(28), 2010, 865-867.

42. Lockhart SR, Roe CC, Engelthaler DM. Whole-genome analysis of cyrptococcus gattii, southeastern United States. Emerg Infect Dis 2016;22(6). https://doi.org/10.3201/eid2206.151455.

43. Stringer JR, Beard CB, Miller RF, Wakefield AE. A New Name (Pneumocystis Jiroveci) for Pneumocystis from Humans. Emerg Infec Dis 2002;8(9):891–4.

44. Carmona EM, Limper AH. Update on the diagnosis and treatment of Pneumocystis pneumonia. Ther Adv Respir Dis 2011;5(1):41–59.

45. Pneumocystis Pneumonia. Centeres for Disease Control and Prevention. 2021. Available at: https://www.cdc.gov/fungal/diseases/histoplasmosis/health-professionals.html. Accessed May 6, 2022.

46. Pereira-Díaz E, Moreno-Verdejo F, de la Horra C, et al. Changing trends in the epidemiology and risk factors of pneumocystis pneumonia in Spain. Front Public Health 2019;7. https://doi.org/10.3389/fpubh.2019.00275.

47. Harris JR, Arunmozhi Balajee S, Park BJ. Pneumocystis Jirovecii Pneumonia: Current Knowledge and Outstanding Public Health Issues. Curr Fungal Infect Rep 2010;4:229–33. https://doi.org/10.1007/s12281-010-0029-3.

Mycobacterial Diseases

Chelsea Ware, MS, PA-C[a], Henry Yoon, MD[a,b],
Eric C. Nemec, PharmD, MEd, BCPS[a,*]

KEYWORDS

- *Mycobacterium tuberculosis* • Mycobacterial disease • Latent tuberculosis
- Antituberculosis medications • COVID-19 • Emerging infectious diseases

KEY POINTS

- Early detection and treatment of latent tuberculosis are essential to meet the World Health Organization's (WHO) goal of reducing deaths and the number of tuberculosis diagnoses.
- Appropriate assessment of associated risk factors to determine if screening is necessary.
- Moving forward, an assessment of funding allocation will be necessary to ensure that research related to tuberculosis treatment, prevention, and socioeconomic impact is essential in furthering the WHO goal of eliminating TB globally.

Mycobacterium infections are a global concern. The *Mycobacterium* genus's 3 major groups of human pathogens include *Mycobacterium tuberculosis* complex (MTC), *Mycobacterium leprae*, and nontuberculosis mycobacteria. The most clinically relevant pathogen and the cause of the disease, tuberculosis (TB), is *M tuberculosis* (*Mtb*), a member of the MTC. These species are all small, aerobic, acid-fast bacilli (AFB) and classified as fast- or slow-growers.[1]

According to the 2021 World Health Organization (WHO) Global TB Report, 5.8 million people were newly diagnosed with TB in 2020, with an estimated 1.3 million deaths among human immunodeficiency virus (HIV)-uninfected individuals and 214,000 HIV-infected individuals, an increase from the 2019 reported deaths.[2] In the United States, 7860 TB cases were reported in 2021[3] and 7163 cases in 2020.[4] The investigators posit that this increase in the United States was exacerbated by the COVID-19 pandemic, which caused a shift in resources, including funding and personnel, to manage the pandemic. This shift, along with mandatory country-wide shutdowns of schools, businesses, and social gatherings and fear of entering health care facilities to avoid COVID-19 infection, may have led to diagnosis and treatment delays and a possible increase in community transmission, leading to the overall increase in the number of infections.[5] The WHO's End TB Strategy has a goal of a 95% decrease in deaths caused by TB by 2035 compared with 2015; however, to

[a] Sacred Heart University, 5151 Park Avenue, Fairfield, CT 06825, USA; [b] Department of Family Medicine, Stamford Hospital, One Hospital Plaza, Stamford, CT 06902, USA
* Corresponding author.
E-mail address: nemece@sacredheart.edu

Physician Assist Clin 8 (2023) 453–465
https://doi.org/10.1016/j.cpha.2023.02.006
2405-7991/23/© 2023 Elsevier Inc. All rights reserved.

physicianassistant.theclinics.com

achieve this, there needs to be an increased interest in clinical trials and funding for new diagnostics and therapeutics.[2] There are many emerging concerns and barriers regarding meeting this goal, including the impact of the COVID-19 pandemic, an increase in cases of multidrug–resistant TB (MDR-TB), the ability of local health departments to provide patient-specific community resources, and increasing the early diagnoses of those with latent TB infection (LTBI), given the disease burden and the WHO goal, new emerging therapies, and new research evaluating the safety and efficacy of new antituberculosis therapies and potential vaccines. This paper describes these areas at a time when mycobacterial infections may be on the increase.

EPIDEMIOLOGY

In 2020, approximately two-thirds of all new cases were in 8 countries: India, China, Indonesia, the Philippines, Pakistan, Nigeria, Bangladesh, and South Africa.[2] Tuberculosis has reemerged over the past few decades due to immigration, drug-resistant TB, and the HIV epidemic.[6] Tuberculosis can affect anyone; however, it disproportionately affects those living in poverty, with greater than 95% of cases and deaths occurring in low-income countries.[7] It is estimated that between 5% and 10% of those infected with *Mtb* will develop active TB infection.[7] Some have an increased risk of developing active TB disease, including those with social or environmental exposures and weakened immune systems. Social and environmental exposures include close contact with a known positive person, being born in an endemic area, and working or living with those at increased risk, including homeless shelters, prisons, and nursing homes. Additional groups include homeless individuals and intravenous drug users. Conditions causing a weakened immune system include: HIV, substance use, silicosis, diabetes mellitus (DM), history of organ transplantation, and corticosteroid use.[8]

CURRENT STANDARDS
Prevention and Screening

Prevention of new TB infections is essential to decreasing TB disease's worldwide burden. Current strategies include vaccination, TB preventive treatment (TPT), and prevention of community transmission. To date, only one vaccine has been developed and used, the Bacillus Calmette-Guerin (BCG) vaccine. This vaccine is effective against severe TB in children and is only recommended in counties with high incidence rates.[9] However, it is less effective against pulmonary TB, which is both more contagious and more common worldwide. TPT is recommended for those infected with TB, or LTBI, or those with a known exposure and considered high risk (**Box 1**).[7,10] Transmission prevention involves knowledge of those at most risk, including environmental and other risks due to weakened immune systems. Screening for active TBI and LTBI is necessary, with antibiotic therapy provided, as required.

Box 1
High risk for active TB development

People living with HIV (PLWH)
Prisoners
Health care workers (HCW)
IVDU
Taking anti-TNF treatments
Receiving dialysis
Organ transplantation

TB screening guidelines involve evaluating TB symptoms and assessing the risk of contracting or progressing to active TB. Symptoms of active TB include cough, hemoptysis, fever, night sweats, and unintentional weight loss, whereas LTBI typically has no symptoms.[11] It is essential to know which diagnostic tools should be used to prevent the development or spread of active TB. To assist, the investigators have developed a decision support tool for the clinical suspicion for tuberculosis (**Fig. 1**). There are 2 screening tests currently available: the tuberculin skin test (TST) and the interferon-gamma release assay (IGRA); both work by detecting memory T-cell response. Screening test recommendations for different populations are described in **Table 1**. Neither test differentiates between LTBI and active TB; therefore, further investigation is necessary for positive screening results. A symptom evaluation and a chest radiography should be performed to exclude active TB.

DIAGNOSIS
Chest Radiography

A chest radiography or chest computerized tomography is necessary for those with a positive TST or IGRA to assess for active TB disease. Those presenting with symptoms concerning for TB disease should have imaging completed. Findings consistent

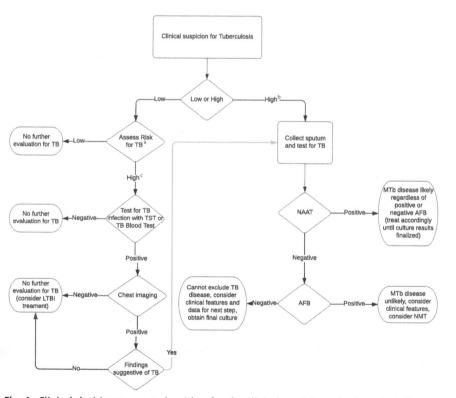

Fig. 1. Clinical decision support algorithm for the clinical suspicion of tuberculosis.[a]https://portal.ct.gov/DPH/Tuberculosis/Tuberculosis-Risk-Assessment-Guide. [b]Until confirmed negative or no longer considered contagious, isolation in negative pressure environment and consultation with infectious disease, pulmonary and/or local public health TB experts should be considered. [c]8–10 weeks post exposure if applicable.

Table 1
Mycobacterium tuberculosis screening tests in specific populations[11]

Mtb Screening Test	Populations
TST	Children <5 year old Those requiring annual testing (ie, HCW)
IGRA	Those >5 years who: Are likely to have *Mtb* infection; Considered low or intermediate risk for disease progression; Testing for LTBI is necessary; History of BCG vaccination; *and/or* Unlikely to return for TST read in 48–72 h
No testing	Individuals determined to be low risk for *Mtb* infection[a]

[a] If required by law, IGRA preferred if 5 y or older, unless univariable, TST is acceptable.

with pulmonary TB disease may include lesions, pleural effusions, and air-space opacities or cavities located in the apical or posterior segment of the upper lobe or the superior aspect of the lower lobes.[12]

Sputum Sample Collection and Testing

Sputum collection should also occur before the initiation of antibiotic therapy. Collection methods include forced and induced sputum production. Some cases may require a bronchoalveolar lavage or fiberoptic bronchoscopy. AFB smear, nucleic acid amplification testing (NAAT), and culture testing should also be performed. Three specimens should be collected, 8 to 24 hours apart, with one sample completed first thing in the morning.[12] Three AFB smears are necessary to confirm pulmonary TB, with increased sensitivity with each specimen. The benefits of AFB microscopy are that they can be resulted within hours and are inexpensive; however, AFB smears cannot differentiate between *Mtb* infection and other mycobacterial infections. According to Infectious Diseases Society of America (IDSA) guidance, AFB smears are recommended if sensitivity is greater than 70% and specificity is greater than 90%. There would be the risk of negative outcomes if a false negative were to occur, which includes additional testing or possible delayed diagnosis. There is a risk of unnecessary antibiotic administration for those with false-positive results.[11]

Mycobacterium tuberculosis Culture

TB diagnosis can occur without a positive culture and be based on clinical symptoms alone; however, a culture should still be attempted. Results may take up to 1 to 2 weeks, with slow-growers potentially taking up to 6 weeks, so additional options for earlier detection are frequently used, including NAAT.[11]

Nucleic Acid Amplification Testing

IDSA recommends NAAT testing on the initial sputum sample in suspected TB, which can provide a result in 24 to 48 hours; however, it does not replace the need for AFB smear and culture.[13] In 2013, the Food and Drug Administration approved the GeneXpert MTB/RIF, which is a cartridge-based NAAT. This rapid test can detect both *Mtb* infection and rifampicin (RIF) resistance. In a systematic review of the Xpert Ultra MTB/RIF, the pooled sensitivity and specificity were 90.9% and 95.6%, respectively, when compared against culture. In RIF resistance detection, pooled sensitivity and specificity were 94.9% and 99.1%, respectively.[14]

TREATMENT

Latent Tuberculosis Infection Disease

Early detection and treatment of LTBI are essential in preventing active TB disease and community transmission of TB. Current CDC guidance offers multiple recommendations for the treatment of LTBI (**Table 2**). Of note, treatment completion rates are higher with shorter duration regimens.[15]

Active Tuberculosis Disease

Once identified as having active TB disease, it is essential to coordinate with infectious diseases, pulmonology, or the local TB control program, ensuring appropriate management occurs. If inpatient, discharge planning should begin as soon as possible in coordination with the TB control program. In addition, consideration of drug susceptibility is essential early on, preventing both drug resistance and disease progression.[16]

Drug-Susceptible Tuberculosis Disease

In drug-susceptible TB disease, treatment duration is lengthy, and adherence to the treatment plan is essential in preventing transmission of disease as well as developing drug resistance (**Table 3**). An intensive and a continuation phase is required, with most regimens requiring 6 to 9 months of therapy. The standard treatment includes

Table 2
Latent tuberculosis infection treatment recommendations[15]

Treatment Regimen	Duration of Therapy	Recommended Populations	Disadvantages
Once weekly isoniazid (INH) plus rifapentine	3 mo	Adults, children >2 y, includes HIV-positive individuals	Increased cost Increased number of pills at one time (10 pills once weekly)
Daily rifampicin (RIF)	4 mo	HIV-negative adults Children of all ages	Drug interactions (warfarin, oral contraceptives, azole antifungals, and HIV antiretroviral therapy) In PLWH with low CD4 count, risk for subclinical TB disease increases
Daily INH plus RIF	3 mo	Conditionally recommended for adults/ children of all ages PLWH (assess for drug-drug interactions)	Hepatotoxicity risk increased when taking both drugs
Daily INH*	6 mo	HIV-negative adults Children of all ages HIV-positive adults/children (conditionally)	Hepatotoxicity
Daily INH*	9 mo	Conditionally for adults and children, all ages, both HIV-negative and -positive	Hepatotoxicity

* Alternative recommended regimens in contrast, the first three rows are preferred regimens.

Table 3
Treatment regimens for drug-susceptible tuberculosis[17]

	Intensive Phase		Continuation Phase		Total Dose Range	Recommended Use
Regimen	Duration/Frequency	Regimen	Duration/Frequency			
INH, RIF, PZA, EMB	8 wk: 7 d/wk x56 doses 5 d/wk x40 doses	INH, RIF	18 wk: 7 d/wk x126 doses 5 d/wk x90 doses	INH, RIF	130–182	Newly diagnosed pulmonary TB
INH, RIF, PZA, EMB	8 wk: 7 d/wk x56 doses 5 d/wk x40 doses	INH, RIF	18 wk: 3x/wk x54 doses		94–110	Alternative regimen Those where frequent DOT in continuation phase is difficult
INH, RIF, PZA, EMB	8 wk: 3x/wk x24 doses	INH, RIF	18 wk: 3x/week x54 doses		78	Caution in PLWH or with cavitary disease—concerns for missed doses and treatment relapse/drug resistance
INH, RIF, PZA, EMB	8 wk: 7 d/wk x14 doses, then 2x/wk x12 doses	INH, RIF	18 wk: 2x/wk x36 doses		62	Do not use in PLWH if smear positive or if there is evidence of cavitary disease

Abbreviation: EMB, ethambutol.

rifampicin (RIF), isoniazid (INH), pyrazinamide (PZA), and ethambutol for 2 months, followed by INH and RIF for 4 to 7 months. The weekly number of doses may vary, as those using directly observed therapy (DOT) can take 5 doses per week, whereas those not using DOT will take 7 doses per week.[17]

Drug-Resistant Tuberculosis

Drug-resistant TB is becoming more common globally, with approximately half a million of those developing TB having RIF resistance in 2019. Resistance can develop at the onset of disease or emerge throughout the treatment course due to inadequate therapy.[18] There are different classifications of resistance (**Table 4**) based on overall susceptibility patterns ranging from MDR-TB to extensively drug-resistant (XDR-TB). MDR-TB has typically required an injectable medication for adequate treatment.

Drug susceptibility testing is beneficial before final selection of antibiotics but may not be available to all patients. Early detection of resistance is of utmost importance, but currently approved rapid diagnostic devices can test only for RIF resistance. By having access to susceptibility testing earlier, we can rely on diagnostic data, rather than relying on known "hotspots" alone for early treatment decision-making. Prevention of drug-resistant TB will require a collaborative public health response, including initiatives encouraging drug adherence, early detection of resistance, and improved treatment regimens.[18]

DISCUSSION
New Developments

Part of the WHO goal to end TB by 2035 includes the need for new diagnostic tools and encouraging clinical research. Although funding remains a primary barrier, there have been many developments in recent years.

In 2020, the WHO recommended an all-oral regimen for drug-resistant TB treatment, with some options significantly shorter than previous regimens used for MDR-TB. For those with RIF resistance and fluroquinolone resistance, the WHO approved the BPaL regimen, which consists of bedaquiline, pretomanid, and linezolid. An open-label, single-group study assessed the efficacy in those with XDR-TB or those with MDR-TB that were nonresponsive to treatment. The study showed that XDR-TB could be effectively treated with BPaL for 26 weeks. They report approximately 90% treatment success, which was defined as favorable outcomes at 6 months posttherapy completion.[19] Additional research is being conducted with novel combinations of drugs in those with drug-susceptible and drug-resistant TB.

Additional recommendations for MDR-TB include the inclusion of a partial lobectomy in conjunction with antimicrobial treatments. The American Thoracic Society recommends an elective partial lobectomy or wedge resection. Evaluation of systematic

Table 4 TB drug resistance[20]	
	Pattern of Drug Resistance
Multidrug-resistant TB (MDR-TB)	INH and RIF
Preextensively drug-resistant TB (Pre-XDR TB)	INH, RIF, and a fluroquinolone (FQ) *or* INH, RIF, and a second-line injectable (amikacin, capreomycin, kanamycin)
Extensively drug-resistant TB (XDR-TB)	INH, RIF, FQ, second-line injectable OR INH, RIF, FQ, and bedaquiline or linezolid

review data showing those who underwent partial lobectomy had higher treatment success. However, this was not consistent in those who underwent a pneumonectomy, with higher reports of death when compared with those who underwent a partial lobectomy. However, the investigators note that surgical intervention versus TB was the cause of death.[20]

In a 2021 WHO update on rapid diagnostics, a new NAAT device met minimal criteria to be recommended as an initial test—the TrueNat point-of-care (POC) assay, which can detect TB and RIF resistance, like the GeneXpert. Data evaluated showed similar sensitivity and specificity for both *Mtb* diagnosis and RIF resistance detection. The benefits of this device include that it is battery-operated and can function at higher temperatures, up to 40°C, which is beneficial to those testing in the field or in developing nations.[21]

In February 2022, the CDC released interim guidance recommending the use of a 4-month daily treatment regimen, which includes high-dose rifapentine (RPT), moxifloxacin, INH, and PZA based on trial results showing this regimen is noninferior to the currently available standard regimen. Important to note, that this regimen is not recommended by the CDC in those weighing less than 40 kg, younger than 12 years, pregnant or breastfeeding, or those with known resistance to any of the regimen antibiotics.[22]

Other recent developments include novel diagnostic tests. In April 2022, the WHO released unpublished data on a new *Mtb* antigen–based skin test, which measures "cell-mediated immunologic response to *Mtb*-specific antigens."[12] Evidence suggests these new tests are accurate, cost-effective, feasible, and safe. Most important is these tests had specificity similar to IGRA tests and better than TST. A formal recommendation by the WHO has not been released; however, they plan to provide updates in late 2022.[23]

SPECIAL POPULATIONS
Health Care Workers

In 2019, TB screening, testing, and treatment of health care workers (HCW) were updated by the CDC. The following guidance is recommended, but organizational requirements may differ.

Baseline screening and testing for those without prior TB disease or LTBI:

- Baseline testing (TST or IGRA) for all HCW
- Complete symptom evaluation
- Individual TB risk assessment

Postexposure screening/testing:

- Symptom evaluation when exposure recognized
- If baseline negative TB test, no history of TB disease, no history of LTBI:
  ○ Perform IGRA or TST at time of exposure identification
  ○ If negative: repeat IGRA/TST 8 to 10 weeks postexposure

Serial screening and testing for HCW without LTBI:

- Not routinely recommended
- Consider for select HCW (those with occupational risks: pulmonologists, respiratory therapists; those in certain settings: ED)
- Annual TB education, including exposure risk information

Evaluation and treatment of positive test result is encouraged for all HCW with untreated LTBI (unless contraindicated).[24]

People Living with Human Immunodeficiency Virus

There is higher mortality of TB infection for those coinfected with HIV. Rapid progression of TB disease is likely because of the effects of HIV on the immune responses that typically restrict TB growth. Patients with TB/HIV co-infection may also present atypically, further delaying diagnosis. The relative risk of active TB disease doubles in year one after initial HIV infection and continues to increase in the following years, as CD4 counts decrease. For this reason, in those with LTBI and HIV, HIV infection will accelerate the progression to active TB disease.[25]

In 2019, results from a randomized controlled trial evaluated the use of a 1-month daily RPT and INH regimen as a preventive treatment in people living with HIV (PLWH). They found this 1-month regimen was noninferior to the standard 9-month regimen. Given the shorter duration of therapy, increased adherence to this regimen was also reported. Currently, this option is only approved for PLWH, as clinical trials have not been conducted in other populations.[26]

Diabetes Mellitus

There has been increasing evidence that DM may be a risk factor for developing active TB. There is speculation, based on animal models, that there is a delay in response of alveolar macrophages, which then impairs the antimicrobial function against TB. Further, there is a delay in response, allowing TB bacilli to replicate, increasing inflammation. The investigators reviewing this increased risk also noted that those with DM were more likely to present with advanced TB. Glycemic control will be essential in these patients to prevent the progression of disease. In addition, they report on a recent study that showed a hemoglobin A1c greater than or equal to 7% may be a risk factor for INH resistance and MDR-TB.[27]

COVID-19 Effects on Tuberculosis

Before the COVID-19 pandemic, tuberculosis was the number one cause of death from a single infectious agent. The pandemic has negatively affected the progress made to combat TB, with the Stop TB Partnership estimating the first year of COVID-19 has pushed TB progress back approximately 12 years.[5] Many resources, including diagnostic tools, workforce, and funding, have shifted to COVID-19. There has also been a disruption in access to care, which included shorter office hours, fewer appointment times, as well as community fear of contracting COVID-19, all contributing to missed or delayed diagnosis of LTBI or active TB infection.[5]

According to the most recent WHO Global Report, there was a reduction in the number of newly diagnosed TB infections, but an increase in the number of individuals who died of TB; this was the first-year increase in TB deaths since 2005. They suspect the impact on TB-related deaths may be larger in 2021, with data unavailable at the time of publication.[2]

In addition, we have yet to see the full extent of the impact COVID-19 will have socioeconomically and on the WHO's End TB Strategy. Given the urgent response needed for COVID-19, health care staff had to shift priorities to COVID-19–related services, which affected the ability to deliver additional TB programs.[28] GeneXpert machines were repurposed in some locations to test for SARS-CoV-2 throughout the pandemic, which limited the number of rapid molecular testing able to be completed.[5] Limited TB services and staffing and the decreased ability to perform rapid testing may lead to significant delays in diagnosis, decrease adherence due to limited follow-up, as well as increase transmission.[28] It is reasonable to suspect that DOT was difficult to implement throughout shut-downs; therefore, electronic directly observed therapy (eDOT) may have been implemented more often in areas where

TB was present. Although there are no current data supporting this throughout the pandemic. There are limitations to the use of eDOT for some individuals, as access to smartphones or the Internet may be a barrier. The true effects of COVID-19 on TB cases and deaths will likely not be seen for years, given the variable duration from initial TB infection to active disease development.

GOALS

End TB 2035

To accomplish the goals of the End TB initiative, the WHO created 3 pillars including patient care and prevention, policies, and supportive systems and research and innovation. Early detection and treatment of LTBI and active infection, as well as a focus on susceptibility testing and contact tracing, collaborative TB/HIV interventions, and implementation of preventive treatment are needed for those at highest risk. Supportive systems focus on community engagement, universal health care coverage, as well as social protection, and improvement of socioeconomic factors that can lead to poverty. In addition, there is a focus on research, encouraging the development of devices, treatments, vaccines, as well as additional interventions and strategies.[29]

Think. Test. Treat. TB

The CDC started the *Think. Test. Treat. TB* campaign in March 2022 to improve testing and treatment of LTBI in the United States.[30] Although cases of active TB in the United States are not as concerning as the global incidence, the CDC estimates that 13 million individuals may be living with latent TB. In the outpatient setting, considering LTBI in those with risk factors for infection is essential in preventing the development of active TB. For those who have increased risk, completing appropriate testing is beneficial, followed by treatment of those who have a positive result.[8]

Barriers to Goals

To meet the goals set forth by the WHO, a significant increase in funding will be necessary. In 2020, funding for TB was US$ 6.5 billion, whereas there is a global goal of US$13 billion per year by 2022.[2] It is estimated that annually US$ 8 billion is necessary to cover the typical cost of case detection and treatment globally. Even before the COVID-19 pandemic, funding became short.[31]

Vaccine Development

As previously stated, we have not had a new vaccine to combat TB in more than 100 years. Many barriers to vaccine creation have been proposed in recent years. As with all aspects of TB, funding and interest have been low, leading to limited ability to invest a significant amount of time in this area. Additional research has shown there may be variability in antigen expression throughout the phases of TB, with some antigen expression only in early latency and others throughout the duration of infection, which may complicate vaccine development. In addition, there are no standardized assays or biomarkers that have proved effective at evaluating vaccine efficacy.[32] Even with limited funding, many clinical trials have been completed or evaluated at many different phases of development, including BCG boosters, messenger RNA vaccines, and a cytomegalovirus-vector vaccine.[33]

SUMMARY

To meet the goals set by the WHO on the global scale, increased funding is essential, as well as ensuring continued interest in the development of new diagnostics, treatments, and preventive measures. Of utmost importance is identifying and treating LTBI; thus, improved diagnostic testing and LTBI treatments will be required. Treating LTBI is significantly more cost-effective than treating active TB.[34] The estimated cost of the treatment of LTBI is around US$500, whereas the treatment of active disease can range from approximately US$20,000 for non-MDR-TB to US$567,000 for XDR-TB.[35,36] In addition, drug-resistant TB is a public health crisis, so we will require improved drug susceptibility testing that can be used globally and treatment regimens that can be universally used for drug-susceptible and drug-resistant TB. The impact of TB will continue to be felt, primarily in underserved communities; however, the emergence of drug-resistant TB should be a concern globally, especially with the recent impact of the COVID-19 pandemic. We have seen what political will can accomplish throughout the urgently needed response to the COVID-19 pandemic; however, TB should not be ignored and should receive the same urgent response.

CLINICS CARE POINTS

- Screening should be completed for all patients who are considered at risk for *Mtb* infection, if asymptomatic, using either the TST or IGRA testing.
- For all positive screening tests, evaluation for active disease is necessary to determine a treatment plan. All those who have LTBI should consider anti-TB treatment.
- Treatment selection should consider the ability to adhere to treatment and to monitoring requirements. The local TB Control Programs should be used in all cases of active TB during outpatient management.
- Those with risk factors for the development of active TB should also be encouraged to manage all comorbid conditions.
- For those at risk for MDR-TB, it is essential that antimicrobial therapies are modified. To prevent MDR-TB, evaluation for treatment adherence should be assessed.

DISCLOSURE

The authors did not receive support from any organization for the submitted work. The authors declare no conflicts of interest.

REFERENCES

1. Riedel S., Hobden J.A., Miller S., et al., eds., Mycobacteria, Jawetz, Melnick, & Adelberg's Medical Microbiology, 28e. McGraw Hill, New York, NY; 2019. Available at: https://accessmedicine.mhmedical.com/content.aspx?bookid=2629&sectionid=217771812. Accessed March 29, 2023.
2. Global tuberculosis report 2021. WHO. Available at: https://www.who.int/publications-detail-redirect/9789240037021 Accessed June 15, 2022.
3. Filardo TD. Tuberculosis — United States, 2021. MMWR Morb Mortal Wkly Rep 2022;71. https://doi.org/10.15585/mmwr.mm7112a1.
4. Deutsch-Feldman M. Tuberculosis — United States, 2020. MMWR Morb Mortal Wkly Rep 2021;70. https://doi.org/10.15585/mmwr.mm7012a1.
5. Wingfield T, Karmadwala F, MacPherson P, et al. Challenges and opportunities to end tuberculosis in the COVID-19 era. Lancet Respir Med 2021;9(6):556–8. https://doi.org/10.1016/S2213-2600(21)00161-2.
6. Borgdorff MW, van Soolingen D. The re-emergence of tuberculosis: what have we learnt from molecular epidemiology? Clin Microbiol Infect 2013;19(10):889–901. https://doi.org/10.1111/1469-0691.12253.

7. Global tuberculosis report 2020. Available at: https://www.who.int/publications-detail-redirect/9789240013131 Accessed June 15, 2022.

8. CDCTB. TB Risk Factors. Centers for Disease Control and Prevention. 2016. Available at: https://www.cdc.gov/tb/topic/basics/risk.htm. Accessed June 15, 2022.

9. Fatima S, Kumari A, Das G, et al. Tuberculosis vaccine: A journey from BCG to present. Life Sci 2020;252:117594.

10. Organizat WH. WHO consolidated guidelines on tuberculosis. Module 1: Prevention. Tuberculosis preventive treatment. Tuberc Lung Dis HIV Infect 2021;(2): 86–92. https://doi.org/10.30978/TB2021-2-86.

11. Lewinsohn DM, Leonard MK, LoBue PA, et al. Official American Thoracic Society/Infectious Diseases Society of America/Centers for Disease Control and Prevention Clinical Practice Guidelines: Diagnosis of Tuberculosis in Adults and Children. Clin Infect Dis 2017;64(2):e1–33. https://doi.org/10.1093/cid/ciw694.

12. Core Curriculum on TB. 2021. Available at: https://www.cdc.gov/tb/education/corecurr/index.htm. Accessed June 15, 2022.

13. Report of an Expert Consultation on the Uses of Nucleic Acid Amplification Tests for the Diagnosis of Tuberculosis. 2020. Available at: https://www.cdc.gov/tb/publications/guidelines/amplification_tests/reccomendations.htm.   Accessed June 15, 2022.

14. Kay AW, Fernández LG, Takwoingi Y, et al. Xpert MTB/RIF and Xpert MTB/RIF Ultra assays for active tuberculosis and rifampicin resistance in children. Cochrane Database Syst Rev 2020;8. https://doi.org/10.1002/14651858.CD013359.pub2.

15. Sterling TR, Njie G, Zenner D, et al. Guidelines for the Treatment of Latent Tuberculosis Infection: Recommendations from the National Tuberculosis Controllers Association and CDC, 2020. MMWR Recomm Rep (Morb Mortal Wkly Rep) 2020;69(1):1–11. https://doi.org/10.15585/mmwr.rr6901a1.

16. Menu of Suggested Provisions for State Tuberculosis Prevention and Control Laws. 2020. Available at: https://www.cdc.gov/tb/programs/laws/menu/treatment.htm. Accessed June 15, 2022.

17. Nahid P, Dorman SE, Alipanah N, et al. Executive Summary: Official American Thoracic Society/Centers for Disease Control and Prevention/Infectious Diseases Society of America Clinical Practice Guidelines: Treatment of Drug-Susceptible Tuberculosis. Clin Infect Dis 2016;63(7):853–67. https://doi.org/10.1093/cid/ciw566.

18. Dean AS, Auguet OT, Glaziou P, et al. 25 years of surveillance of drug-resistant tuberculosis: achievements, challenges, and way forward. Lancet Infect Dis 2022. https://doi.org/10.1016/S1473-3099(21)00808-2.

19. Conradie F, Diacon AH, Ngubane N, et al. Treatment of Highly Drug-Resistant Pulmonary Tuberculosis. N Engl J Med 2020;382(10):893–902. https://doi.org/10.1056/NEJMoa1901814.

20. Nahid P, Mase SR, Migliori GB, et al. Treatment of Drug-Resistant Tuberculosis. An Official ATS/CDC/ERS/IDSA Clinical Practice Guideline. Am J Respir Crit Care Med 2019;200(10):e93–142. https://doi.org/10.1164/rccm.201909-1874ST.

21. Penn-Nicholson A, Gomathi SN, Ugarte-Gil C, et al. A prospective multicentre diagnostic accuracy study for the Truenat tuberculosis assays. Eur Respir J 2021;58(5). https://doi.org/10.1183/13993003.00526-2021.

22. Carr W. Interim Guidance: 4-Month Rifapentine-Moxifloxacin Regimen for the Treatment of Drug-Susceptible Pulmonary Tuberculosis — United States, 2022. MMWR Morb Mortal Wkly Rep. 2022;71. doi:10.15585/mmwr.mm7108a1

23. Rapid communication: TB antigen-based skin tests for the diagnosis of TB infection. Available at: https://www.who.int/publications-detail-redirect/WHO-UCN-TB-2022.1. Accessed June 15, 2022.

24. Sosa LE. Tuberculosis Screening, Testing, and Treatment of U.S. Health Care Personnel: Recommendations from the National Tuberculosis Controllers Association and CDC. MMWR Morb Mortal Wkly Rep 2019;68. https://doi.org/10.15585/mmwr.mm6819a3.

25. Kwan CK, Ernst JD. HIV and Tuberculosis: a Deadly Human Syndemic. Clin Microbiol Rev 2011;24(2):351–76. https://doi.org/10.1128/CMR.00042-10.

26. Swindells S, Ramchandani R, Gupta A, et al. One Month of Rifapentine plus Isoniazid to Prevent HIV-Related Tuberculosis. N Engl J Med 2019;380(11):1001–11. https://doi.org/10.1056/NEJMoa1806808.

27. Antonio-Arques V, Franch-Nadal J, Caylà JA. Diabetes and tuberculosis: A syndemic complicated by COVID-19. Med Clin Engl Ed 2021;157(6):288–93. https://doi.org/10.1016/j.medcle.2021.04.006.

28. Fuady A, Houweling TAJ, Richardus JH. COVID-19 and Tuberculosis-Related Catastrophic Costs. Am J Trop Med Hyg 2021;104(2):436–40. https://doi.org/10.4269/ajtmh.20-1125.

29. The end TB strategy. Available at: https://www.who.int/publications-detail-redirect/WHO-HTM-TB-2015.19. Accessed June 15, 2022.

30. CDCTB. Think. Test. Treat TB Campaign. Centers for Disease Control and Prevention. 2022. Available at: https://www.cdc.gov/thinktesttreattb/index.html. Accessed June 15, 2022.

31. Raviglione M, Sulis G. Tuberculosis 2015: Burden, Challenges and Strategy for Control and Elimination. Infect Dis Rep 2016;8(2):6570. https://doi.org/10.4081/idr.2016.6570.

32. Zhu B, Dockrell HM, Ottenhoff THM, et al. Tuberculosis vaccines: Opportunities and challenges. Respirology 2018;23(4):359–68. https://doi.org/10.1111/resp.13245.

33. Heaton PM. Challenges of Developing Novel Vaccines With Particular Global Health Importance. Front Immunol 2020;11. Available at: https://www.frontiersin.org/article/10.3389/fimmu.2020.517290. Accessed June 15, 2022.

34. Holland DP, Sanders GD, Hamilton CD, et al. Costs and Cost-effectiveness of Four Treatment Regimens for Latent Tuberculosis Infection. Am J Respir Crit Care Med 2009;179(11):1055–60. https://doi.org/10.1164/rccm.200901-0153OC.

35. CDC Estimates for LTBI Treatment Costs. Published April 13, 2022. Available at: https://www.cdc.gov/tb/publications/infographic/ltbi-treatment-costs.htm. Accessed June 15, 2022.

36. CDC Estimates for TB Treatment Costs. 2021. CDC Estimates for LTBI Treatment Costs. Available at: https://www.cdc.gov/tb/publications/infographic/appendix.htm. Accessed March 29, 2023.

A Review and Update of Emerging and Re-emerging Spirochetal Diseases in the United States

Check for updates

Peter A. Young, MPAS, PA-C[a,b],*, Sampath Wijesinghe, DHSc, PA-C[c],
Claire Liepmann, MD[d], Gordon H. Bae, MD[b]

KEYWORDS

- Spirochetal diseases • Syphilis • Lues venerea
- Emerging and reemerging infectious diseases • Lyme disease • Lyme borreliosis
- *Borrelia burgdorferi*

KEY POINTS

- Untreated syphilis is highly transmissible through body fluids and may lead to severe morbidity or mortality.
- Prevalence and geographical spread have increased in the United States.
- Men who have sex with men are also disproportionately affected, representing the majority of US cases.
- Due to the potential for false-positive screening test results, 2 antibody tests are needed for diagnosis: a nontreponemal test such as rapid plasma reagin or Venereal Disease Research Laboratory and a treponemal test, such as *Treponema pallidum* particle agglutination assay.
- Parenteral penicillin G has been used effectively for healing syphilitic lesions, preventing transmission, and preventing late sequelae.

PART 1: SYPHILIS

He who knows syphilis, knows medicine.

—*Sir William Osler, MD.*

[a] Department of Dermatology, The Permanente Medical Group, 2345 Fair Oaks Boulevard, Sacramento, CA 95821, USA; [b] Department of Dermatology, Stanford University School of Medicine, Redwood City, CA, USA; [c] Department of PA Education, Stanford University School of Medicine, Stanford, CA, USA; [d] Department of Infectious Diseases, Indiana University School of Medicine, Maywood, IL, USA
* Corresponding author.
E-mail address: payoung@stanford.edu

Physician Assist Clin 8 (2023) 467–481
https://doi.org/10.1016/j.cpha.2023.02.007
2405-7991/23/© 2023 Elsevier Inc. All rights reserved.

physicianassistant.theclinics.com

INTRODUCTION

Syphilis is an ancient disease; a chronic bacterial infection caused by *Treponema pallidum*, subspecies *pallidum*,[1] which may have emerged in humans as early as 7000 BC.[2] In Europe and the Americas, syphilis rates have fluctuated periodically, increasing in association with precipitating crises of war, poverty, and mass migration; declining during periods of strengthened preventive efforts by public health campaigns. Its clinical presentation varies significantly from asymptomatic to dramatic, sometimes involving multiple organ systems and/or displaying polymorphic cutaneous lesions, earning syphilis the nickname of the great imitator. Clinicians must be familiar with the disease because untreated syphilis remains highly transmissible through bodily fluids and may lead to severe morbidity or mortality.[1] Between 2010 and 2019, syphilis prevalence in the United States has increased 2.67-fold.[3] Confronting syphilis with updated knowledge is as important now as ever, despite its status as a stigmatized disease not discussed openly.[2,4] Herein, we review syphilis in general and the most relevant recent literature.

HISTORY

Multiple theories exist as to the origins of syphilis, the most popular of which is the Columbian hypothesis; this posits that Christopher Columbus brought the disease from the Americas to Europe on his return in 1493. Radiocarbon dating has shown that human bones from the Americas, but not Europe, exhibited syphilitic lesions before 1492. A Spanish physician present for Columbus' return from the New World has written that multiple crew members suffered from syphilis on their return voyage to Spain, a disease "so far not seen and never described."[2]

In late 1494, France invaded Italy with an army composed largely of mercenaries from neighboring European states including Spain. In 1495, Italian physicians wrote descriptions of a terrifying and sometimes fatal sexually transmissible disease, seen as a generalized pustular eruption on the bodies of invading soldiers. The war lasted 30 years, during which time there was extensive rape, prostitution, and marriages between locals and mercenaries, many of whom brought the disease to their homelands on return from the war.[2]

The first written appearance of the word Syphilis appeared in 1530, when Italian physician Girolamo Fracastoro authored a poem about a fictitious shepherd named Syphilus who suffered from the disease. In 1546, Fracastoro published a treatise on infectious diseases, in which he consistently refers to the disease as syphilis. Although Fracastoro's inspiration for the name is not known, the popularity of his poem and scientific writings resulted in its widespread use as a sort of eponym.[5] Syphilis has also been called lues venera, from Latin *lues* meaning pest or plague and *venereus*, relating to sexual intercourse.

In 1905, Germany's Fritz Schaudinn and Erich Hoffmann, a zoologist and dermatologist, respectively, discovered syphilis' causative spirochete by microscopic examination of fresh, Giemsa-stained specimens collected from skin lesions, which they subsequently named *T pallidum*.[6–8]

For centuries, treatment of syphilis was aimed at eliminating the illness via induction of perspiration, diarrhea, urination, and salivation; achieved with various ingested substances including Guaiacum Officinale, mercurous chloride, and bismuth salts. The 1908 Nobel Prize in physiology and medicine was awarded to German physician Paul Ehrlich, for his discovery that arsphenamine, an arsenical compound, exerted antibiotic activity against *T pallidum*. In 1927, Austrian physician Julius Wagner-Jauregg received the Nobel Prize for discovering that neurosyphilis symptoms could be alleviated by intentionally infecting patients with *Plasmodium vivax* to induce severe fever paroxysms, then injecting quinine to treat the iatrogenic malaria.[2] The veneration of these barbaric treatments should illuminate for posterity the desperation of sufferers to find any relief from this devastating disease.

In 1928, Scottish physician Sir Alexander Fleming discovered penicillin, the world's first broadly effective antibiotic, for which he shared the 1945 Nobel Prize with pharmacologist Howard Florey and biochemist Sir Ernst Chain.[6,7] To date, penicillin remains the recommended first-line treatment of syphilis.

EPIDEMIOLOGY

Syphilis is distributed worldwide and disproportionately affects populations with limited socioeconomic privilege. In the United States, Native Americans, Pacific Islanders, African Americans, and Hispanic populations experience the highest rates.[9] Men who have sex with men (MSM) are also disproportionately affected, representing the majority (56%) of US cases in 2019.[3]

Following AIDS prevention campaigns in the 1980s, the United States saw a dramatic reduction in sexually transmitted bacterial diseases,[10] with syphilis rates reaching an all-time low in the 1990s.[11] Starting in 1995, several countries began to see increasing syphilis rates with a proportionate shift toward the MSM population.[12–14] In the early 2000s, the US rate of syphilis increased by 62% in men, leading to an overall increase despite a 53% decrease among women. This may be partially attributable to the increased availability of preexposure prophylaxis antiretroviral therapy for HIV around the same time, which has been associated with reduced use of condoms in MSM.[12,15–17]

In 2020, sexually transmitted diseases reached an all-time high in the United States for the seventh consecutive year, when there were 133,945 reported cases of syphilis.[9,18] Between 2010 and 2019, the US syphilis rate increased 2.67-fold, from 15 to 40 per 100,000.[3] During this time, syphilis among women of reproductive age doubled. Congenital syphilis (CS) and its associated mortality have also steadily increased from 2011 to 2020, representing 7% of cases. The geographic spread and density of infections have both increased, with 32 US states and the District of Columbia reporting increased congenital cases from 2019 to 2020.[9] One possible explanation for the recent rapid increase is what a former Centers for Disease Control and Prevention (CDC) director calls "a deadly cycle of panic and neglect," in which public health crises, in general, propel government officials to scramble and provide funding to control and prevent diseases only after a delayed process of outbreaks being characterized by scientists, who then mount lobbying efforts to garner overdue resources.[19]

PATHOGENESIS

Syphilis is caused by *T pallidum*, subspecies *pallidum*, a slow-growing spirochetal bacterium measuring 0.15 μm in diameter and 6 to 15 μm in length. *T pallidum* has more than 99% DNA homology to *T pallidum* subspecies *pertenue* and *Treponema carateum*, the spirochetal bacteria causative of yaws and pinta, respectively.[1]

With the exception of CS, which is transmitted vertically from mother to fetus, the disease is primarily spread through direct contact with syphilitic lesions. Historically a small number of cases have been contracted via blood transfusions or needle sharing during illicit drug use.[1] Syphilis enhances the spread of HIV, owing to ulcerative skin having a compromised epidermal barrier and increased the presence of macrophages and T-cells with HIV receptors.[17]

Because of *T pallidum*'s slow growth rate, infection has a long incubation period, taking 3 weeks to manifest initial lesions at the site of inoculation. If untreated, the spirochete spreads hematogenously to internal organs, the skin, and the central nervous system (CNS).[20]

CLINICAL PRESENTATION

Syphilis is a chronic disease, with 3 stages: primary, secondary, and tertiary (also called latent). Following exposure and a roughly 3-week incubation period, primary syphilis begins as a painless, indurated, usually solitary ulcer at the inoculation site (a chancre). Adjacent lymphadenopathy may be present, with or without tenderness. The chancre is often seen on the glans penis but may also appear in visually occult sites such as the vagina, cervix, rectum, perirectal skin, and oropharynx. Chancres have also been reported on the fingers and neck. Untreated, primary lesions self-resolve in 3 to 6 weeks without scarring, with treatment they will resolve in under a week.[1]

Syphilis is most diagnosed in its secondary stage, when systemic infection manifests as cutaneous lesions that are the most variable and polymorphous of any known infectious disease. The skin eruption may be localized or generalized and classically consists of numerous, painless, dusky-red macules and patches up to 2 cm in diameter, which often involve the mucous membranes, palms, and soles. Lesions may also be pustular, papular, or scaly, sometimes mimicking papulosquamous dermatoses such as pityriasis rosea or psoriasis. Verruciform skin lesions may appear in moist areas, referred to as condyloma lata. Without treatment, the cutaneous lesions of secondary syphilis may resolve spontaneously without scarring, over 3 to 12 weeks. Additional manifestations of secondary syphilis may include nephrotic syndrome, hepatosplenomegaly, hepatitis, and diffuse lymphadenopathy.[1]

After resolution of secondary syphilis, the disease enters a variable asymptomatic latent phase in which diagnosis can only be made by serologic tests. Within 1 to 2 years, about 25% of patients will experience a recurrence of signs and symptoms typical of secondary syphilis during which time they are again very contagious. This latent phase is divided into early (within 1 year) and late (over a year) subtypes, which differ in the management strategies.[21,22] Left untreated, one-third of these patients develop tertiary syphilis 15 to 30 years later, manifesting as cardiovascular syphilis (including aortitis) or gummatous syphilis (soft, noncancerous, granulomatous lesions that destroy tissue). Neurosyphilis can occur at any stage of infection.[23]

The most common form of neurosyphilis is tabes dorsalis (from Latin *tabes*, literally "wasting away," and *dorsalis* referring to the chiefly affected spinal components). This usually begins as chronic spirochetal meningitis lasting 1 to 2 decades, which leads to severely damaged dorsal roots, dorsal root ganglia, and posterior columns producing a constellation of characteristic sequelae. Sacral root damage can result in bladder hypotonia with overflow incontinence, constipation, and impotence. Partial loss of small myelinated and unmyelinated fibers may cause coldness, numbness, or tingling, with associated impaired sensations of light touch, pain, and temperature. Loss of proprioceptive fibers causes ataxia (impaired motor coordination) with a high-stepping gait and slapping of the ground with each step. Recurrent episodes of sudden, brief stabbing pain may occur, usually in the legs, called lightning pains.[24]

Syphilitic lesions of the brainstem may affect the efferent pupillary fibers associated with the light reflex, while sparing fibers associated with the accommodation reflex, resulting in Argyll Robertson pupils. The pupil will constrict in response to light, that is, they accommodate but not in response to a close object, that is, they are nonreactive.[25,26] Additional sequelae of late neurosyphilis may include sudden epigastric pain (visceral crisis), areflexia, Charcot joints, and trophic ulcers.[24]

DIAGNOSTIC TESTS

Confirming a diagnosis of syphilis is complex. Live culture of *T pallidum* is not possible, and traditionally diagnosis was made by direct visualization with dark field microscopy of ground lesional exudate, although this can be done on nasal discharge or tissue as well. This is the only test offering immediate diagnosis, expediting treatment, and minimizing partner transmission.[27] However, accurate results depend on a high level of skill and experience not available to many modern clinics.[28] *T pallidum* may also be visualized in skin biopsy specimens using treponemal fluorescent antibody stains or silver stains.[29,30] There are no commercially available blood tests that directly detect *T pallidum*, thus clinicians rely on antibody tests.

Serologies must be interpreted cautiously because they may result in false negatives up to 3 weeks after appearance of a primary chancre[30]; high-risk patients should be rechecked. Due to the potential for false-positive screening test results, 2 antibody tests are needed for diagnosis: a nontreponemal test such as rapid plasma reagin (RPR, 92.7% sensitive) or Venereal Disease Research Laboratory (VDRL, 72.5% sensitive) and a treponemal test, such as *T pallidum* particle agglutination assay, microhemagglutination assay for *T pallidum* antibodies, fluorescent treponemal antibody absorbed test (FTA-ABS, 98.2% sensitive), or treponemal-specific enzyme immunoassay (TP-EIA, comparably sensitive to FTA-ABS).[22,31] False-positive nontreponemal results can be caused by viral infections (Epstein-Barr virus, hepatitis, HIV, varicella, measles), lymphoma, tuberculosis, malaria, endocarditis, connective tissue disease, pregnancy, older age, injection drug abuse, or technical errors.[23]

Traditional serologic testing algorithms involve initial screening with a nontreponemal test, such as RPR, which, if reactive, is then confirmed with a treponemal test such as FTA-ABS. In general, an asymptomatic patient requires no further testing if the nontreponemal test is negative. An increasingly popular algorithm reverses the order, using a treponemal test such as TP-EIA for screening, followed by a nontreponemal test for confirmation if positive. This is often preferred as treponemal testing has been automated and is therefore less expensive than RPR testing. Although the reverse screening method has a higher false-positive rate compared with the traditional algorithm, it can detect some syphilis cases that otherwise would have been missed.[31]

In neurosyphilis patients, cerebrospinal fluid (CSF) may be checked and may be normal or show mild lymphocytic pleocytosis (10–50 cells/μL) and elevated protein (45–75 mg/dL). A quarter of these patients have nonreactive CSF-VDRL.[24]

Treponemal antibodies remain positive indefinitely in most patients even after effective treatment. Thus, a positive treponemal serology may not differentiate between a current or former infection, and treatment decisions may require in-depth review of patient medical records. Health departments may be of assistance because they maintain records of positive serologies for reportable diseases including syphilis.[4] The need for 2 tests and sometimes discordant results can be confusing to health professionals.[32] When interpreting results, clinicians should not hesitate to consult with appropriate specialists if necessary.

Nontreponemal titers should decrease after treatment and are checked at regular intervals. Adequate response to treatment is considered a 4-fold decrease of nontreponemal antibody titer within 6 to 12 months after therapy.[22]

SYPHILIS AND PREGNANCY

Pregnancy adds a layer of complexity to diagnosing and managing syphilis. Due to immune system alterations, more false negatives and false positives occur from nontreponemal[33] and treponemal[34] tests, respectively. Women should be screened early in pregnancy and again at 28 weeks and at delivery if they are at high risk for infection. Treatment is safe during pregnancy, and although sometimes challenging to interpret, posttreatment nontreponemal titers are important to follow. Specialist involvement for individualized care may be necessary.[4]

CONGENITAL SYPHILIS

Maternal syphilis may cause spontaneous abortion (10%), stillbirth (10%), infant death (20%), a healthy child (40%), or CS (20%).[17] If early syphilis in the mother is untreated, the risk of fetal transmission is estimated to be 70% to 100%, and usually occurs after 16-week gestation.[35] Spirochetes can cross the placenta and infect a fetus from about 14-week gestation, and the risk of infection increases with gestational age if the mother is infected during pregnancy. Thus, infection at an early stage in pregnancy, if treated, should not affect the pregnancy.

The clinical manifestations of CS are described as early or late (appearing before or after 2 years of age, respectively). Symptoms can manifest at birth or within the first 2 months of life, often as cachexia and skin lesions. Early CS skin lesions appear as small dark red-copper macules that are most severe on the hands and feet. These are infectious and may resemble acquired secondary syphilis, although they are more severe, more generalized, persist longer, and may be bullous or erosive.[17,35] Infants with early CS may also have bloody or purulent nasal discharge (snuffles), perioral or perianal fissures, lymphadenopathy, and hepatosplenomegaly. Osteochondritis may occur and cause severe pain, reducing extremity movements, resulting in pseudoparalysis of Parrot. Affected infants may also manifest anemia, hepatitis, syphilitic pneumonitis, nephropathy, and thrombocytopenia. They may have neural involvement at birth but most neurosyphilis symptoms are considered late manifestations.

Late manifestations of untreated CS in a child or adolescent include bone and joint, tooth, eye, skin, and CNS involvement. This stage is usually noninfectious and corresponds to adult tertiary syphilis; the sequelae are the consequences of inflammation at sites of earlier treponemal infection. Interstitial keratitis is seen in one-third of affected children and often takes many years to manifest. If present along with characteristic dental abnormalities (peg-shaped central incisors) and neural deafness (eighth cranial nerve damage), these findings are called the Hutchinson triad. Other typical late manifestations include anterior bowing of the shins, frontal bossing, Mulberry molars, saddle nose, rhagades (perioral fissures) and Clutton joints (symmetric painless knee swelling).[17,23]

All infants born to mothers with positive serologies for syphilis should be carefully evaluated and the treatment of the mother reviewed. All infants being evaluated for syphilis should have a thorough physical examination, complete blood count (CBC) with differential, and CSF VDRL/cell count/protein; other testing may be clinically indicated including chest or long bone x-rays, eye examination, liver function tests, neuroimaging, and auditory brainstem response. Infants suspected of having CS should undergo thorough physical and ophthalmologic examination, serologic tests, CSF-VDRL and cellular/protein analysis, long bone and chest x-rays, complete blood cell and platelet count, and liver function tests. Nontreponemal and treponemal antibodies may be passively transferred from mother to fetus, thus, laboratory tests in newborns must be interpreted carefully. If passive antibody transfer occurs, the neonatal titer should become negative in 4 to 6 months. If the mother is infected late during pregnancy, both may be nonreactive at delivery, and subsequent clinical signs and titers will confirm the diagnosis.[35] At the author's institution (CL), treponemal antibodies are rechecked at 18 to 24 months to confirm the resolution of maternal antibodies.

Diagnosis of CS can be challenging and given the possible sequelae treatment may be given even when suspicion is low. Providers should not hesitate to contact a pediatric infectious disease specialist for help interpreting serologies and determining management. Because of the challenges around diagnosis of CS, infants are typically categorized into "proven or highly probable CS," "possible CS," "CS less likely," and "CS unlikely treatment is determined based on risk of CS." Preferred treatment is parenteral penicillin G. Infants should be monitored closely in follow-up, with evaluations at 1, 2, 3, 6, and 12 months of age, and nontreponemal blood tests at 2 to 4, 6, and 12 months after treatment. This should continue until results become nonreactive, or the titer has decreased 4-fold.[35] If nontreponemal serologies are not decreasing by 6 to 12 months, the child should be reevaluated and possibly retreated.

SKIN LESION HISTOLOGY

Histologic findings of skin biopsies vary between primary syphilitic chancres, secondary syphilis, and tertiary syphilis. When stained with hematoxylin and eosin (H&E), chancre classically exhibits ulceration and granulation tissue with numerous plasma cells beneath. The surface shows a zone of necrosis, fibrin, and neutrophils. These findings are similar to chancroid, therefore differentiation typically requires serology, special stains, and culture (to rule out other causative organisms). Immunostains or silver stains may reveal spirochetes.[29]

Secondary syphilis is nearly as variable microscopically as it is clinically. Sections stained with H&E may show neutrophils in the stratum corneum and vacuolar interface dermatitis with either effacement of the rete ridges or slender, "icicle-like" psoriasiform acanthosis. The dermis seems hypercellular or "busy," due to interstitial infiltration with perivascular histiocytes and lymphocytes containing visibly excessive pink cytoplasm. Vessels may lack visible lumen due to obliteration by endothelial swelling. Plasma cells are present in about two-thirds of cases. Gummas of tertiary syphilis may show granulomatous dermatitis with plasma cells on H&E, and spirochetes are generally not visible.[29]

DIFFERENTIAL DIAGNOSIS

The differential diagnosis of primary syphilis chancre may include herpes simplex virus, chancroid (*Haemophilus ducreyi*), lymphogranuloma venereum (*Chlamydia trachomatis*), granuloma inguinale (*Klebsiella granulomatis*), ecthyma (*staphylococci and/or streptococci*), bullous fixed drug eruption, Bechet disease, ulcerative squamous cell carcinoma, and calciphylaxis. Secondary syphilis skin lesions may resemble pityriasis rosea, pityriasis rubra pilaris, early guttate psoriasis, disseminated lichen planus, drug eruption, reactive arthritis. Cutaneous lesions of tertiary syphilis should be differentiated from sarcoidosis, granuloma annulare, lupus vulgaris, malignancies, cutaneous T-cell lymphoma, and other cutaneous proliferative T-cell disorders.

MANAGEMENT

Parenteral penicillin G has been used effectively for healing syphilitic lesions, preventing transmission, and preventing late sequelae. However, no comparative trials have been conducted to guide selection of an optimal penicillin regimen, and even fewer data evaluate nonpenicillin regimens.[36] Of note, treatment of early syphilis can lead to acute onset of fever, headache, and myalgias (Jarisch–Herxheimer reaction); this is due to release of tumor necrosis factor-alpha (TNF-α) when spirochetes are phagocytosed.[17]

For primary or secondary syphilis in nonpregnant adults, the recommended regimen is a single 2.4 million unit dose of intramuscular (IM) benzathine penicillin G.[36] Additional doses of benzathine penicillin G, amoxicillin, or other antibiotics do not enhance efficacy of this regimen for primary and secondary syphilis among persons with HIV.[37–39] In pregnancy, treatment can vary depending on the stage.

For infants and children aged 1 month or older, primary, secondary, and early latent syphilis should be treated with a single dose of IM benzathine penicillin G, dosed at 50,000 units/kg body weight (up to the adult dose of 2.4 million units). Infants and children should be managed by pediatric infectious disease and evaluated for sexual abuse through consultation with child protective services. Birth and maternal records should be reviewed to determine whether they have congenital or acquired syphilis.[36]

Clinical and serologic evaluation should be performed at 6 and 12 months after treatment; more frequent evaluation might be prudent if opportunity for follow-up is uncertain or if repeat infection is a clinical concern. Serologic response (ie, titer) should be compared with the titer at the time of treatment. However, assessing serologic response to treatment can be difficult, and definitive criteria for cure or failure by serologic criteria have not been well established. In addition, nontreponemal test titers might decrease more slowly for persons previously treated for syphilis.[36,40,41]

The preferred treatment of neurosyphilis is intravenous penicillin G, 2 to 4 million units every 4 hours for 10 to 14 days. CSF examination 6 months after treatment should demonstrate a normal cell count and decreasing protein content. If not, a second course of therapy is indicated. The CSF examination should be repeated every 6 months for 2 years or until the fluid normalizes.[24]

PART 2: LYME BORRELIOSIS
Introduction

In the United States, Lyme disease is the most common vector-borne disease and is caused by the spirochetal bacteria *Borrelia burgdorferi sensu stricto* (ss).[42] It is transmitted to humans through the bite of infected *Ixodes* (blacklegged) ticks. Symptoms may include fever, headache, fatigue, and a characteristic targetoid skin eruption–erythema migrans (EM). If untreated, Lyme can progress to involve the joints, heart, and nervous system. Lyme borreliosis is usually diagnosed clinically, and most cases can be successfully treated with oral antibiotics. Patients should be counseled on preventive methods, such as applying insect repellent, self-checking for ticks, applying pesticides, and reducing exposure to tick habitat.[43]

History

The causative organism of Lyme disease is estimated to be 60,000 years old.[44] The first known occurrence of human borreliosis was written by Herxheimer and Hartmann in 1902, in their description of acrodermatitis chronica atrophicans (ACA), although the cause remained unknown for 80 years. In 1909, Afzelius described the first case of EM, hypothesizing it was caused by his patient's recent tick bite. In 1968, the first American with EM was described: a physician bitten by a tick while hunting, who for 3 months experienced fever, headache, and dull radiating hip pain. He was cured within 48 hours of administering parenteral penicillin.[45]

In 1975, an outbreak of a mysterious illness in Old Lyme, Connecticut, prompted investigation by health authorities. More than 50 residents had been diagnosed with juvenile or idiopathic arthritis, a quarter of whom described EM-like skin lesions. Afflicted patients lived almost exclusively in wooded areas and onset occurred primarily during summer months but arthritis had not hitherto been described as having geographic or seasonal tendencies. In 1977, serologic evidence surfaced in support of an infectious cause, and in 1980, it was shown that systemic antibiotics shorten the EM lesion and prevent or lessen arthritic sequelae.[45] In 1982, entomologist Willy Burgdorfer isolated the causative organism, which now bears his name.[46]

Epidemiology

During the twentieth century, *Ixodes* ticks were mostly confined to temperate climates in the northern hemisphere.[42] However, climate change is expanding *Ixodes* tick habitat and lengthening their active warm season, spreading borreliosis.[44,47–49] In North America, geographic distribution of high incidence areas is growing: US counties with an incidence of 10 or more confirmed cases per 100,000 persons increased 33% from 2008 to 2019.[43] In 2019, 34,945 cases of Lyme disease were reported to the CDC, 4% more than in 2018. The actual US incidence is likely 10 times higher than reported, and is thought to exceed 300,000 cases annually.[50]

Cause

The spirochetal bacteria causing Lyme borreliosis, *B burgdorferi*, is a member of the family Spirochaetaceae.[51] Nine genospecies of *B burgdorferi* sensu lato (sl) complex may cause Lyme disease[42,52] but the exclusive cause in the United States is *B burgdorferi* sensu stricto (ss), with European cases also being caused by *Borellia garinii* and *Borellia afzelii*.[53] *B burgdorferi* is maintained in an enzootic transmission cycle consisting of *Ixodes* (black legged) ticks and vertebrate hosts including humans.[54]

Reservoirs

In the northeastern United States, white-footed mice, white-tailed deer, and racoons are the reservoirs for *Ixodes scapularis*. In western states, the wood mouse and western fence lizard are reservoirs for *Ixodes pacificus*. Small mammals such as the white-footed mouse are important in the transmission cycle because they can remain asymptomatic while infected with *B burgdorferi*, thereby serving as reservoirs from which serial generations of ticks acquire the disease.[51]

Vectors

Ixodes ticks mature through 4 developmental stages during 2 years: egg, larva, nymph, and adult. Larvae hatch from eggs in the late summer to feed on small animals such as mice, from whom they may contract *B burgdorferi*. Larvae grow to nymphs and feed during spring or early summer, maturing into adults in the fall or winter. Adult female ticks continue feeding, primarily on large animals.[51]

Transmission to Humans

About 12% to 15% of *Ixodes* ticks carry *B burgdorferi*,[42] transmitting the infection while feeding on hosts, causing symptomatic disease in humans about 1% to 3% of the time.[42,51] Tick bites often go unnoticed because of their small size, and secretions, which prevent itching or pain in the host. Infected ticks must remain attached for at least 1 day to transmit the infection, with the most effective transmission occurring 2 to 3 days after attachment. Human infection depends on outdoor activities and inadequate protective garments, and tick factors such as geography and seasonal variations in infectivity.[51]

Microbiology

B burgdorferi features antigenic surface lipoproteins in place of a lipopolysaccharide membrane, which promote its transmission and survival across various environments. Following transmission from tick to host via bite, plasmin protein secreted in tick saliva shields the spirochete from recognition by host immune cells. The immune response is further confounded by the spirochete's ability to reduce expression of surface proteins that could be targeted by anti-*B burgdorferi* antibodies. This effectively renders complement and other immune defenses moot, allowing evasion of *B burgdorferi*.[51]

Cutaneous Findings

The most common sign of Lyme disease is EM: an erythematous to violaceous targetoid patch that expands over several days to weeks, which occurs in up to 90% of patients.[51] The (perhaps overtaught) morphology of a bright red outer ring with a central clearing is more typical of *B afzelii* infections in Europe, with homogeneous EM being more typical of US patients, where *B burgdorferi* ss predominates. Half of patients with EM do not recall a tick bite; 18% of EM cases show multiple skin lesions.[42]

Cutaneous Findings Endemic to Europe

European borreliosis manifests signs and symptoms not seen in America, owing to the region's greater etiologic diversity. Borrelial lymphocytoma (BL) is a B-cell pseudolymphoma commonly seen in endemic regions of Europe. BL results from *B burgdorferi* antigen in the skin and appears in children as a solitary, soft, nontender, well-demarcated bluish-red nodule or plaque ranging 1 to 5 cm in diameter. ACA is a late-stage cutaneous borreliosis lesion caused by *B afzelii*, which is absent from North America. ACA classically affects the extensor surfaces of distal extremities in elderly females and may be preceded by EM near the site months or years prior. ACA progresses slowly over weeks to months from an inflammatory phase, in which lesions are edematous and bluish-red, to a chronic atrophic phase, characterized by skin atrophy with visible telangiectasias. Two-thirds of ACA patients have associated peripheral neuropathy. In Austria and Germany, *B burgdorferi* may also be responsible for some cases of morphea.[51]

Systemic Manifestations

Hematogenous spread of *Borrelia* spp may affect the joints, nervous system (neuroborreliosis), and heart. Lyme arthritis typically presents 3 to 6 months after infection, as afebrile oligoarthritis or monoarthritis, often involving the knee. If untreated, chronic intermittent pain and swelling may persist for years. If *Borrelia* is eradicated with antibiotics, most Lyme arthritis patients are cured but may require anti-inflammatory therapy to control proliferative synovitis for years.[42]

Neuroborreliosis occurs in about 10% of Lyme disease patients, presenting days to weeks after a tick bite as lymphocytic meningitis, cranial neuritis, or radiculoneuritis. When present, cranial neuritis usually affects the facial nerve, and is bilateral in a quarter of affected patients. Other cranial nerves may be affected, resulting in diplopia, pain, hearing loss, or vertigo. Lyme radiculitis has been reported, which mimics spinal disc herniation: neuropathic pain is present in a dermatomal distribution, sometimes with sensory defects and paresis.[42]

Cardiac involvement may occur during early disseminated infection, manifesting as atrioventricular conduction defects, acute myopericarditis, or cardiomyopathy.[42] A recent investigation showed that more than one-third of 113 studied patients with atrial fibrillation had a history of *Borrelia* infection, the authors positing that the spirochete may contribute to chronic cardiac inflammation.[52]

Pregnancy Considerations

In the acute phase of *Borrelia* infection, the disease is vertically transmissible from mother to fetus transplacentally. Studies evaluating for fetal harm when mothers are infected with Lyme borreliosis have had variable results, with some showing fewer adverse birth outcomes in mothers treated with antibiotics,[55] and others showing no difference.[56]

Diagnostic Confirmation

Clinical signs often precede antibody response by several weeks, therefore serologies may be falsely negative during early disease. In the presence of EM, a clinical diagnosis should be made, and empiric treatment given.

In the absence of EM, the variable presentation and differential diagnosis of Lyme disease may warrant serologic testing. Typically 2-tiered testing is performed, where positive ELISA-based screening tests are confirmed with another ELISA, a Western blot, or immunoblot. Background seroprevalence exists and ranges from 5% to 50%. Serum borrelia IgG may persist for decades, thus serology cannot be used to monitor disease activity or eradication.[42]

Polymerase chain reaction (PCR) has reasonable sensitivity on skin and synovial samples but low sensitivity on CSF. PCR is not accurate in other materials such as blood and urine. PCR has limited utility in monitoring treatment response, as Borrelia DNA may be detected after successful antibiotic treatment.[42]

CSF culture is similar to PCR, in having low yield for *Borrelia* spp. Diagnosis relies on indirect measures of meningeal inflammation: pleocytosis, intrathecal antibody production. Intrathecal *Borrelia* antibody is measured by calculating the CSF:serum antibody index and has been shown to persist for years after successful treatment, thus cannot be used to monitor treatment.[42]

Skin Histology

The diagnosis is usually made clinically in part because histologic features of EMs are nonspecific. Perivascular infiltrate may be present; it is highly variable but often superficial and deep lymphoid. There may be plasma cells or eosinophils; silver-stained sections may show spirochetes around vessels of the superficial dermis.[29]

Differential Diagnosis

EM may resemble tinea corporis, Southern Tick Associated Rash Illness, erythema annulare centrifugum, and fixed drug eruption. Many patients with Rocky Mountain spotted fever may also exhibit a rash and systemic symptoms similar to Lyme disease.

Management

For localized EM or early disseminated disease, the recommended first-line therapy is oral doxycycline 100 mg twice daily. Randomized trials have shown equal efficacy and sequelae prevention at 2.9 years for 10 days of this treatment compared with 15 or 21 days.[42] For children aged younger than 8 years, amoxicillin 50 mg/kg/d divided in 3 daily doses for 14 days is recommended. A 2018 network meta-analysis of 2532 patients showed no significant differences in treatment response by antibiotic agent, dose, or duration; the antibiotics investigated were doxycycline, cefuroxime axetil, ceftriaxone, amoxicillin, azithromycin, penicillin V, and minocycline.[57]

Lyme neuroborreliosis is usually treated with intravenous ceftriaxone for at least 2 weeks, resulting in slow recovery. Symptoms persist in up to half of patients after 30 months, leading some clinicians to extend ceftriaxone therapy to 4 weeks. Oral doxycycline has been shown in a European trial to be as effective as ceftriaxone, including for long-term outcomes such as neurologic sequelae, quality of life, fatigue, and cognition; for this reason, many guidelines consider doxycycline a reasonable treatment option.[42]

Lyme arthritis may be treated with 30 days of oral doxycycline or amoxicillin, which resolves about 90% of cases. Approximately 10% to 20% of patients develop antibiotic refractory arthritis, a proliferative synovitis that requires intra-articular steroid injections, oral non-steroidal anti-inflammatory drug (NSAIDs), immunosuppressants, or synovectomy.[42]

ACA requires 4 weeks of doxycycline therapy, and may take months after therapy for resolution; neuropathy and dermal atrophy are often permanent.[42]

ACKNOWLEDGMENTS

The authors are indebted to the following exceptional medical librarians, without whom this study would not be possible: Ana Macias, Melissa Spangenberg, and Morgan Brynnan.

CONFLICTS OF INTEREST

The authors declare no conflicts of interest or relevant disclosures.

FUNDING

This work was made possible in part by a mentorship grant from the Dermatology Education Foundation, awarded to PA Young and G.H. Bae. No other funding sources or disclosures.

REFERENCES

1. Hook EW 3rd. Syphilis. Lancet 2017;389(10078):1550–7.
2. Tampa M, Sarbu I, Matei C, et al. Brief history of syphilis. J Med Life 2014; 7(1):4–10.
3. Centers for Disease Control and Prevention. Sexually transmitted disease surveillance 2019. Atlanta: U.S. Department of Health and Human Services; 2021. Available at: https://www.cdc.gov/std/statistics/2019/default.htm. Accessed April 8, 2022.
4. Machefsky AM, Loosier PS, Cramer R, et al. A new call to action to combat an old nemesis: addressing rising congenital syphilis rates in the United States. J Womens Health (Larchmt) 2021;30(7):920–6.
5. Stratman-Thomas WK. The Lure of Medical History: Girolamo Fracastoro and Syphilis. Cal West Med 1930;33(4):739–42.
6. Forrai J. History of different therapeutics of venereal disease before the discovery of penicillin. In: Sato NS, editor. Syphilis - recognition, description and diagnosis. Intech; 2011. p. 37–9.
7. Sefton AM. The Great Pox that was...syphilis. J Appl Microbiol 2001;91(4):592–6.
8. De Souza EM. A hundred years ago, the discovery of Treponema pallidum. An Bras Dermatol 2005;80:547–8.
9. Centers for Disease Control and Prevention. Congenital syphilis preliminary 2020 data. US Department of Health and Human Services. Available at: https://www.cdc.gov/std/statistics/2020/Congenital-Syphilis-preliminaryData.htm. Accessed April 8, 2022.

10. van Duynhoven YT. The epidemiology of Neisseria gonorrhoeae in Europe. Microbes Infect 1999;1(6):455–64.
11. US Centers for Disease Control and Prevention. Summary of notifiable diseases: United States, 2003. MMWR Morb Mortal Wkly Rep 2005;52:1–85.
12. US Centers for Disease Control and Prevention. Outbreak of syphilis among men who have sex with men: Southern California, 2000. MMWR Morb Mortal Wkly Rep 2001;50:117–20.
13. Nicoll A, Hamers FF. Are trends in HIV, gonorrhoea, and syphilis worsening in western Europe? BMJ 2002;324(7349):1324–7.
14. Tichonova L, Borisenko K, Ward H, et al. Epidemics of syphilis in the Russian Federation: trends, origins, and priorities for control. Lancet 1997;350(9072): 210–3.
15. Peterman TA, Heffelfinger JD, Swint EB, et al. The changing epidemiology of syphilis. Sex Transm Dis 2005;32(10 Suppl):S4–10.
16. Fenton KA, Lowndes CM. Recent trends in the epidemiology of sexually transmitted infections in the European Union. Sex Transm Infect 2004;80(4):255–63.
17. Stary G, Stary A. Sexually transmitted infections. In: Bolognia J, Schaffer JV, Cerroni L, editors. Dermatology. 4th edition. Elsevier; 2017. p. 1448–58.
18. Centers for Disease Control and Prevention. Syphilis – CDC Fact Sheet Available at: https://www.cdc.gov/std/syphilis/stdfact-syphilis-detailed.htm. Accessed May 16, 2022.
19. Chen C. Syphilis is resurging in the U.S., a sign of public health's funding crisis. Morning Edition, National Public Radio. 2021. Available at: https://www.npr.org/sections/health-shots/2021/11/01/1050568646/syphilis-std-public-health-funding. Accessed May 16, 2022.
20. Sparling PF, Swartz MN, Musher DM, et al. Clinical manifestations of syphilis. In: Holmes KK, Sparling PF, Stamm WE, et al, editors. Sexually transmitted diseases. 4th ed. New York: McGraw Hill; 2008. p. 661–84.
21. Gjestland T. The Oslo study of untreated syphilis: an epidemiologic investigation of the natural course of syphilitic infection based on a restudy of the Boeck-Bruusgaard material. J Chronic Dis 1955;2:311–44.
22. Workowski KA, Bolan GA, Centers for Disease Control and Prevention. Sexually transmitted diseases treatment guidelines, 2015. MMWR Recomm Rep (Morb Mortal Wkly Rep) 2015;64(RR-03):1–137.
23. Committee on Infectious Diseases. Red book: 2021–2024 report of the committee on infectious diseases. 32nd edition. American Academy of Pediatrics; 2021. p. 729–44.
24. Jankovic J. Disorders of nerve roots and plexuses. In: Daroff R, Jankovic J, Mazziotta J, et al, editors. Bradley and daroff's neurology in clinical practice. 8th edition. Elsevier; 2022. p. 1829–52.
25. Thompson HS, Kardon RH. The argyll robertson pupil. J Neuro Ophthalmol 2006; 26(2):134–8.
26. Pearce JM. The argyll robertson pupil. J Neurol Neurosurg Psychiatr 2004;75(9): 1345.
27. Wheeler HL, Agarwal S, Goh BT. Dark ground microscopy and treponemal serological tests in the diagnosis of early syphilis. Sex Transm Infect 2004;80(5): 411–4.
28. Rogstad KE, Simms I, Fenton KA, et al. British Cooperative Clinical Group of the British Association for Sexual Health and HIV. Screening, diagnosis and management of early syphilis in genitourinary medicine clinics in the UK. Int J STD AIDS 2005;16(5):348–52.

29. Elston DR. Bacterial, spirochete, and protozoan infections. In: Elston DM, Ferringer T, editors. Dermatopathology. 3rd edition. Elsevier; 2019. p. 301–4.

30. Lautenschlager S. Cutaneous manifestations of syphilis : recognition and management. Am J Clin Dermatol 2006;7(5):291–304.

31. Hicks CB, Clement M. Syphilis: Screening and diagnostic testing. In: UpToDate. Wolters Kluwer. 2022. Available at: https://www.uptodate.com/contents/syphilis-screening-and-diagnostic-testing. Accessed May 16, 2022.

32. Mmeje O, Chow JM, Davidson L, et al. Discordant syphilis immunoassays in pregnancy: perinatal outcomes and implications for clinical management. Clin Infect Dis 2015;61(7):1049–53.

33. Liu LL, Lin LR, Tong ML, et al. Incidence and risk factors for the prozone phenomenon in serologic testing for syphilis in a large cohort. Clin Infect Dis 2014;59(3): 384–9.

34. Park IU, Chow JM, Bolan G, et al. Screening for syphilis with the treponemal immunoassay: analysis of discordant serology results and implications for clinical management. J Infect Dis 2011;204(9):1297–304.

35. Paller AS, Mancini AJ. Congenital infections of the newborn. In: Paller AS, Mancini AJ, editors. Hurwitz clinical pediatric dermatology. 5th edition. Elsevier; 2016. p. 33–5.

36. Centers for Disease Control and Prevention. Sexually transmitted infections treatment guidelines, 2021. US Department of Health and Human Services. Available at: https://www.cdc.gov/std/treatment-guidelines/toc.htm. Accessed April 11, 2022.

37. Rolfs RT, Joesoef MR, Hendershot EF, et al. The Syphilis and HIV Study Group. A randomized trial of enhanced therapy for early syphilis in patients with and without human immunodeficiency virus infection. N Engl J Med 1997;337:307–14.

38. Yang CJ, Lee NY, Chen TC, et al. One dose versus three weekly doses of benzathine penicillin G for patients co-infected with HIV and early syphilis: a multicenter, prospective observational study. PLoS One 2014;9:e109667.

39. Ganesan A, Mesner O, Okulicz JF, et al. Infectious Disease Clinical Research Program HIV/STI Working Group. A single dose of benzathine penicillin G is as effective as multiple doses of benzathine penicillin G for the treatment of HIV-infected persons with early syphilis. Clin Infect Dis 2015;60:653–60.

40. Seña AC, Wolff M, Martin DH, et al. Predictors of serological cure and serofast state after treatment in HIV-negative persons with early syphilis. Clin Infect Dis 2011;53:1092–9.

41. Ghanem KG, Erbelding EJ, Wiener ZS, et al. Serological response to syphilis treatment in HIV-positive and HIV-negative patients attending sexually transmitted diseases clinics. Sex Transm Infect 2007;83:97–101.

42. Kullberg BJ, Vrijmoeth HD, van de Schoor F, et al. Lyme borreliosis: diagnosis and management. BMJ 2020;369:m1041.

43. Centers for Disease Control and Prevention. Lyme Disease Data and Surveillance. US Department of Health and Human Services. Available at: https://www.cdc.gov/lyme/index.html. Accessed April 12, 2022.

44. Walter KS, Carpi G, Caccone A, et al. Genomic insights into the ancient spread of Lyme disease across North America. Nat Ecol Evol 2017;1(10):1569–76.

45. Dammin GJ. Erythema migrans: a chronicle. Rev Infect Dis 1989;11(1):142–51.

46. Burgdorfer W, Barbour AG, Hayes SF, et al. Lyme disease-a tick-borne spirochetosis? Science 1982;216(4552):1317–9.

47. Bhate C, Schwartz RA. Lyme disease: Part I. Advances and perspectives. J Am Acad Dermatol 2011;64(4):619–36 [quiz: 637–8].

48. Sprong H, Azagi T, Hoornstra D, et al. Control of Lyme borreliosis and other Ixodes ricinus-borne diseases. Parasit Vectors 2018;11(1):145.

49. Lindgren E, Tälleklint L, Polfeldt T. Impact of climatic change on the northern latitude limit and population density of the disease-transmitting European tick Ixodes ricinus. Environ Health Perspect 2000;108(2):119–23.

50. Kuehn BM. CDC estimates 300,000 US cases of Lyme disease annually. JAMA 2013;310(11):1110.

51. Heymann WR, Ellis DL. Borrelia burgdorferi Infections in the United States. J Clin Aesthet Dermatol 2012;5(8):18–28.

52. Szymanska A, Platek AE, Dluzniewski M, et al. History of lyme disease as a predictor of atrial fibrillation. Am J Cardiol 2020;125(11):1651–4.

53. Stanek G, Reiter M. The expanding Lyme Borrelia complex–clinical significance of genomic species? Clin Microbiol Infect 2011;17(4):487–93.

54. Spielman A, Wilson ML, Levine JF, et al. Ecology of Ixodes dammini-borne human babesiosis and Lyme disease. Annu Rev Entomol 1985;30:439–60.

55. Waddell LA, Greig J, Lindsay LR, et al. A systematic review on the impact of gestational Lyme disease in humans on the fetus and newborn. PLoS One 2018;13(11):e0207067.

56. Lakos A, Solymosi N. Maternal Lyme borreliosis and pregnancy outcome. Int J Infect Dis 2010;14(6):e494–8.

57. Torbahn G, Hofmann H, Rücker G, et al. Efficacy and safety of antibiotic therapy in early cutaneous lyme borreliosis: a network meta-analysis. JAMA Dermatol 2018;154(11):1292–303.

Mpox (Formally Known as Monkeypox)

Molly O'Neill, PA-C[a], Tricia LePage, PA-C[a], Vanessa Bester, EdD, PA-C[b,*],
Henry Yoon, MD[a], Frederick Browne, MD[a,c], Eric C. Nemec, PharmD, MEd, BCPS[a]

KEYWORDS

- Mpox (Monkeypox) • Smallpox • *Orthopoxvirus* • Transmission
- Clinical presentation • Prevention • Treatment • Outbreak

KEY POINTS

- In late 2022, the WHO and CDC moved to change the name of Monkeypox to Mpox, to reduce racial stigma associated with the original name.
- Human Mpox, a zoonosis, originates from the Mpox virus, a double-stranded DNA virus, which belongs to the *Orthopoxvirus* genus of the Poxviridae family.
- The modes of transmission are currently limited to animal-to-human transmission and human-to-human transmission. It remains under investigation whether the virus can be transmitted through a sexual route via seminal or vaginal fluids; therefore, Mpox is not defined as a sexually transmitted infection.
- The clinical features of Mpox consists of a prodromal stage, consisting of fevers, headaches, myalgias, and lethargy; followed by a rash that evolves from macules, to papules, to vesicles, to pustules, to scabs, to depigmented scars; and with a distinguishing feature of severe lymphadenopathy.
- Since September 2022, there have been confirmed cases in 96 nonendemic countries with approximately 21,504 cases in the United States.

INTRODUCTION: THE EPIDEMIOLOGY OF MPOX

Mpox originates from the Mpox virus, which belongs to the *Orthopoxvirus* genus of the Poxviridae family.[1–3] Other *Orthopoxvirus* species include the variola virus (the now eradicated smallpox virus), vaccinia virus (a virus used in the creation of the smallpox vaccine), and cowpox virus.[1–3] The identified clades consist of the West African clade and the Congo Basin clade, each with varying fatality rates of 1% and 10%, respectively.[1–4] Since the eradication of smallpox in 1980, the Mpox virus has emerged as the most relevant *Orthopoxvirus* infection in humans.

---

[a] Sacred Heart University PA Program, College of Health Professions, Sacred Heart University, 5151 Park Avenue, Fairfield, CT 06825, USA; [b] Augsburg University PA Program, 2211 Riverside Avenue, CB149, Minneapolis, MN 55454, USA; [c] Griffin Hospital, 130 Division Street, Derby, CT 06418, USA
* Corresponding author.
E-mail address: besterva@augsburg.edu

Physician Assist Clin 8 (2023) 483–494
https://doi.org/10.1016/j.cpha.2023.02.008
2405-7991/23/© 2023 Elsevier Inc. All rights reserved.

physicianassistant.theclinics.com

The double-stranded DNA virus was first discovered in 1958 at a research facility in Denmark when a group of laboratory monkeys from Africa developed vesicular lesions, consequently terming the virus as "Mpox."[1,2] The name remains a misnomer because rodents, including squirrels and rats, account for the largest known reservoir for the disease, whereas monkeys are considered hosts for the disease, similar to humans.[1] The virus did not demonstrate animal-to-human zoonotic transmission until 1970, when a 9-month-old boy also developed vesicular lesions in Bukenda, now a province of the Democratic Republic of Congo.[1–4]

Since its discovery, the virus mainly had been contained within Central and West Africa with a limited number of cases elsewhere that were linked to either international travel through Africa or African animal imports.[2] The vaccinia virus provided cross-immunity to the recipients for Mpox. However, the cessation of vaccination efforts following the eradication of smallpox and zoonotic spillover contributed to the virus's continual re-emergence.[3,4] The once neglected zoonotic disease has recently garnered attention after outbreaks have been reported in 73 nonendemic countries, including the United States.[5]

TRANSMISSION

The modes of transmission are currently limited to animal-to-human transmission and human-to-human transmission. Transmission from animal-to-human occurs through contact with an infected animal's skin lesions, bodily fluids, or respiratory droplets. The virus then enters the human body through a break in the skin barrier, the respiratory tract, or mucous membranes.[1,2] The virus then rapidly replicates at the inoculation site and disperses to nearby lymph nodes. Once infected, human-to-human transmission may subsequently follow. Direct transmission may occur through contact with skin lesions, bodily fluids, and respiratory droplets, whereas indirect transmission may occur through contact with infected materials, such as clothing or linens, because the virus survives outside the body for long periods of time.[2,4] There have also been cases of mother-to-child transmission through the placenta, known as congenital Mpox, contact during delivery, and close contact following the birth.[2]

It remains under investigation whether the virus is transmitted through a sexual route via seminal or vaginal fluids. Data do not definitively support this mode of transmission at this time.[2,4] Consequently, Mpox is not classified as a sexually transmitted infection. Lesions found on the perigenital, perianal, and perioral regions are a common occurrence in Mpox and skin-to-skin contact during sexual encounters can assist in transmission of the virus; however, it is important to emphasize that transmission can occur with nonsex-related lesions.[4]

CLINICAL PRESENTATION

The disease characteristics of Mpox reflects that of the infamous smallpox in terms of symptom onset and dermatologic findings. Similarly to smallpox, the incubation period may last 7 to 21 days with a prodromal stage of pyrexia, cephalgias, myalgias, and lethargy.[1,2] The distinguishing feature from smallpox seems to be the associated lymphadenopathy. Lymphadenopathy affects more than 90% of patients with Mpox and presents either unilaterally or bilaterally, primarily affecting the postauricular, submandibular, cervical, axillary, and inguinal lymph nodes.[1,4] The smallpox-like rash appears 1 to 2 days following the onset of lymphadenopathy. The rash traditionally begins with an enanthem, a lesion that develops on the tongue or mouth.[5] Within 24 hours, a macular rash presents on the face and disseminates caudally to the rest of the body in a centrifugal distribution.[1,5] By the third day, the rash evolves into maculopapular lesions, approximately 2 to 5 mm in diameter.[4,5] By the fourth and fifth day, the maculopapular lesions become vesicular.[4,5] The vesicles then turn into pustules over the course of 2 days and remain for approximately 5 to 7 days.[4,5] By the end of the second week, the pustules desquamate and scab. The scabs typically remain for 1 week before they resolve, leaving behind a depigmented scar.[4,5] The infectious period of Mpox remains until all of the scabs have fallen off.[5] However, the total duration of signs and symptoms may last 2 to 5 weeks in its entirety.[1]

Mpox presents more mildly with better-predicted outcomes compared with smallpox; however, the virus is not negligible. The fatality rate of Mpox ranges from 1% to 10% depending on the specific clade, primarily affecting children, young adults, and the immunocompromised.[1,2,4] In endemic countries, traditional risk factors for contracting the disease consist of being of the male sex, living in forested regions, being younger than 15 years of age, and never being inoculated with a smallpox vaccination.[1] In addition to fatality, numerous complications have been reported with Mpox, including secondary bacterial infections, sepsis, respiratory distress, bronchopneumonia, encephalitis, corneal infections with subsequent blindness, gastrointestinal involvement with emesis and diarrhea, and spontaneous abortions during pregnancy.[1,3,4]

DIAGNOSIS

There are several factors to take into consideration when making the diagnosis. A few of the most important include the patient's risk factors, history, clinical manifestations, and possible exposures. By taking a thorough history and physical examination it can help focus on whether the patient is at high risk for having Mpox and can also help rule in or out other viral rashes. It is also important to consider the patient's vaccination history. This is helpful information in determining which laboratory test to perform and also determining their overall risk for developing the illness.[6]

Similar to other viral infections, there are several laboratory methods to diagnose the condition (**Table 1**). The most accurate diagnosis is performed from obtaining a culture of lesion material because the lesion material itself has the highest viral quantity. Fluid from a lesion or vesicle if available for collection is an efficient sample for testing, although dried crusts, the roof of a lesion, or blood are also acceptable options.[7] Once the lesion material is obtained, the most current guidelines recommend placing it in a dry, sterile tube as opposed to a viral transport media, and keeping the specimen cold.[7] Because of high accuracy and sensitivity, polymerase chain reaction is the preferable method of diagnosis. Several department guidelines require results to be reported to local and national health departments; as stated by the Centers for Disease Control and Prevention (CDC), positive results need to be reported within 24 hours.[5] It is extremely important that personnel handling specimens due so with caution to avoid accidental exposure.[8]

MANAGEMENT/TREATMENTS

There are currently two vaccines approved for preexposure prophylaxis: ACAM2000 and JYNNEOS. These vaccines were initially created to combat smallpox but have been found to reduce the rate of contracting Mpox by 85%.[4] ACAM2000 is a live replication-competent *Vaccinia virus*, which means that the vaccine contains virus particles capable of infecting cells and replicating. It was derived from the same strain used to manufacture the Dryvac vaccine, the vaccine previously used to eradicate smallpox.[9] The vaccine requires one percutaneous dose and is administered with a bifurcated needle through multiple punctures. The replication-competent component of the vaccine is associated with increased adverse events, including progressive

Table 1		
Summary of diagnostic methods[6]		
Test	**Advantages**	**Disadvantages**
Viral culture (obtained from patient specimen)	• Most reliable method • Can provide definitive classification	• Slow turnaround time • Risk of contaminated specimen • Further viral characterization required
Electron microscopy (produces a "brick-shaped particle")	• Can identify viral particles in specimens obtained via biopsy, viral culture, fluid from vesicles • Ability to differentiate between Orthopoxvirus and herpes virus	• Inability to differentiate between orthopoxviruses
Immunohistochemistry	Identifies antigens in biopsy specimens to rule out other agents	• Unable to identify Mpox specifically
Polymerase chain reaction	If the specimen is handled properly, it can diagnose Mpox virus specifically from taking material from a lesion on a patient with an active infection	• Risk of contamination
Anti-Orthopoxvirus IgG	Can identify previous Orthopoxvirus infection or smallpox vaccination	• Not specific to Mpox virus • False-positive if previously vaccinated against smallpox
Anti-Orthopoxvirus IgM	• Can identify recent Orthopoxvirus exposure • Useful diagnostic tool for patients with a prior smallpox vaccination	• Not specific to Mpox virus
Tetracore Orthopox Biothreat Alert	Can identify an active case when obtained from lesion specimen	• Not specific to Mpox • Less sensitive than polymerase chain reaction

vaccinia, eczema vaccinatum, and myocarditis.[9] These detrimental adverse events lead to death among 1 of every 1 million persons vaccinated.[4] Therefore, contraindications for this vaccine include patients with a severe allergy to a vaccine component, a history of eczema or similar variant, cardiac disease, immunocompromising conditions, pregnancy, or breastfeeding.[9] However, JYNNEOS is a live replication-deficient vaccine that does not replicate in cells. The vaccine requires two subcutaneous doses administered 28 days apart from each other.[4,9] Unlike ACAM2000, JYNNEOS has a limited number of adverse effects, and it is only contraindicated in patients with a severe allergy to a vaccine component. It can safely be used in patients with eczema and those who are immunocompromised.[9]

The Advisory Committee on Immunization Practices (ACIP) initially recommended inoculation with ACAM2000 as preexposure prophylaxis in 2015, when that vaccine was the only vaccine on the market. However, ACIP changed its stance in 2021 when evidence suggested that JYNNEOS provided a slight increase in disease prevention compared with ACAM2000. The ACIP now recommends JYNNEOS for primary vaccination and booster doses and 461,049 doses have been reported to be administered in the United States as of September 6, 2022.[9,10]

The current recommendations state that preexposure vaccination should be administered to certain laboratorians studying orthopoxviruses, health care personnel at risk for occupational exposure, veterinarians, animal controllers, designated *Orthopoxvirus* response teams, certain US military personnel, and those who care for patients infected with orthopoxviruses.[4,9] At this time, there are currently insufficient data on the effectiveness of the vaccines on the current Mpox outbreak. However, the Strategic National Stockpile currently possesses both vaccines. It has been distributing the vaccines to various jurisdictions throughout the United States to combat Mpox and protect those currently at risk.

In addition to preexposure prophylaxis, the vaccines can also be administered for postexposure prophylaxis to stop the Mpox virus from causing illness. The CDC recommends administering the vaccine within 4 days of exposure to prevent the disease. If given between 4 and 14 days from exposure, the vaccine may reduce the symptoms of the disease, but it may not prevent it entirely.[4,10] The current outbreak has led public health officials to extend the reach of postexposure prophylaxis to slow the disease's widespread progression with an approach called "PEP++." PEP++ intends to protect individuals with certain risk factors through vaccination, whether or not they have had a documented exposure to Mpox.[10] Coupled with self-isolation, postexposure prophylaxis would assist in providing optimal outcomes and preventing the spread of the disease.

Supportive care currently remains the treatment of choice for Mpox to manage symptoms, treat secondary bacterial infections and other complications, and prevent the virus's spread.[1] In addition to supportive care, tecovirimat and brincidofovir may be recommended for patients with severe cases of Mpox.[4] These antivirals were designed to protect against smallpox; however, the genetic similarities of the smallpox virus and Mpox virus allow protection against both diseases.

The Food and Drug Administration (FDA) approved tecovirimat for the treatment of smallpox in June 2018 for adults and children weighing more than 13 kg.[11] The FDA Animal Rule authorized the use of the drug based on the efficacy observed in animal trials.[11–13] The effectiveness in humans has not yet been determined because trials have not been feasible, and inducing smallpox in humans to study the drug would be considered unethical. However, clinical trials of the drug on people without *Orthopoxvirus* proved safe with minimal side effects.[12,14] As a result, the CDC granted expanded access protocol to allow the administration of tecovirimat to treat Mpox.[13] Tecovirimat inhibits the *Orthopoxvirus* VP37 protein, consequently impeding the production of egress-competent enveloped virions necessary for the virus's circulation within the host.[11,14] The purpose of the drug is to ultimately reduce viremia, leading to quicker recovery, specifically for patients with weakened immune systems.

The FDA additionally approved brincidofovir for the treatment of smallpox in adults and children, including neonates, in June 2021.[12,13] Brincidofovir works by converting to cidofovir intracellularly, which then phosphorylates to cidofovir diphosphate. Cidofovir diphosphate inhibits *Orthopoxvirus* DNA polymerase, reducing the rate of viral DNA synthesis.[15] Similarly to tecovirimat, the FDA approved the drug under the Animal Rule because it proved to be efficacious in treating orthopoxviruses in animals and because studies in human trials were neither feasible nor ethical.[12,16] During a 24-week trial, brincidofovir demonstrated an increased incidence of mortality compared with the placebo when it was evaluated using a different disease, cytomegalovirus.[13,15,16] Consequently, brincidofovir comes with a black box warning, and it is solely approved for the treatment of smallpox.[15] There are currently no data on the effectiveness of brincidofovir in the treatment of Mpox; however, it has proven to be efficacious against orthopoxviruses in in vitro and animal studies.[13] Consequently, the CDC is working on granting expanded access for the use of brincidofovir in the treatment of Mpox.[13]

PREVENTION

Prevention strategies for the general public are similar to other common illnesses and infectious diseases. People should avoid close contact with anybody that has a rash resembling Mpox. They should also avoid close contact with possible fomites of those who have Mpox; this includes bedding, blankets, towels, and clothing. Frequent hand-washing using warm water and soap or an alcohol-based hand sanitizer also assists in preventing the spread of the virus.[17] In such places as Central and West Africa, it is recommended to avoid contact with certain animals, such as rodents and primates, to avoid the risk of animal-to-human transmission.[18]

Guidelines regarding infection prevention within the health care setting are frequently changing and often vary depending on local and hospital-based protocols. Many general recommendations can be applied and are discussed here. When a patient presents with suspected Mpox, infection prevention should be notified as soon as possible.[18] Patients with confirmed and/or suspected Mpox should be placed in a single room with a private bathroom. Confirmed cases are placed together if a single room is unavailable. When transported outside of the room, patients should wear a well-fitted surgical mask with all lesions covered with a blanket or clothing to avoid spreading. Because of the risk of resuspension and spread of dried lesion materials, such tasks as vacuuming, sweeping, dusting, and portable fan use must be avoided in rooms where a patient with suspected Mpox was present. All intubation and extubation procedures should take place in an isolation room designated for airborne infection.[17]

Regarding appropriate personal protective equipment, health care personnel and caregivers providing care to suspected or confirmed Mpox patients should be wearing a gown, gloves, goggles or face shield, and an N95 mask or similarly approved respirator.[17] All US Department of Transportation Hazardous Materials Regulations should be followed regarding disposal of patient materials, soiled personal protective equipment, dressing, storage, and handling. Current guidelines vary depending on the virus strain. Materials of the West African clade should be disposed of and managed as UN3291 Regulated Medical Waste and handled as potentially infectious medical waste. The Congo Basin clade should be handled as Hazardous Material Regulations Category A.[18] As of current guidelines in the 2022 outbreak, patients must be assessed by a clinical provider and a public health figure to determine if the patient has any epidemiologic risk factors for the Congo Basin clade. If it is determined that the patient does not, then the waste should be managed as regulated medical waste. Cleaning and disinfection should be performed using the facilities' standard disinfection procedures.[18]

For nonhospitalized patients, isolation is the recommended procedure for those with suspected or confirmed Mpox. The precautions' duration varies and depends on state and local health department guidelines. In general, precautions and isolation should be in place until all lesions have crusted over, separated, and new skin has formed. Droplet and contact precautions are recommended. If varicella zoster virus is also suspected, then airborne precautions should be initiated until varicella is ruled out.[18]Additionally, for sexually active populations, patients with Mpox must avoid any sexual encounters until all skin lesions have crusted, fallen off, and new skin has formed. It is recommended that on resolution of symptoms, condoms should be used for all sexual activity for 12 weeks. Patients should also be evaluated for coinfection with sexually transmitted infections. Suspected Mpox patients who also have HIV should be closely monitored because of the risk of more severe infection.[17]

In addition to the prevention strategies previously discussed for the general public and health care workers collaborating with individuals who have suspected or confirmed Mpox, primary prevention and proper education are also extremely important. With skin-to-skin contact being the driving form of transmission, people should be advised to avoid and, at the least, practice caution in crowded areas of close contact with others. People should also be advised to practice frequent hand washing and avoid sharing blankets, pillows, clothing, and towels with others.[5] High-risk populations, such as men who have sex with men (MSM), people with multiple sexual partners, and individuals that attend large close contact gatherings, such as concerts, raves, and festivals, should exercise an even higher level of caution. Individuals partaking in these activities should increase their handwashing, wear long pants and sleeves to avoid exposed skin, avoid kissing, and avoid sharing beverages or other items.[19] Further information on secondary and tertiary prevention is discussed regarding vaccines in the treatment section.

CURRENT OUTBREAK

Over the years, the United States has not been immune to the Mpox virus. In 2003, several Midwesterners contracted Mpox after exposure to infected pet prairie dogs. The virus then spread expeditiously with cases identified in six states, including Illinois, Indiana, Kansas, Missouri, Ohio, and Wisconsin.[1] An investigation discovered that the virus was imported to the United States from Ghana through a shipment containing infected African rodents. During the shipment, the infected rodents were residing near the prairie dogs, later sold as pets.[1] In 2021, the Mpox virus revealed itself twice in the United States. It re-emerged in two individuals who returned from trips to Nigeria, one who returned to Texas in July 2021 and the other who returned to Washington, DC, in November 2021.[2] Unfortunately, that was not the last that the United States would see of Mpox.

In May 2022, an individual returning from Nigeria exhibiting signs and symptoms of Mpox was the first confirmed case in the United Kingdom. Soon after, five different continents confirmed cases unrelated to the case in the United Kingdom. It soon became apparent that there had been multiple introductions from Africa.[4] Since August 2022, there have been confirmed cases in 73 nonendemic countries, with approximately 5811 cases in the United States.[5] Its widespread presence has now made itself known as the largest Mpox outbreak outside of endemic Africa. As a result, the World Health Organization (WHO) Director-General declared that the Mpox outbreak constitutes a Public Health Emergency of International Concern on July 23, 2022.[20]

The current outbreak demonstrates a high prevalence of Mpox in men, particularly MSM. For instance, 336 laboratory cases of Mpox in the United Kingdom were confirmed by June 8, 2022, and 311 of the confirmed cases were determined to be male, with three confirmed cases determined to be female (gender information was not available for the remaining 25 cases).[21] Researchers at the UK Health Security Agency conducted questionnaires, received responses from 152 confirmed cases, and published a technical briefing on June 10, 2022. The briefing revealed that out of the 152 responses, 151 patients stated that they belonged to the MSM community and the remaining patients chose not to answer the question.[21] The UK Health Security Agency retrospectively reinterviewed in an attempt to understand transmission patterns better. Of the 42 participants, 44% reported more than 10 sexual partners in the previous 3 months, and 44% reported group sex during incubation.[21] Although this briefing includes only a small subset of those infected, Mpox seems to be spreading through the sexual and social networks of the MSM community. The virus found this particular niche during Pride month, when the LGBTQ+ community gathers for large events in celebration, possibly allowing the virus to take advantage of this specific group opportunistically. However, the risk of contracting Mpox is not limited to MSM because viruses do not infect people based on sexuality. The virus can infect men, women, transgender, nonbinary people, and others alike.[22] Therefore, it is of the utmost importance not to stigmatize a community based on sexual practices and repeat past mistakes when addressing certain diseases.

LESSONS LEARNED FROM PREVIOUS DISEASE-ASSOCIATED STIGMATIZATION

The WHO defines health-related stigma as a negative association between a group of people and a specific disease.[23,24] Stigma has unfortunately been a common theme related to disease outbreaks throughout history, causing people to place blame on a foreign "other."[25,26] It has precipitated animosity, crime, health disparities, financial inequities, and social inequalities for centuries.[27] Stigmatization can even be traced back to one of the oldest infectious diseases known to human history: leprosy (otherwise known as Hansen disease). During ancient times, people believed Hansen disease was a repercussion for sinful ways. Afflicted persons were consequently treated inhumanely, isolated from society, and exiled to quarantine colonies to avoid contagion.[28] The powerful stigma associated with Hansen disease forced infected persons to wear noisy bells and cautionary garments to alert the public of their presence in society.[28] The disease also caused infected persons to lose their families and jobs and destroyed their property and homes.[28] Hansen disease provides an archaic example of how misconceptions and fear have fueled stigmatizing acts against groups of people, leading to detrimental consequences that affect employment opportunities, housing, and access to medical care.[27] Although Hansen disease may have been one of the first stigmatized diseases, it certainly has not been the last. As a result, it is essential to reflect on past disease-associated stigmas to derive their origin and decimate their formation.

The COVID-19 pandemic currently exemplifies the blatant stigmatization and discriminatory behaviors brought on by a present-day viral outbreak. During the height of COVID-19, the Asian community, people of low socioeconomic status, and health care workers were commonly stereotyped as disease carriers, leading to avoidance and social ostracization.[29] Stigmatization was particularly evident toward the Asian community because they were forced to endure acts of violence and intolerance because of the coronavirus being titled the "Chinese" or "Wuhan" virus.[25] In March 2020, a national survey of 1141 US residents revealed that 40% of Americans participated in at least one discriminatory behavior toward an Asian person.[30] In June 2020, the Pew Research Center conducted surveys involving 9654 US residents that revealed that 31% of Asians had been subjected to slurs because of their ethnicity, 26% of Asian Americans confirmed that they were fearful of someone threatening or physically attacking them, and 40% of US residents agreed that it had become more commonplace for people to express racist views toward Asians.[30]

Unfortunately, the spread of COVID-19 does not mark the first time the Asian community has been unfairly targeted and vilified. Throughout history, people of Asian ethnicity have been stereotyped as the "perpetual foreigner" and caricatured as the "yellow peril," which portrays people of Asian descent as a threat to European-

American norms with the inability to conform to society.[31] These xenophobic stereotypes have historically contributed to discriminatory immigration policies geared toward Asian Americans and the establishment of internment camps during World War II.[31] These longstanding anti-Asian sentiments were only exacerbated by the fear and uncertainty brought on by the novel coronavirus, the possible origin of the COVID-19 virus, the misleading media coverage, and the derogatory language used by public leaders.[30] The measures used to contain the virus, such as social distancing, lockdowns, travel restrictions, and misinformation, contributed to xenophobia and prejudice.

Social distancing and quarantines were enforced as part of the contagion mitigation strategies; however, these practices also reduced interactions with the stigmatized persons and instilled the idea of "others" being the disease carriers.[26] In addition, the travel restrictions implemented to prevent the spread of COVID-19 helped facilitate the idea that the virus was a foreign invader, reinforcing the fear of the "other."[26] The psychological impact of being a disease carrier significantly impacts public health. For instance, evidence indicates that the rate of suicidal ideation and attempts were heightened because of stigma during the COVID-19 pandemic.[23] Along with increased suicidality, stigma also led to the concealment of illness and avoiding medical treatment. The implications associated with COVID-19 caused people to hide their symptoms and relevant medical history to prevent stigmatization. This avoidant behavior resulted in delayed health care, poor outcomes, and fatalities.[23] Stigmatization only assists the spread of the pandemic and does nothing to thwart it, ultimately affecting people socially, mentally, and physically.

Similar to the Asian community, the Mpox outbreak is not the first time the MSM community has been stigmatized. In the 1980s, the HIV/AIDS epidemic swept the nation, primarily affecting the MSM community. At the time, HIV/AIDS represented a perplexing and misunderstood disease, leading to the stigmatization that resulted in violence, avoidance, and discrimination. Despite progress in managing and treating HIV/AIDS, stigma continues to act as a barrier to accessing prevention, care, and treatment services.[32–34] Within 40 years since the beginning of the epidemic, more than 700,000 people have died of AIDS. Thirty-four quantitative and qualitative studies analyzing MSM living with HIV showed that HIV stigma corresponded with increased HIV-transmission risk behaviors and poorer self-reported health.[32] As a result, stigma instigates the transmission of the virus and consequently forges adverse health outcomes.

With the current Mpox outbreak, it is time to encourage infected individuals to safely quarantine, encourage preexposure and postexposure vaccinations as needed, and implement contract tracing programs to contain the virus and prevent its spread. With the current outbreak predominantly affecting the MSM community, strategies need to be implemented immediately to prevent the spread of misinformation. This requires social mobilization and community engagement.[13] Community leaders and health care providers can accomplish this by using inclusive language when discussing the virus not to stigmatize the MSM community and not create a false sense of immunity in members outside the MSM community.[35] They should become well-versed in the epidemiology, clinical presentation, and treatment of the virus to ensure the health of all and not promote discriminatory practices. Images shared of the rash by community leaders and health care providers should illustrate the appearance of the current outbreak and avoid images depicting extreme cases to negate fear and avoid homophobic or racist stereotypes.[35] They should also work to get information out to their citizens and patients regarding how to seek help and where they can access preexposure and postexposure vaccinations. In previous pandemics, the media reported misinformation, spread fear, promoted xenophobia, created stigma, and pointed fingers. It is vital to hold the media accountable to disentangle the stigma from particular groups. This is achieved by circulating authentic information and conducting fact-checks on false information.[24] Along with the media, the public should also be educated on the consequences of consuming and sharing illegitimate information.[24] Although sometimes contributing to misinformation, social media is a powerful tool to destigmatize the virus and provide helpful resources. It is a platform that allows people to express their personal experiences with Mpox, making the virus more relatable and eradicating unnecessary fear.[35] Social media also works as an avenue to reach a broader audience and inform the public of vaccination sites and other preventative measures. As seen in previous viral outbreaks, stigmatization can worsen the spread of a virus. As a result, people need to be conscious of inequities and preexisting stereotypes to combat them.[24] Most importantly, the public needs to learn from previous mistakes to prevent the past from repeating itself.

SUMMARY

As of September 2022, the current Mpox outbreak has established itself as a public health emergency by the WHO. Currently affecting 96 nonendemic countries, now is the time to act to stop the spread of the virus. However, as the world moves to prevent the spread of Mpox, it is imperative to fight stigma. When reflecting on past pandemics, the creation of stigma by the public almost seems to be a visceral reaction. The world now belongs to the twenty-first century, making it time to practice critical thinking, empathy, and self-awareness. In this way, the world has the potential to eradicate Mpox and improve health care for all. Although new to nonendemic countries, Mpox is not a new virus. Existing for nearly half a century, Mpox has an advantage compared with previous viral outbreaks in the way that it is already equipped with vaccines and treatments. It is hoped that this can help mitigate the fear and panic associated with viral outbreaks and allow the world to come together to stop the spread of the virus.

CLINICS CARE POINTS

- When evaluating a patient with a vesicular viral exanthem preceded by generalized lymphadenopathy, a thorough travel history, sick contact, and/or known exposure to Mpox is necessary.

- In suspected cases of Mpox, initiate immediate droplet and contact precautions; cover exposed, open lesions; and mask the patient to prevent additional spread.

- Confirmed exposure to Mpox requires a 21-day monitoring period (overseen by public health authorities) for symptom development.

DISCLOSURE

The authors declare no competing interests.

REFERENCES

1. Petersen E, Kantele A, Koopmans M, et al. Human Mpox: epidemiologic and clinical characteristics, diagnosis, and prevention. Infect Dis Clin North Am 2019; 33(4):1027–43.

2. Kumar N, Acharya A, Gendelman HE, et al. The 2022 outbreak and the pathobiology of the Mpox virus. J Autoimmun 2022;102855.
3. Sklenovská N, Van Ranst M. Emergence of Mpox as the most important orthopoxvirus infection in humans. Front Public Health 2018;6:241.
4. Quarleri J, Delpino MV, Galvan V. Mpox: considerations for the understanding and containment of the current outbreak in non-endemic countries. GeroScience 2022. https://doi.org/10.1007/s11357-022-00611-6.
5. CDC. Mpox in the U.S. Centers for Disease Control and Prevention. 2022. Available at: https://www.cdc.gov/poxvirus/Mpox/lab-personnel/report-results.html. Accessed July 25, 2022.
6. McCollum AM, Damon IK. Human Mpox. Clin Infect Dis 2014;58(2):260–7.
7. Mpox. Available at: https://www.who.int/news-room/fact-sheets/detail/Mpox. Accessed July 25, 2022.
8. Laboratory testing for the Mpox virus: Interim guidance. Available at: https://www.who.int/publications-detail-redirect/WHO-MPX-laboratory-2022.1. Accessed July 25, 2022.
9. Rao AK, Petersen BW, Whitehill F, et al. Use of JYNNEOS (Smallpox and Mpox Vaccine, Live, Nonreplicating) for preexposure vaccination of persons at risk for occupational exposure to orthopoxviruses: recommendations of the Advisory Committee on Immunization Practices — United States. MMWR Morb Mortal Wkly Rep 2022;71(22):734–42.
10. Considerations for Mpox Vaccination | Mpox | Poxvirus | CDC. 2022. Available at: https://www.cdc.gov/poxvirus/Mpox/considerations-for-Mpox-vaccination.html. Accessed July 13, 2022.
11. Hoy SM. Tecovirimat: first global approval. Drugs 2018;78(13):1377–82.
12. Treatment | Smallpox | CDC, 2021. Available at: https://www.cdc.gov/smallpox/clinicians/treatment.html. Accessed July 13, 2022.
13. Treatment Information for Healthcare Professionals | Mpox | Poxvirus | CDC. 2022. Available at: https://www.cdc.gov/poxvirus/Mpox/clinicians/treatment.html. Accessed July 25, 2022.
14. TPOXX (tecovirimat) Label. Available at: https://www.accessdata.fda.gov/drugsatfda_docs/nda/2018/208627Orig1s000TOC.cfm. Accessed July 18, 2022.
15. TEMBEXA (brincidofovir) Label. Available at: https://www.accessdata.fda.gov/drugsatfda_docs/label/2021/214460s000. Accessed July 18, 2022.
16. Research C for DE and. FDA approves drug to treat smallpox. FDA 2021. Available at: https://www.fda.gov/drugs/news-events-human-drugs/fda-approves-drug-treat-smallpox. Accessed July 18, 2022.
17. Clinical management and infection prevention and control for Mpox: Interim rapid response guidance, 10 June 2022. Available at: https://www.who.int/publications-detail-redirect/WHO-MPX-Clinical-and-IPC-2022.1. Accessed July 14, 2022.
18. Infection Control: Healthcare Settings | Mpox | Poxvirus | CDC. Published 2022. https://www.cdc.gov/poxvirus/Mpox/clinicians/infection-control-healthcare.html. Accessed July 14, 2022.
19. Social Gatherings, Safer Sex, and Mpox | Mpox | Poxvirus | CDC. 2022. Available at: https://www.cdc.gov/poxvirus/Mpox/specific-settings/social-gatherings.html. Accessed July 26, 2022.
20. Second meeting of the International Health Regulations (2005) (IHR) Emergency Committee regarding the multi-country outbreak of Mpox. Available at: https://www.who.int/news/item/23-07-2022-second-meeting-of-the-international-health-regulations-(2005)-(ihr)-emergency-committee-regarding-the-multi-country-outbreak-of-Mpox. Accessed July 26, 2022.

21. Investigation into Mpox outbreak in England: technical briefing 1. GOV.UK. Available at: https://www.gov.uk/government/publications/Mpox-outbreak-technical-briefings/investigation-into-Mpox-outbreak-in-england-technical-briefing-1. Accessed July 14, 2022.

22. Cahill, S. Mpox and Gay and Bisexual Men: Fact Sheet. 2022. Available at: https://fenwayhealth.org/wp-content/uploads/TFIR-337_Mpox-Fact-Sheet2.pdf. Accessed July 18, 2022.

23. Peprah P, Gyasi RM. Stigma and COVID-19 crisis: a wake-up call. Int J Health Plann Manage 2021;36(1):215–8.

24. Chopra KK, Arora VK. Covid-19 and social stigma: role of scientific community. Indian J Tuberc 2020;67(3):284–5.

25. Logie CH. Lessons learned from HIV can inform our approach to COVID-19 stigma. J Int AIDS Soc 2020;23(5):e25504.

26. Logie CH, Turan JM. How do we balance tensions between COVID-19 public health responses and stigma mitigation? Learning from HIV research. AIDS Behav 2020;24(7):2003–6.

27. Pettit ML. Disease and stigma: a review of literature. Health Educ 2008; 40(2):70–6.

28. Santacroce L, Del Prete R, Charitos IA, et al. *Mycobacterium leprae*: a historical study on the origins of leprosy and its social stigma. Infez Med 2021;29(4): 623–32.

29. Khoo EJ, Lantos JD. Lessons learned from the COVID-19 pandemic. Acta Paediatr Oslo Nor 1992 2020;109(7):1323–5.

30. Wu C, Qian Y, Wilkes R. Anti-Asian discrimination and the Asian-white mental health gap during COVID-19. Ethn Racial Stud 2021;44(5):819–35.

31. Nadler JT, Voyles EC, Minorities M, et al. Stereotypes of Asian Americans. In: Nadler JT, Voyles EC, editors. Stereotypes: the incidence and impact of Bias. Santa Barbara, CA: ABC-CLIO; 2020. p. 300–6.

32. Babel RA, Wang P, Alessi EJ, et al. Stigma, HIV risk, and access to HIV prevention and treatment services among men who have sex with men (MSM) in the United States: a scoping review. AIDS Behav 2021;25(11):3574–604.

33. Mahajan AP, Sayles JN, Patel VA, et al. Stigma in the HIV/AIDS epidemic: a review of the literature and recommendations for the way forward. AIDS Lond Engl 2008; 22(Suppl 2):S67–79.

34. Sullivan PS, Satcher Johnson A, Pembleton ES, et al. Epidemiology of HIV in the USA: epidemic burden, inequities, contexts, and responses. Lancet Lond Engl 2021;397(10279):1095–106.

35. Reducing Stigma in Mpox Communication and Community Engagement | Mpox | Poxvirus | CDC. 2022. Available at: https://www.cdc.gov/poxvirus/Mpox/reducing-stigma.html. Accessed July 19, 2022.

Severe Acute Respiratory Syndrome Associated Infections

Brent Luu, PharmD, BCACP[a],*,
Virginia McCoy-Hass, DNP, MSN, RN, FNP-C, PA-C[a],
Teuta Kadiu, RN, MSL[a], Victoria Ngo, PhD[a], Sara Kadiu, PharmD[b],
Jeffrey Lien, PharmD[c]

KEYWORDS

- Coronavirus • SARS-CoV2 • MERS • Influenza • Severe acute respiratory syndrome

KEY POINTS

- Despite advancements in vaccines and antimicrobial development, life-threatening pathogens continue to emerge and reemerge globally.
- Globalization, climate change and human encroachment into nature accelerate emergence, and spread of infectious diseases.
- Microbial adaptation and breakdown of public health measures are also major drivers for emergence and reemergence of human pathogens.
- An integrated approach to global surveillance, vector control, early detection, drug and vaccine development, public hygiene and sanitation, public education and health policy interventions will be essential.
- Pandemic preparedness plans should be developed at all levels to facilitate rapid responses, prevent spread, and reduce morbidity and mortality.

INTRODUCTION

Viral infections are a source of respiratory illness in pediatric and adult populations worldwide. Influenza and coronaviruses (CoV) are some of the most common viral pathogens leading to respiratory illness and death. Prevalence of mortality rates from influenza range from 291,243 to 645,832 per year worldwide[1,2] and 12,000 to 52,000 in the United States (US).[3] More recently, respiratory illness from CoV severe acute respiratory syndrome (CoV-SARS) accounts for more than 1 million deaths in the United States alone.[4] Although infections with respiratory viral pathogens are not

[a] UC Davis Betty Irene Moore School of Nursing, 2450 48th Street, Sacramento, CA 95817, USA;
[b] Partners Pharmacy, 181 Cedar Hill Road Suite 1610, Marlborough, MA 01752, USA;
[c] Walgreens, 227 Shoreline Highway, Mill Valley, CA 94941, USA
* Corresponding author.
E-mail address: brluu@ucdavis.edu

Physician Assist Clin 8 (2023) 495–530
https://doi.org/10.1016/j.cpha.2023.03.002
2405-7991/23/© 2023 Elsevier Inc. All rights reserved.

Abbreviations	
ORFs	Open reading frames
NSPs	Nonstructural proteins
NP	Nasopharyngeal
OP	Oropharyngeal
CT	Computed tomography
CRP	C-reactive protein
CXR	Chest x-ray

selective, they are most detrimental to vulnerable populations such as the very young, elderly, and those with comorbid conditions. Generally, viral pathogens cause respiratory symptoms such as cough and shortness of breath but other organ systems can become compromised. Treatment is primarily supportive with antivirals and anti-inflammatory pharmacotherapeutics. However, vaccination is the best method for preventing disease complications and death. This article will explore the epidemiology, pathogenesis, diagnosis, treatment, and prevention of severe acute respiratory syndrome caused by coronavirus 2 (SARS-CoV2), and Middle Eastern respiratory syndrome (MERS).

SEVERE ACUTE RESPIRATORY SYNDROME-CORONAVIRUS 2 (SARS-COV2)
Prevalence and Mortality

The global and US incidence and prevalence of SARS-CoV2 varies due to population demographics, individual comorbidities, as well as emergence of new viral strains. Currently, the US Centers for Disease Control and Prevention (CDC) reports a total of approximately 89.1 million cumulative cases since the initial occurrence of the virus in the US, with a daily average of more than 126,000 cases per 7-day moving average as of July 2022.[4,5] Although death counts from SARS-CoV2 vary on a weekly basis, common risk factors include patient demographics such as age 60 years and older (85%), male gender (66%), history of smoking, as well as comorbid conditions including hypertension, diabetes, heart disease, chronic kidney or lung disease, and malignancy.[6] Patients reporting a history of smoking are more likely to experience acute respiratory distress, which is a primary cause of death in hospitalized patients with SARS-CoV2. Social isolation among both community-dwelling and hospitalized individuals infected with SARS-CoV2 presents a significant psychological concern. Additionally, their loss from the workforce, and the resulting decline in productivity, negatively influences national and global economies.

Pathogenesis

SARS-CoV2 is a member of the Coronaviridae family. It is an enveloped positive-stranded RNA virus containing a large genome, ranging from 26 to 32 kilobases.[7,8] The virion is spherical in shape with a core shell and luminous surface protein projections that give it the appearance of a solar crown (Latin: corona = crown). The genome contains 14-open reading frames (ORFs) that encode for 27-proteins.[9] The 5'-terminus of the genome encodes for 15-nonstructural proteins (NSPs), which are responsible for the transcription and replication of the SARS-CoV2 genome.[9] The 3'-terminus of the genome contains genes that encode for the 4-surface structural proteins, as well as 8-other proteins with unknown functional purpose.[9] The function of the 4-structural proteins is as follows: the N-protein is responsible for the viral replication as well as the host's response to the virus; the S-protein facilitates viral binding to susceptible host cells; the M-protein aids in creating networks within the host cell that produce viral particles; the E-protein assists with the production and release of viral particles into the host cell.[7,9,10]

SARS-CoV2 enters the host by attaching to receptors in cells that express angiotensin-converting enzyme 2 (ACE-2). SARS-CoV2 affinity for human ACE-2 cells is greater than that of SARS-COV.[8] Cells that express ACE-2 can be found in the lungs, gastrointestinal (GI) tract, medullary sections of the brain, epithelial cells, as well as cardiovascular, and immune systems; therefore, symptoms can indicate single or multiple system compromise (**Table 1**). However, most of the pathologic findings indicate respiratory compromise. Early lung changes include pulmonary edema, protein exudation, vascular congestion, pneumocyte hyperplasia, and interstitial thickening. Late pulmonary changes may include injury of alveoli, formation of fibrous exudates, desquamation, and hyaline membrane formation (ie, acute respiratory distress syndrome [ARDS]).[10] Respiratory failure without subjective perception of dyspnea (silent hypoxemia) has been reported, and is associated with hypocapnia caused by compensatory hyperventilation.[11]

The virus may also infiltrate occasional lymphocytes in the esophageal squamous epithelium, as well as plasma cells and lymphocytes in the lamina propria of the stomach, duodenum, and rectum.[10,12]

Risk Factors and Complications

Risk factors for SARS-CoV2 include older age, gender, and presence of comorbid conditions. Although most patients infected with the virus are reported to be aged between 30 and 79 years, poor prognosis and death is more common in the elderly (ie, aged 80 years or older).[6] Being male has also been associated with greater risk for infection, although no causative link has been reported thus far. Additionally, comorbid conditions associated with greater risk for SARS-CoV2 infection include diabetes, chronic lung disease, cardiovascular disease, immunocompromising conditions, chronic kidney disease, and obesity.[6] Careful history taking can identify patients at greatest risk and prevent complications.

Table 1
Symptoms of severe acute respiratory syndrome caused by coronavirus 2 infection[10,13]

Organ System	Common Symptoms	Severe Symptoms
Systemic	Fever/chills Fatigue Myalgias	
Respiratory	Cough Shortness of breath Sputum production Chest tightness Congestion or runny nose Sore throat	Dyspnea Hemoptysis Hyperventilation Severe respiratory distress
Cardiovascular	Not commonly present	Disseminated thrombosis Acute ischemic stroke
Neurologic	Headache New loss of sense of taste or smell Foggy mentation (COVID brain)	Altered consciousness Neurologic deficits
Gastrointestinal	Nausea/vomiting Diarrhea Anorexia	Abdominal pain
Skin		Rash (purpuric vascular, urticarial, vesicular)[14]

SARS-CoV2 complications include multisystem organ failure including ARDS and respiratory failure, sepsis and septic shock, arrhythmia, acute cardiac injury, myocarditis, heart failure, cardiac tamponade, coagulopathy, and acute renal injury.[15] Heart failure, myocardial infarction, arrhythmias, and cardiac arrest occur more frequently in patients with associated pneumonia. Coagulopathy such as acute venous thromboembolism, deep vein thrombosis, and pulmonary embolism have been reported in patients with SARS-CoV2 infection.[15] Analysis suggests multifactorial causes of coagulopathy in these patients including older age, more severe illness, more chronic illness, stasis, and high thrombotic and inflammatory abnormalities.[16] In severe COVID-19 disease, hypercoagulability can be stimulated by endothelial cell dysfunction, increased blood viscosity from hypoxia.[15] Additionally, patients who concomitantly experienced an acute ischemic stroke were found to have an elevated d-Dimer, fibrinogen, and the presence of antiphospholipid antibodies, although the mechanism of action has yet to be determined.[13]

Screening and Diagnosis

The preferred standard method for detecting the presence of SARS-COV2 is the reverse transcriptase polymerase chain reaction test (RT-PCR).[17] The RT-PCR is a version of nucleic acid amplification testing (NAAT) used to amplify the genetic material of the collected sample to detect presence of viral RNA.[18] Recommendations for aspirate collection include nasopharyngeal (NP) and oropharyngeal (OP) swabs for asymptomatic persons, and bilateral anterior nares collection for those who are symptomatic. Other recommended aspirates for diagnosis include tracheal or bronchoalveolar lavage aspirates. However, because the use of bronchoscopy poses the risk for exposure to patients and health-care providers, it is recommended only for intubated patients and if diagnosis, using upper airway aspirate, is uncertain.[11] Overall sensitivity (Sn) of RT-PCR tests for SARS-CoV2 is reported in the 45% to 60% for nasal and NP specimens.[19] A major reason for the high rate of false-negative RT-PCR results is the timing of sampling relative to the onset of symptoms. Studies have shown that the median false-negative rate decreases from 67% 1 day before symptom onset to 38% on the day of symptom onset and to 20% by days 3 and 4 postonset of symptoms. Thereafter, Sn declines and the false-negative rate is 100% by day 8 to 14. Therefore, the optimal days for RT-PCR testing via nasal or NP swab are days 3 to 4 after symptom onset, and asymptomatic testing can be expected to have a significantly high rate of false-negative results. Thus, clinical and epidemiologic data should be factored into clinical decision-making, and if there is a high index of suspicion for SARS-CoV2, a negative RT-PCR alone cannot rule out infection. Repeat testing over several days is recommended to improve test sensitivity. According to the US Food and Drug Administration, the specificity (Sp) of available RT-PCR tests for SARS-CoV2 is 100%.[18]

Antigen tests are immunoassays that detect the presence of the viral antigen, indicating current infection with SARS-CoV2. Antigen tests currently include point-of-care, laboratory-based, and self-tests.[17] Antigen tests can be used at point-of-care because they produce results in 15 to 30 minutes. Similar to RT-PCR and other NAAT tests, antigen tests require the collection of NP, nasal, or saliva specimens from symptomatic persons. However, antigen tests are less sensitive than NAAT tests, meaning they should be used with caution in asymptomatic individuals. The Sn of antigen tests for SARS-CoV2 varies considerably between asymptomatic and symptomatic persons (58.1% and 72%, respectively).[18] Similarly, Sn is also highly variable between brands, ranging from 34.1% to 88.1%. Average Sp is high among all patients and brands at 99.6%.[18] Studies have shown some antigen tests to be as effective as viral culture in detecting the presence of SARS-CoV2.[20] Thus, they may be useful as a biomarker to detect contagiousness.

However, they may provide false-negative results early in the disease process and are not used routinely for this purpose in clinical practice.

Antibody tests, such as the SARS-CoV2 rapid IgG–IgM combined antibody test, can be used to detect antibodies against the virus in persons who have been previously infected or vaccinated. Antibody tests are not recommended for the diagnosis of acute SARS-CoV2 but can be used to identify an earlier infection. However, antibody testing is not recommended to determine immunity to SARS-CoV2 due to either an earlier infection or vaccination. Indeed, new strains of the virus may predispose individuals to become infected or require booster vaccination to sustain immunity against the virus.[21] Antibody testing may be used to support the presumptive diagnosis of COVID-19 in persons who present with SARS-CoV2 symptoms greater than 8 days after onset.[21] Available antibody tests include chemiluminescence assay (CLIA), enzyme-linked immunosorbent assay (ELISA) and lateral flow immunoassay (LFIA). CLIA has the highest Sn/Sp (92% and 99%), followed by ELISA (86% and 99%), and then LFIA (78% and 98%).[22] **Table 2** reviews the advantages and disadvantages of tests for SARS-CoV2 infection. **Figs. 1** and **2** illustrate the optimal timing of diagnostic tests for SARS-CoV2 infection and algorithms for SARS-CoV2 testing in symptomatic and asymptomatic persons.

Other Diagnostic Testing

Laboratory testing, chest x-ray, and chest computed tomography (CT) are useful diagnostic tests in the evaluation of confirmed or suspected SARS-CoV2 infection.[8] A study of almost 1100 hospitalized patients with SARS-CoV2 showed variable white blood cell count. Leukopenia ($<4000/mm^3$) was identified in 33.7%, normal leukocyte counts ($4000–10,000/mm^3$) in 60.4%, and leukocytosis ($>10,000/mm^3$) in 5.9%. Lymphopenia ($<1500/mm^3$) occurred in 83.2%. Thrombocytopenia was identified in 36.2% of the cases. The most common abnormal serologic findings in this study were elevated C-reactive protein (CRP; 60.7% of patients), elevated lactase dehydrogenase (41.0%), and increased d-Dimer (46.4%).[24] A meta-analysis of 43 studies including 3600 patients showed the most common abnormal laboratory findings were elevated CRP (68.8%), lymphopenia (57.4%), and elevated lactate dehydrogenase (LDH) (51.6%).[25] Leukopenia, lymphopenia, thrombocytopenia, elevated CRP, elevated LDH, and increased d-Dimer were all more prevalent in patients with severe disease versus patients with non-severe disease.[24,25]

Chest CT has been found to have moderate-to-high Sn (67%–100%) but low Sp (25%–80%) for the diagnosis of SARS-CoV2. Chest x-ray is less sensitive than CT, with a reported Sn of 69%.[26] However, CT is not available in all parts of the world, and the use of chest CT in cases of suspected SARS-CoV2 infection is associated with higher radiation exposure, infection control issues related to patient transport, and delays due to the need for CT room decontamination. Therefore, the American College of Radiology recommends that CT should not be used as a first-line test for the diagnosis of SARS-CoV2 and should be reserved for hospitalized, symptomatic patients with specific clinical indications for CT.[27]

Chest x-ray (CXR) remains the primary imaging modality used in the diagnosis and evaluation of patients with SARS-CoV2; and positive chest x-ray findings can preclude the need for chest CT.[28] The most common chest x-ray and CT findings in SARS-CoV2 infection are lung consolidation and ground glass opacities. These findings typically have a bilateral, peripheral, and lower lung distribution.[28] Ground glass densities observed on CT may often have a correlate that is difficult to detect on CXR (**Fig. 3**). One of the most specific features of SARS-CoV2 pneumonia is the high prevalence of peripheral lung opacities (present in 33%–86% of patients), which often are multifocal

Table 2
Advantages and disadvantages of tests to detect the presence of severe acute respiratory syndrome caused by coronavirus[11,17–23]

Test	Use	Advantages	Disadvantages
Molecular test (RT-PCR, NAAT)	• Within 2 wk of symptom onset • To detect viral RNA • Within 2 wk of symptom onset • Asymptomatic screening • NP or OP swab for asymptomatic patients • Bilateral NP or nasal swab for symptomatic patients • Bronchoscopy (intubated patients only) if diagnosis uncertain	• Most Sn and Sp method to confirm acute infection	• Expensive • Requires specialized skills and equipment (must be run in a laboratory) • Results take 24–48 h
Antigen rapid detection tests	• Within 2 wk of symptom onset • To detect viral protein if molecular testing not available or rapid results needed • NP or OP swab	• Rapid results (15–30 min) • Can be done at point-of-care, including self-tests • Requires minimal training • Less expensive than molecular tests	• Less Sn than molecular tests • Variable quality, especially with self-tests • If test negative, must repeat sample for molecular testing
Antibody test	• More than 2 wk after symptom onset • To establish late or retrospective diagnosis if molecular and antigen tests negative • Primarily used in the inpatient setting or to identify antibody donors • Used in combination with molecular and antigen tests • Blood test	• Rapid antibody tests can provide results in 15–20 min	• Laboratory-based assays can take 24 h for results • May be nonspecific (false-positive result) • Does not distinguish between natural or vaccine-induced seropositivity • Not used for diagnosis of acute infection

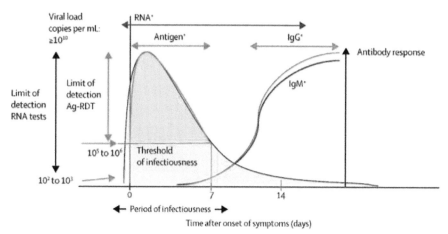

Fig. 1. The viral dynamics of, and antibody response to, SARS-CoV-2 infection in a patient who is symptomatic, and the optimal timeframe for deployment of different types of tests. *Reprinted* with permission from Elsevier. The Lancet, 2022, 399: 757-68.

and can be readily seen on chest radiograph (**Fig. 4**). Lung opacities can rapidly evolve into a diffuse pattern within weeks after symptom onset, often peaking at around 6 to 12 days (**Fig. 5**) and may result in diffuse air space disease (ARDS; **Fig. 6**).[28]

Pharmacologic Management of COVID-19

Clinical management of patients with COVID-19 is based on determination of outpatient versus inpatient treatment, disease severity, and the patient's risk of disease progression. Disease severity is classified as asymptomatic/presymptomatic, mild, moderate, severe, and critical illness (**Box 1**).[29]

The clinical course is asymptomatic or mild in 80% to 90% of cases. Early in the COVID-19 pandemic (January 2019 to April 2020), the progression to severe disease occurred in about 10% of cases, and critical (life-threatening) illness developed in around 5% of cases. Vaccination is highly effective against COVID-19 associated hospitalization and death. During the first 11 months (December 2020 to October 2021) following the availability of SARS-CoV2 vaccines, the rates of severe COVID-19-associated outcomes and death dropped to 0.015% and 0.0033%, respectively.[30] Death, when it occurs, is usually caused by the progression to ARDS and multiorgan failure.[11] Early in the clinical course, the primary pathogenic process is driven by the replication of SARS-CoV2. In later stages and severe disease, a dysregulated immune/inflammatory response to SARS-CoV2 drives tissue damage. Based on this pathogenesis, therapies that directly target SARS-CoV2 are anticipated to have the greatest efficacy early in the course of the disease, and immunosuppressive/anti-inflammatory therapies are likely to be more useful in the later stages.[31]

Our scientific understanding of SARS-CoV2 continues to evolve and many of the therapeutic agents used to treat COVID-19 have not been compared side by side in clinical trials. Clinical guidelines for the management of patients with SARS-CoV2 infection have been promulgated and are under frequent revision as new data become available. Clinicians should refer to the most recent version of the guidelines for up-to-date information. For detailed information please visit https://www.covid19treatmentguidelines.nih.gov/.

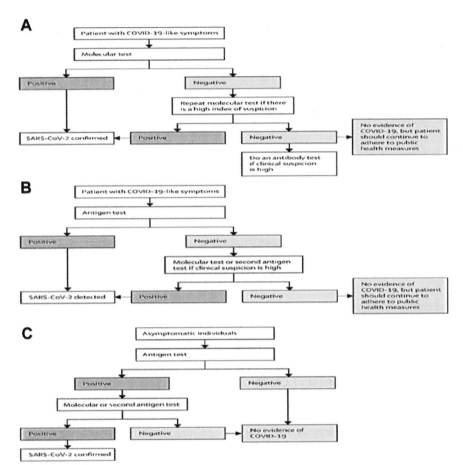

Fig. 2. Algorithms for testing to detect SARS-CoV-2 in symptomatic and asymptomatic individuals. (*A*) Preferred testing algorithm for individuals with COVID-19-like symptoms. (*B*) Testing algorithm for individuals with COVID-19-like symptoms when molecular testing is not available, or results are delayed. (*C*) Testing algorithm for COVID-19 case finding among asymptomatic individuals. *Reprinted* with permission from Elsevier. The Lancet, 2022, 399: 757-68.

Management of Nonhospitalized Patients

Most patients with COVID-19 have asymptomatic or mild illness and do not require targeted pharmacologic intervention. All symptomatic patients should receive supportive management, including the use of over-the-counter antipyretics, antitussives, and analgesics.[31] Nonpharmacological treatments may also be used, including drinking fluids, pulmonary hygiene, and resting in a prone position.[32] Patients who suffer from moderate illness and/or those who are at high risk of disease progression may require pharmacologic intervention. Considerations when selecting a pharmacologic agent are the potential for drug–drug interactions, the ability to administer intravenously (IV) medications, and the prevalent variants of concern in the region.

In nonhospitalized patients who do not require supplemental oxygen and are at high risk of disease progression, ritonavir-boosted nirmatrelvir or remdesivir is recommended as first-line therapy. Ritonavir-boosted nirmatrelvir is administered orally (PO) and

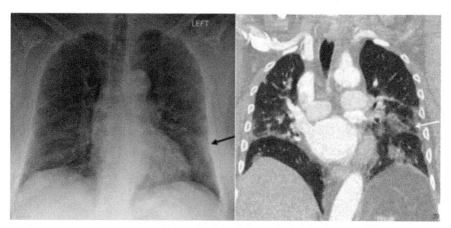

Fig. 3. CXR (*left*) with patchy peripheral left mid to lower lung opacities (*black arrow*) corresponding to ground glass opacities (*white arrow*) on coronal image from contrast-enhanced the contemporaneous chest CT (*right*). (*Reprinted from* Jacobi, et al.[28])

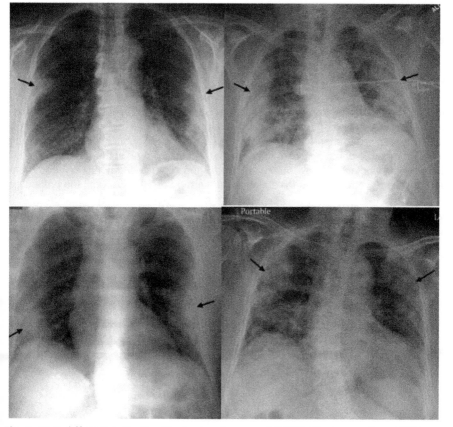

Fig. 4. Four different patients with varying degrees of COVID-19 pneumonia on CXR predominantly involving the peripheral lungs bilaterally (*black arrows*). (*Reprinted from* Jacobi, et al.[28])

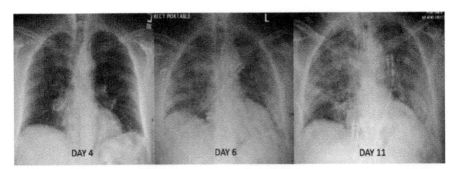

DAY 4   DAY 6   DAY 11

Fig. 5. Serial radiographs during 7 days in a patient with COVID-19 infection depicting the progression of diffuse lung disease that ultimately required intubation. (*Reprinted from* Jacobi, et al.[28])

is therefore preferred over remdesivir, which is administered IV. Ritonavir-boosted nirmatrelvir has significant drug–drug interactions and must be monitored carefully. Alternative therapy, such as molnupiravir should be reserved for cases where ritonavir-boosted nirmatrelvir and remdesivir are unavailable or their use is clinically inappropriate[32] (note: bebtelovimab is no-longer authorized for use in the US due to poor infectiveness toward the major circulating Omicron subvariants in the country).[33] The routine use of systemic corticosteroids is not recommended and should be reserved for cases where another indication warrants their use.[32]

   Table 3 provides an overview of the mechanisms of actions, dosing, adverse drug reactions, monitoring, and clinical pearls for the use of pharmacologic agents used in the treatment of COVID-19.

   In previously hospitalized patients after discharge, the guidelines recommend against continuing treatment with remdesivir, baricitinib, or dexamethasone if the patient is stable and *does* not require oxygen supplementation. There is currently insufficient data to recommend for or against the use of these agents in patients requiring supplemental oxygenation postdischarge. In patients being discharged from the ED despite a new or increasing requirement for oxygen supplementation, it is recommended to start dexamethasone for a maximum duration of 10 days, until the patient no

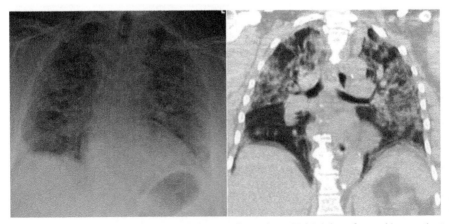

Fig. 6. CXR (*left*) and subsequent coronal image from chest CT (*right*) performed in a patient with COVID-19 and diffuse ground glass and consolidative opacities throughout both lungs. (*Reprinted from* Jacobi, et al.[28])

Box 1	
Clinical spectrum of COVID-19 illness[29]	
Severity	**Criteria**
Asymptomatic/ presymptomatic	Positive test, no symptoms consistent with COVID-19
Mild	Any COVID-19 symptoms *without* shortness of breath, dyspnea, or abnormal chest imaging
Moderate	Evidence of lower respiratory disease on imaging or examination and $SpO_2 \geq 94\%$ on room air
Severe	$SpO_2 < 94\%$ on room air, $Pao_2/Fio_2 <300$ mm Hg, respiratory rate >30 breaths/min, or lung infiltrates >50%
Critical	Respiratory failure, septic shock, and/or multiorgan failure

longer requires oxygen supplementation. Additionally, remdesivir can be used in this subset of patients; however, its use may be limited due to its parenteral administration, and availability of home infusion resources.[32]

Management of Hospitalized Patients

Patients with moderate illness who are at risk for progression to higher severity and those with severe disease (see **Box 1**) should be hospitalized. Inpatient treatment of COVID-19 involves the use of anti-inflammatory, immunosuppressive, and in certain cases, antithrombotic therapies. Treatment is determined based on the patient's oxygen requirements. In hospitalized patients who *do not* require supplemental oxygen, corticosteroid therapy is *not* recommended based on the results from the Randomized Evaluation of COVID-19 Therapy (RECOVERY) trial, showing no benefit in this population. Currently, there is insufficient evidence for or against the use of remdesivir in patients not requiring supplemental oxygen (level of evidence: BIII). The use of remdesivir in these patients should be determined using clinical judgment and reserved for patients at risk of progressing to severe disease.[46]

Patients requiring supplemental oxygenation are subdivided into 3 treatment groups:[46]

- Patients requiring low-flow oxygen
- Patients requiring high-flow oxygen or noninvasive ventilation (NIV)
- Patients requiring mechanical ventilation (MV) or extracorporeal membrane oxygenation (ECMO)

Treatment for patients who require low flow supplemental oxygen consists of the use of one of the following therapies: remdesivir monotherapy, dexamethasone plus remdesivir, or dexamethasone monotherapy. Because early COVID-19 is characterized by rapid viral replication, the use of remdesivir is likely to be most effective in the first 10 days after symptom onset. In the later course of disease, corticosteroids may be beneficial in decreasing a potential systemic inflammatory response. Corticosteroid monotherapy may be used in certain cases. However, immunosuppressive effects of steroids may reduce viral clearance when used without an antiviral.[46] In patients with rapidly increasing supplemental oxygen requirements, adding another immunomodulatory agent (eg, baricitinib, or tocilizumab) to dexamethasone, or remdesivir monotherapy, or combination therapy of remdesivir and dexamethasone is recommended. Overall, this group should be monitored closely for disease progression and increasing oxygen requirements, and the treatment should be adjusted accordingly. If disease progression occurs during remdesivir therapy, the full course of treatment should be completed.[46] When selecting immunomodulatory agents,

Table 3
Pharmacologic agents used in the treatment of severe acute respiratory syndrome caused by coronavirus

Drug	Mechanism of Action	Dosing	Adverse Drug Reactions	Monitoring	Clinical Pearls
Antivirals					

Ritonavir-boosted Nirmatrelvir (Paxlovid)[34]	• Ritonavir: CYP 3A4 inhibitor, inhibiting nirmatrelvir metabolism
	• Nirmatrelvir: protease inhibitor, inhibiting the viral protease MPRO (aka 3CLpro)
		• eGFR ≥60 mL/min: nirmatrelvir 300 mg + ritonavir 100 mg PO BID ×5 d
		• eGFR ≥30 to <60 mL/min: nirmatrelvir 150 mg + ritonavir 100 mg PO BID ×5 d
		• eGFR <30 mL/min or Child-Pugh Class C: not recommended
			• Dysgeusia
			• Diarrhea
			• Hypertension
			• Myalgia
				• Drug–Drug interactions resulting in:
				  ○ Clinically significant adverse reactions, severe, life-threatening, or fatal events from greater exposures of concomitant medications or Paxlovid
				  ○ Loss of therapeutic effect of Paxlovid and possible viral resistance
				• Paxlovid is a strong CYP3A inhibitor
				• Concomitant use with drugs metabolized by CYP3A or initiation of medications metabolized by CYP3A in patients already receiving Paxlovid, may increase plasma concentrations of medications metabolized by CYP3A
					• For use in adults and pediatric patients ≥12 y or older and 40 kg or more
					• Start within 5 d of symptom onset

Drug	Mechanism	Dose	Adverse effects	Monitoring	Comments
Remdesivir[35]	Adenosine analog inhibits RNA-dependent RNA polymerase causing premature termination of viral transcription	• Pediatric 28 d and older, 3–39 kg: Dose: 5 mg/kg ×1, then 2.5 mg/kg/dose q 24 h × 2 d • Pediatric 28 d and older, >40 kg and adults: Dose: 200 mg IV × 1, then 100 mg IV q 24 h × 2 d • Course may be longer for severe COVID-19 (ie, 4–9 d) • Each dose infused during 30–120 min	• Nausea • Hypersensitivity and infusion reactions • Increased PT (with normal INR) • Increased transaminases	• Observation for ≥1 h after infusion for hypersensitivity reactions • Before initiation and during treatment: eGFR, liver function, PT tests • Drug interaction with chloroquine and hydroxychloroquine: decreased remdesivir antiviral activity	• FDA-approved drug for the treatment of COVID-19 • For use in adults and pediatric patients aged 28 d and older • Start within 7 d of symptom onset • Consider d/C if ALT >10× ULN • d/C if ALT elevated with signs and symptoms of liver inflammation
Molnupiravir[36]	Prodrug Cytidine analog incorporated into viral RNA leading to accumulation of errors, resulting in inhibition of viral replication	• 800 mg PO BID ×5 d	Rash Hypersensitivity	N/A	• For use in adults ≥18 y • Start within 5 d of symptom onset • Do not use if pregnant • Effective contraception should be used: • Female: during and 4 d after treatment • Male: during and 3 mo after treatment • Avoid breastfeeding during use and for 4 d after treatment • Do not use if < 18 y old (bone/cartilage toxicity)

(continued on next page)

Table 3
(continued)

Drug	Mechanism of Action	Dosing	Adverse Drug Reactions	Monitoring	Clinical Pearls
Monoclonal Antibodies					
Bebtelovimab[37] (*NIH expert panel recommended against use of this drug for the treatment of COVID-19*)[33]	Neutralizes the viral spike protein, blocking its attachment to human ACE2 receptors	175 mg IV ×1 dose (injected during ≥30 s)	• Hypersensitivity and infusion reactions • Pruritus • Rash • Nausea/vomiting	• Observation for ≥1 h after injection • Clinical worsening of COVID-19	• Start within 7 d of symptom onset • Adults and pediatric patients ≥12 y old and ≥40 kg • Has not been studied in patients hospitalized due to COVID-19 • Monoclonal antibodies may be associated with worse clinical outcomes when administered to hospitalized patients with severe COVID-19
Tixagevimab/cilgavimab (Evusheld)[38] As of January 26, 2023, Evusheld is no longer authorized for emergency use due to its low effectiveness against the major variants circulating in the US[39]	Targets SARS-CoV2 spike protein-directed attachment	• Initial dose: 300 mg of tixagevimab and 300 mg of cilgavimab administered as 2 individual intramuscular injections • Repeat dose: 300 mg of tixagevimab and 300 mg of cilgavimab every 6 mo, as indicated, timed from	• Most common adverse events (all grades, incidence ≥3%) are headache, fatigue, and cough • Serious hypersensitivity reactions, including anaphylaxis, have been observed	• Clinically monitor for hypersensitivity reactions after injections and observe for at least 1 h • For individuals with a history of severe hypersensitivity reaction to a COVID-19 vaccine, consider consultation with an allergist-immunologist before administration	• For the pre-exposure prophylaxis of COVID-19 in adults and pediatrics ≥12 y weighing at least 40 kg who have NOT had a known recent exposure to an individual infected with SARSCoV-2 *and* have moderate to severe immune compromise *or* for

Drug	Mechanism	Dosing	Adverse effects	Monitoring	Comments
		the date of the most recent dose • For individuals who initially received 150 mg tixagevimab and 150 mg cilgavimab (eg, as part of a clinical trial): • Initial dose ≤3 mo prior: 150 mg tixagevimab and 150 mg cilgavimab • Initial dose >3 mo prior: 300 mg tixagevimab and 300 mg cilgavimab			whom COVID-19 vaccination is not recommended due to a history of severe adverse reaction • Caution for use in individuals at high risk for cardiovascular events
Sarilumab[40,41] *(NIH expert panel recommended against the use of this drug for the treatment of COVID-19)*[33]	Binds IL-6, inhibits IL-6-mediated proinflammatory signaling	• 400 mg IV infusion once (infused over 1 h)	• Most common adverse reactions (incidence at least 3%) are neutropenia, increased ALT, injection site erythema, upper respiratory infections and urinary tract infections • Thrombocytopenia • Lipid abnormalities • Serious infections (with long-term use) • GI perforation (with long-term use) • Hypersensitivity reaction	• Liver function tests • CBC	• Only used in combination with corticosteroids • Use as alternative to tocilizumab

(continued on next page)

Table 3 (continued)					
Drug	Mechanism of Action	Dosing	Adverse Drug Reactions	Monitoring	Clinical Pearls

Tocilizumab[42]	• Binds IL-6, inhibiting IL-6-mediated proinflammatory signaling	Weight-based dosing: Patients <30 kg: 12 mg/kg IV infusion ×1 Patients ≥30 kg: 8 mg/kg IV infusion ×1 Maximum dose = 800 mg Use actual body weight If no improvement, may repeat dose in 8 h	• Most common adverse reactions (incidence ≥3%) are constipation, anxiety, diarrhea, insomnia, hypertension, and nausea
			• Serious AEs:
			• Serious infections
			• Gastrointestinal perforation
			• Neutropenia
			• Thrombocytopenia
			• Altered lipid profile
			• Elevated liver enzymes
			• Hypersensitivity reactions
				• Liver function tests
				• CBC
					• Approved by the FDA for treatment of COVID-19 in hospitalized patients
					  ○ Adults and pediatric patients aged ≥2 y
					  ○ Only used in combination with corticosteroids

JAK Inhibitors

Drug	Mechanism	Dosing	Adverse Effects	Monitoring	Comments
Baricitinib[43]	• Blocks IL-6-mediated inflammatory response • Possible antiviral activity by blocking viral entry into lung cells	• eGFR ≥60 mL/min: 4 mg PO once daily • eGFR 30 to <60 mL/min: 2 mg PO once daily • eGFR 15 to <30 mL/min: 1 mg PO once daily • eGFR <15 mL/min: not recommended • In pediatric patients ≥2 y to <9 y: 2 mg PO once daily • Duration of therapy: 14 d or until discharge	• Infections • Venous thrombosis	• eGFR • CBC • AST and ALT	• Approved by the FDA for treatment of COVID-19 in hospitalized patients • For use in adults and pediatric patients aged ≥2 y • Only used as combo therapy with corticosteroids • For patients unable to swallow tablets: crush and disperse in water
Tofacitinib[44]	Blocks signaling from cytokines Inhibits inflammatory response	• eGFR ≥60 mL/min/1.73 m²: 10 mg PO twice daily • eGFR <60 mL/min/1.73 m²: 5 mg PO twice daily • Duration of therapy: 14 d or until discharge	• Infections • Malignancies • Hyperlipidemia • MI, stroke • Thrombosis • Anemia	• CBC • LFTs • Platelets • Hgb/Hct	• Only used in combination with corticosteroids • *Use as alternative to baricitinib*

Corticosteroid

Drug	Mechanism	Dosing	Adverse Effects	Monitoring	Comments
Dexamethasone[45]	Anti-inflammatory	• 6–12 mg IV or PO 1 to 3 times daily • Duration: up to 10 d	• Adrenal suppression • Hyperglycemia • Infections • Impaired wound healing • Psychosis	• Blood glucose • Blood pressure • Potassium	• An alternative corticosteroid may be used if dexamethasone is not available

the clinical benefits versus the potential increased the risk of infection, including opportunistic infections must be considered. The level of evidence supporting the addition of an immunomodulatory agent to dexamethasone in this subgroup of patients is weak (ie, BIIa).[46]

Treatment for patients requiring supplemental oxygen using a high-flow device or NIV consists of dexamethasone plus oral baricitinib, or plus intravenous tocilizumab, or monotherapy. Remdesivir may be added to one of these options in certain patients.[47] Remdesivir monotherapy in this population may be clinically inadequate and should therefore not be used. Immunomodulatory agents may be added to dexamethasone in patients with rapidly increasing oxygen need because clinical benefit has been demonstrated in multiple trials for this patient subgroup. The Randomized, Embedded, Multi-factorial, Adaptive Platform Trial for Community-Acquired Pneumonia trial showed ~22% reduction in mortality in patients receiving tocilizumab versus usual care. In the RECOVERY trial, there was a 14% reduction in all-cause mortality by day 28 in patients receiving tocilizumab plus dexamethasone versus usual care. A Study of Baricitinib in Participants With COVID-19 (COV-BARRIER) showed a 48% reduction in all-cause mortality in this subgroup.[46]

An open label, randomized controlled trial comparing baricitinib and tocilizumab in patients with COVID-19 showed that baricitinib was noninferior to tocilizumab for the time to hospital discharge within 28 days. The percentage of patients discharged alive for the baricitinib group was reported at 58.4% versus 52.4% for the tocilizumab group, with a *P*-value less than .001 for noninferiority.[48] Therefore, the selection of these therapies is based on availability and patient-specific factors. In cases where baricitinib or tocilizumab are unavailable or their use is inappropriate, second-line options are oral tofacitinib (a JAK inhibitor) or IV sarilumab (an IL-6 receptor antagonist). JAK inhibitors and IL-6 receptor antagonists should *not* be used together due to an increased risk of serious infection and lack of supporting data.[46]

Treatment for patients requiring MV or ECMO must be provided in a critical care setting. At this stage of disease, patients are experiencing a systemic inflammatory response that can lead to multiorgan dysfunction syndrome. To limit damage due to inflammation, guidelines recommend starting dexamethasone plus IV tocilizumab or PO baricitinib is recommended. If baricitinib, tofacitinib, tocilizumab, or sarilumab is not available or not feasible to use, dexamethasone monotherapy should be started. Remdesivir monotherapy for critically ill patients is contraindicated due to studies showing possible increased mortality, and no improvement in recovery rate. However, for patients already receiving remdesivir who subsequently require MV or ECMO, remdesivir treatment should be continued until completion.[46] Additional considerations in the treatment of hospitalized patients may be found in **Box 2**. See **Box 3** for additional consideration in the treatment of special populations with COVID-19.

Box 2
Additional considerations in the treatment of hospitalized patients with COVID-19[46]

- Equivalent dose of other corticosteroid such as prednisone, methylprednisolone, or hydrocortisone may be used if dexamethasone is not available.

- Baricitinib or tocilizumab should only be given as *dual therapy* with dexamethasone (or another corticosteroid at an equivalent dose).

- The combination of dexamethasone and a JAK inhibitor or IL-6 receptor antagonist increases the risk of opportunistic infections or reactivation of latent infections. For patients from *Strongyloides* endemic areas, antiparasitic prophylaxis (such as ivermectin) is indicated.

Box 3	
Additional considerations in the treatment of special populations with COVID-19[49]	
Pregnancy	• Increased risk of severe disease from SARS-CoV2 infection in pregnant persons
	• Use shared decision-making to discuss the use of investigational drugs or drugs approved for other indications as treatments for COVID-19 in pregnant or lactating patients
	• In general, treatment options for pregnant patients with COVID-19 should be the same as for nonpregnant patients
	• The COVID-19 Treatment Guidelines Panel recommends *against* withholding treatment for COVID-19 and SARS-CoV2 vaccination from pregnant or lactating persons due to theoretic safety concerns
Children	• Infection is *generally* milder than in adults, most children do not require specific therapy
	• Children with comorbid conditions (eg, neurologic impairment developmental syndromes, obesity, immune impairment, diabetes, and so forth) as well as non-White children and older teens may be at an increased risk for severe COVID-19 disease
	• Consultation with a pediatric infectious disease specialist is recommended for hospitalized children with COVID-19 who require supplemental oxygen, are at increased risk for severe disease, or who require treatment with remdesivir or dexamethasone
	• Multisystem Inflammatory Syndrome in Children (MIS-C) is a serious delayed complication of SARS-CoV2 infection that may develop in a small subgroup of children and young adults
Cancer or immuno-compromised	• Patients who are undergoing active cancer treatment or are immunocompromised are at high risk of progression to severe COVID-19 disease
	• Vaccination is the best first-line prevention of COVID-19 in these populations. However, vaccine response rates may be lower
	• They *may* be eligible to receive antiSARS-CoV2 monoclonal antibodies as preexposure prophylaxis (PrEP)
	• Treatment of COVID-19 in these patients is the same as the general population
	• Multiple drug–drug interactions may occur, consult with hematology-oncology or other specialties as appropriate
Transplant	• These patients are eligible to receive the anti-SARS-CoV-2 monoclonal antibodies tixagevimab plus cilgavimab (Evusheld) as PrEP
	• If SARS-CoV2 is detected or strongly suspected, transplantation should be deferred, if possible
	• The optimal management and therapeutic approach to COVID-19 in these populations is unknown. At this time, the procedures for evaluating and managing COVID-19 in transplant candidates are the same as those for nontransplant candidates
	• Multiple drug–drug interactions may occur, consult with transplant specialist before initiation of therapy
HIV	• COVID-19 vaccines should be given regardless of CD4 T lymphocyte (CD4) cell count or HIV viral load because the potential benefits outweigh the potential risks
	• The Advisory Committee on Immunization Practices recommends that people with advanced or untreated HIV should receive a 3-dose series of

| | an mRNA COVID-19 vaccine, with the third dose at least 28 d after the second dose
• Monoclonal antibodies (tixagevimab plus cilgavimab) can be used as PrEP in people with advanced or untreated HIV
• The triage, management, and treatment of COVID-19 in people with HIV is generally the same as for the general population
• Opportunistic infections should also be considered in the differential diagnosis of febrile illness
• Ritonavir-boosted nirmatrelvir (Paxlovid) may be combined with ritonavir-based or cobicistat-based antiretroviral therapy
• Multiple drug–drug interactions may occur, consult with HIV specialist before initiation of therapy |
| Influenza | • Influenza vaccine and COVID-19 vaccine may be administered concurrently at different injection sites
• For patients with active COVID-19 infection who have not received influenza vaccine:
 ○ If asymptomatic or mildly ill: May be vaccinated when isolation period completed or if in a health-care setting for another reason
 ○ If moderately to severely ill: Defer vaccine until isolation completed and no longer moderately or severely ill
• During periods when influenza is circulating, patients hospitalized with severe respiratory illness should be tested for both influenza and COVID-19
• Coinfection with SARS-CoV2 does not alter influenza treatment
• Empiric treatment with oseltamivir should be started as soon as possible in hospitalized patients with suspected influenza |

Fig. 7 provides an algorithm for the treatment of nonhospitalized and hospitalized patients with COVID-19.

Antithrombotic therapy in patients with COVID-19

Acute thrombosis/thromboembolism may be a complication of SARS-CoV2 infection. Patients who experience sudden loss of peripheral perfusion, or rapid deterioration of pulmonary, cardiac, or neurologic function should be evaluated for thromboembolic disease. See **Box 4** for key points in the evaluation and management of this population.

Prevention of COVID-19 infection

The most effective primary prevention of COVID-19 infection is vaccination. Mitigating the spread of COVID-19 can be achieved through hand hygiene, mask wearing, and social distancing. The outbreak of COVID-19 infection caused by the SARS-CoV2 virus is a unique pandemic with global impact. In December 2020, the United States implemented an Emergency Use Authorization (EUA) for a newly developed COVID-19 vaccine that boasted high efficacy. Since the introduction of COVID-19 vaccines, FDA has granted EUA to 4 vaccines, including the approval of 2 of them for use in specific age groups. This process continues to evolve and clinicians should find up-to-date information on FDA approval for COVID-19 vaccines at: https://www.fda.gov/emergency-preparedness-and-response/counterterrorism-and-emerging-threats/coronavirus-disease-2019-covid-19. As of September 2022, 4 countries have approved mucosal vaccines for SARS-CoV2. Phase III trial data for these vaccines have not been published as of this writing, although Phase II trial data of the inhaled

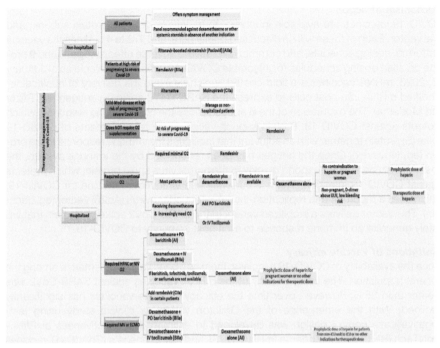

Fig. 7. Algorithm for treatment of nonhospitalized and hospitalized patients with COVID-19.[32,46,49,51]

vaccines (i.e from CanSino Biologics in Tianjin) showed significantly higher blood-serum antibody levels compared with booster by injection.[52] Theoretically, mucosal vaccines could prevent viral transmission from person to person (so-called "sterilizing immunity"), which is not conferred by injected COVID-19 vaccines. Currently, there are more than 100 mucosal SARS-CoV2 vaccines in development, with more than 20 already in human trials. Mucosal COVID-19 vaccines could facilitate access to vaccines and reduce viral transmission. However, further research is needed to confirm their long-term efficacy.[52,53]

Box 4
Antithrombotic therapy in patients with COVID-19[47,50]

- Prophylactic dose of heparin:
  - Hospitalized patients with mild-to-moderate COVID-19 and at high risk of progressing to severe disease, unless contraindicated (AI).
  - Pregnant patients (BIII)
  - Patients without indication for therapeutic anticoagulation
  - Patients transferred from a non-ICU unit to ICU and have no other indications for therapeutic anticoagulation (BIII)

- Therapeutic dose of heparin:
  - Nonpregnant patients with d-Dimer level above the ULN without increased bleeding risk (CIIa)

- Guidelines are continuously evolving based on current new data

- Consult with a specialist for further guidance in the management of these populations

Mechanism of action

COVID-19 vaccines are available in several formulations: mRNA, protein subunit, and viral vector. Each of these will be discussed briefly here, and **Table 4** outlines the vaccine platforms, dosing schedule, and common and severe adverse effects. **Figs. 8** and **9** provide detailed dosing schedules for injectable COVID-19 vaccines available as of January 27, 2023. mRNA vaccines are lipid coated, which facilitate the delivery of nucleoside-modified mRNA into host cells to express the SARS-CoV2 spike (S) antigen (eg, Pfizer and Moderna). The expression of the S antigen elicits the host immune response, which protects against COVID-19. Protein subunit vaccines contain fragments of COVID-19 spike (S) protein together with an adjuvant that facilitates the immune response to the protein (eg, Novavax). Once the antigen has been recognized by the immune system, the host will then be able to respond quickly to the actual virus spike protein, which protects against COVID-19 infection. There is currently one viral vector vaccine for COVID-19, which uses a recombinant, replication-incompetent adenovirus (Ad26) vector (eg, Janssen). This vector delivers a stabilized variant of the SARS-CoV2 spike (S) protein that will safely generate an immune response to elicit host immunity to COVID-19.[54]

Limitations of vaccine efficacy

Since the availability of COVID-19 vaccines, there has been varied acceptance among the general population. The initial efficacy of the mRNA vaccines against SARS-CoV2 was greater than 95%; however, over time the efficacy of these vaccines has significantly declined. With the emergence of the Omicron variant, a clinical study using test-negative case control design was developed to estimate the effectiveness of Pfizer-BioNTech (BNT162b2), Moderna (mRNA-1273), and AstraZeneca's (ChAdOx1) vaccines against the Omicron and the Delta variants in England. Compared with the preclinical trials that displayed an initial 95% efficacy for individuals receiving a primary series of BNT162b2, this study reported vaccine efficacy of 65.5% at 2 to 4 weeks, with decrease to 8.8% after 10 weeks.[55] In the population that received a booster dose, vaccine effectiveness was only 39.6% at an interval of 10 or more weeks.[55] The best results were recorded when a primary course of BNT162b2 was followed by a booster of mRNA-1273 which reported vaccine effectiveness of 73.9% at 2 to 4 weeks, and 64.4% at 5 to 9 weeks.[55]

The methodology of using vaccines from multiple platforms in a vaccine series for the prevention of a specific disease is not novel. Current practice globally to address vaccine shortages includes using crossover of COVID-19 vaccine types/manufacturers based on availability.[56] Mixing vaccines of different platforms has been demonstrated to result in a stronger cellular immune response, higher IgG and neutralizing antibodies.[57–60]

COVID-19 vaccination schedule recommendations are published by the CDC and are determined by age, immune status, and the specific vaccine type (see **Figs. 8** and **9**).

In August 2022, the US FDA announced the EUA of bivalent formulations of the Moderna and Pfizer-BioNTech COVID-19 vaccines for use as a single booster dose at least 2 months following primary or booster vaccination. These "updated boosters" contain 2 mRNA components of SARS-CoV2, one from the original strain and one that is found in both the BA.4 and BA.5 lineages of the Omicron variant.

SUMMARY

Global trends indicate that COVID-19 is transitioning from a pandemic to an endemic phase. As the SARS-CoV2 virus continues to evolve, our understanding and the body of literature will continue to rapidly expand. Clinicians are encouraged to review the most up-to-date information regarding variants of concern, vaccines, and treatment options.

Table 4
Injectable COVID-19 vaccinations[63-66]

	Pfizer/BioNTech	Moderna	Johnson & Johnson/ Janssen	Novavax	AstraZeneca
FDA status	Approved	Approved	EUA only as of August 2022	EUA only as of August 2022	Not approved as of August 2022
Vaccine platform	mRNA	mRNA	Recombinant DNA vector	rS viral protein plus Matrix-M™ adjuvant	Recombinant DNA vector
CDC recommended dosing schedule	See **Figs. 8** and **9**	See **Figs. 8** and **9**	See **Figs. 8** and **9**	See **Figs. 8** and **9**	See package insert
Common adverse effects	• Injection site reaction • Fatigue • Headache • Myalgias • Joint pain • Fever • Chills	• Injection site reaction • Fatigue • Headache • Myalgias • Joint pain • Fever • Chills	• Injection site reaction • Fatigue • Headache • Myalgias • Joint pain • Fever • Chills	• Injection site reaction • Fatigue • Headache • Myalgias • Joint pain • Fever • Chills • Nausea/vomiting • Anorexia	• Injection site reaction • Fatigue • Headache • Myalgias • Joint pain • Fever • Chills • Nausea/vomiting
Serious adverse effects	• Hypersensitivity reaction	• Hypersensitivity reaction	• Hypersensitivity reaction • Thrombosis and thrombocytopenia (Rare) • Guillain-Barre syndrome (Rare)	• Hypersensitivity reaction • Myocarditis • Pericarditis • Lymphadenopathy	• Hypersensitivity reaction • Thrombosis and thrombocytopenia (Rare) • Demyelinating disorders (Rare)

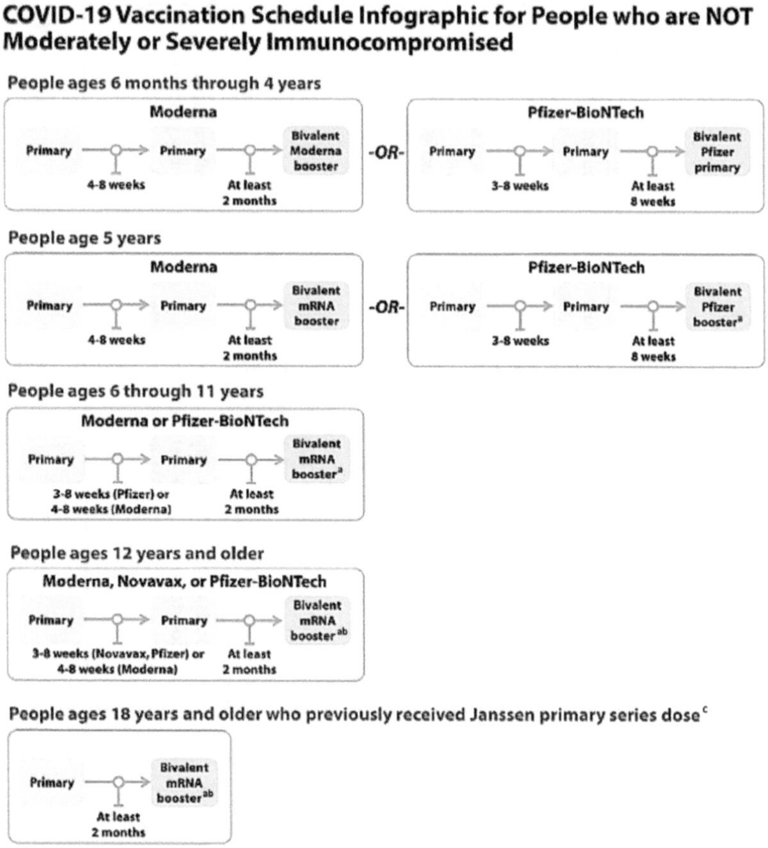

COVID-19 Vaccination Schedule Infographic for People who are NOT Moderately or Severely Immunocompromised

People ages 6 months through 4 years

People age 5 years

People ages 6 through 11 years

People ages 12 years and older

People ages 18 years and older who previously received Janssen primary series dose[c]

Fig. 8. COVID-19 vaccine schedule for people who are *not* immunocompromised. [a]For people who previously received a monovalent booster dose(s), the bivalent booster dose is administered at least 2 months after the last monovalent booster dose. [b]A monovalent novamax booster dose may be used in limited situations in people ages 18 years and older who completed a primary series using any COVID-19 vaccine, have not received any previous booster dose(s), and are able unable or unwilling to receive an mRNA vaccine. The monovalent Novavax booster dose is administered at least 6 months after completion of a primary series. [c]Janssen COVID-19 vaccine should only be used in certain limited situations. See https://www.cdc.gov/vaccine/covid-19/clinical-consideration/interlm-considerations-us-appendix,html#.appendix-a. (*Adapted from* Centers for Disease Control and Prevention.[61,62])

MIDDLE EAST RESPIRATORY SYNDROME
Prevalence, Mortality, and Economic Burden

The Middle East Respiratory Syndrome coronavirus (MERS-CoV) is one of the significant emerging viral infections in the twenty-first century. This infection is caused by a single-stranded positive-sense RNA virus,[67] which was first officially reported in Saudi Arabia in September 2012. However, it was later traced back to the first case in Jordan in April of the same year.[68,69] Since the identification of this new viral infection, it has spread through travel to many countries around the globe including the United States (US). Two confirmed cases in the US were reported in May 2014 from Indiana and Florida. These cases were among health-care workers who stayed and worked in Saudi Arabia.[67]

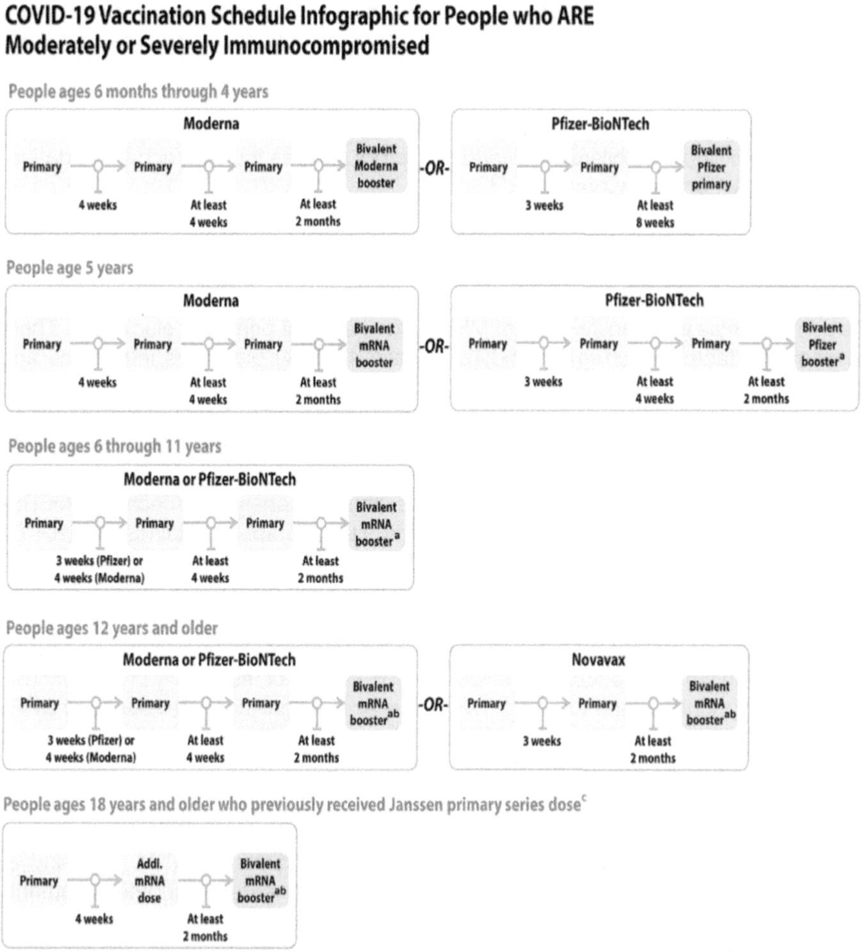

COVID-19 Vaccination Schedule Infographic for People who ARE Moderately or Severely Immunocompromised

People ages 6 months through 4 years

People age 5 years

People ages 6 through 11 years

People ages 12 years and older

People ages 18 years and older who previously received Janssen primary series dose[c]

Fig. 9. COVID-19 vaccine schedule for people who are moderately or severely immunocompromised. [a]For people who previously received a monovalent booster dose is administered at least 2 months after the last monovalent booster dose. [b]A monovalent novamax booster dose may be used in limited situations in people ages 18 years and older who completed a primary series using any COVID-19 vaccine, have not received any previous booster dose(s), and are able unable or unwilling to receive an mRNA vaccine. The monovalent Novavax booster dose is administered at least 6 months after completion of a primary series. [c]Janssen COVID-19 vaccine should only be used in certain limited situations. See https://www.cdc.gov/vaccine/covid-19/clinical-consideration/interlm-considerations-us-appendix,html#.appendix-a. (*Adapted from* Centers for Disease Control and Prevention.[61,62])

The original source of this viral infection has been linked to dromedary camels, from which the virus has jumped to humans perhaps during calving season.[70] Studies have suggested that MERS coronavirus is exclusively maintained in camels and the spread of the virus between humans has been poor.[70] In other words, the transmission from camels to humans has occurred many times, whereas the subsequent transmission from human to human has been limited.[71] Unfortunately, in 2015, a widespread outbreak occurred in South Korea.[71] This observed outbreak involved human-to-human transmission in a hospital setting, which led to 185 secondary cases from a single index case.[71] According to the World Health Organization (WHO), the worldwide total of laboratory-confirmed cases of MERS as of July 2022 was reported at 2591, including 894 fatalities, which translated to a case fatality rate of 37.2%.[72]

The economic impact of MERS has been very significant. The estimated loss reported from the South Korea outbreak within 1 year was on the order of hundreds of millions to billions of dollars from various sectors such as tourism, accommodation, food, beverage, and transportation.[73]

PATHOGENESIS AND COMPLICATIONS
Progression of Infection

The pathogenesis and transmission of MERS-CoV have not been fully elucidated. There are many host factors, such as dipeptidyl peptidase-4 (DPP4), proteases, interferons, and sialic acids that have been identified in vitro to potentially affect the infection process.[74] In particular the DPP4, also known as CD26,[75] has been known to play an important role as the functional receptor for MERS-CoV.[74,75] This enzyme could either be expressed on the cell surface or in aqueous solution, which is involved in many pathways cleaving various substrates, such as chemokines, neuropeptides, and hormones. The infection of MERS-CoV in human hosts is mediated by the interaction of the viral spike protein (S1) with DPP4 on the cell surface and the $\alpha2,3$-sialic acids.[74] There are other pathways that could potentially involve in virus–host interactions; however, they have been less studied. Once the virus has entered the host cell, it initiates transcription and translation of viral proteins within the host's cytoplasm to generate new viral particles. In human hosts, MERS-CoV replication primarily occurs in the lower respiratory tract, especially in the epithelial cells of the bronchioles and alveoli.[74] This is due to the significant prevalence of DPP4 in the lower pulmonary tract and its absence in the nasal epithelium.[74]

Transmission, Manifestations, and Risk Factors

MERS-CoV is an airborne infectious disease, which can be transmitted by inhaling the infectious respiratory droplets spread from infected individuals while coughing or sneezing.[76] Many human-to-human transmissions have occurred in inpatient settings, such as intensive care (ICU), or other ambulatory care settings such as dialysis centers. Transmission may also occur through fomites such as contaminated surfaces, devices, or equipment. Once exposed, the incubation period averages 5 to 12 days.[76]

The symptoms of MERS-CoV infection include rhinorrhea, fever, cough, fatigue, nausea, vomiting, GI symptoms, myalgia, splenic atrophy, lymphadenopathy, seizures, hepatic dysfunction, shortness of breath, and respiratory failure.[67,76] Nevertheless, the manifestation of the infection in human hosts may range from severe pneumonia to no significant symptoms.[74] Risk factors that could contribute to more severe disease are chronic kidney disease, diabetes, pulmonary diseases, or immune compromise.[76] Patients who have history of smoking or preexisting pneumonia were also found to have a higher rate of mortality.[77] In addition, patients diagnosed with chronic obstructive pulmonary disease have been shown to express higher levels of DPP4 in their lung tissue, subsequently increasing the susceptibility of MERS-CoV infection.[74,78] According to the autopsy data from human as well as animal models, the pathogenesis of severe MERS-CoV infection was highly associated with the upregulation of DPP4, especially in type 1 pneumocytes, which accounted for 95% of the total surface area of the alveoli. Damage of this pulmonary cell type caused by the viral infection eventually leads to significant morbidity.[66] Other risk factors of more severe disease also include advanced age and the inadequate or delayed response of type 1 interferon, which is a cytokine that functions as an inhibitor of viral replication in susceptible cells.[66]

Laboratory testing and diagnosis

The diagnosis of MERS-CoV infection may be achieved by obtaining a complete clinical history and diagnostic laboratory tests.[61,79] Clinical diagnosis involves a thorough medical history of clinical signs and symptoms as well as history of close contact and traveling to and from outbreak areas, which helps to rapidly screen and triage suspected cases. Since the symptomatic presentations of MERS are nonspecific, clinical history alone is not adequate. Further laboratory testing is required to confirm MERS-CoV infection. According to the CDC, these laboratory tests are categorized into either *molecular* or *serology* tests. The *molecular* tests are indicated for patients with active infection. These include real-time reverse-transcription polymerase chain reaction (rRT-PCR) assays. These molecular tests detect viral genetic material (ie, RNA) in collected specimens. As of this writing, there is no officially FDA-approved test available for MERS-CoV infection; however, there is one current rRT-PCR test available under EUA for the detection of MERS. When a suspected case of MERS-CoV presents, an rRT-PCR that detects at least 2 viral genetic targets should be ordered. The usual recommended genetic targets are the conserved domains ORF 1a and 1b or other targets including the regions upstream of gene E (upE), which is responsible for viral assembly; or gene S, which encodes for the spike protein that facilitates the binding of viral particles to the host cell; or gene N, which encodes the N protein that helps to regulate the viral replication.[79] In fact, WHO has recommended rRT-PCR that targets both the upE and ORF-1a regions because this test can detect as low as 5 copies of RNA from MERS-CoV.[80] In addition, the sensitivity and Sp of this test has also been reported at 95% and 100%, respectively.[79] Meanwhile, the sensitivity may range from 55% to 100% and Sp of 33% to 100% for tests that used the N gene as a target.[79]

The CDC also recommends collection of samples from multiple locations, including the upper respiratory tract by using NP or OP swabs; or lower respiratory tract by collecting sputum and/or tracheal aspirates; or serum; or stool samples.[67] Studies have suggested that the RNA of MERS-CoV may be detected in blood, stool, upper and lower pulmonary tracts, and urine.[67] Viral loads from the pulmonary specimens usually peak during the second week after the onset of symptoms.[67] Further, the positive rate from the cotton swab of the upper respiratory tract was up to 88.2%, which is lower than those samples from sputum or tracheal aspirate (ie, 100%).[67] Serum samples show approximately 33% of positivity for MERS-CoV RNA at initial diagnosis. Seropositivity has been shown to be associated with poorer outcomes.[81] The CDC recommends collection of collect samples of 2 to 3 mL of tracheal aspirate, or pleural fluid into a sterile collecting cup. The specimen may be stored at 2°C to 8°C up to 72 hours; otherwise, they may be stored at -70°C for a longer time. Of note, the NP and OP specimens may be collected and stored in the single vial under the same specified conditions.[68] Clinicians should consult with local laboratories for specific specimen collection and handling guidelines. There is an increasing number of commercially available tests for MERS-CoV; however, their performance may have not been validated and compared with the reference PCR testing.[71] In a patient who is under investigation for MERS-CoV, a single negative result of the rRT-PCR test confirms no current *active* MERS-CoV infection. Nevertheless, additional testing of other specimens should be completed to confirm negative results.[67] In a patient with confirmed MERS-CoV infection, the CDC recommends 2 consecutive negative rRT-PCR tests on all specimens to ensure clearance of the infection.[67] **Fig. 10** provides an algorithm for laboratory testing in suspected MERS-CoV infection.

When the result of rRT-PCR test is positive, it confirms MERS-CoV infection. However, if the result is negative, then the test should be repeated. If the repeat test result is positive, it also confirms the diagnosis. However, if the result of the second rRT-PCR

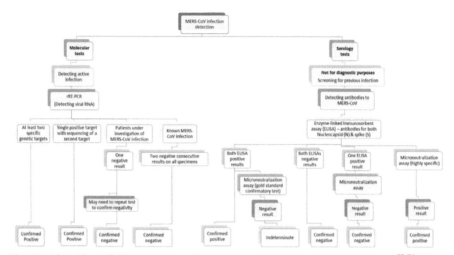

Fig. 10. Algorithm of CDC recommendations for suspected MERS-CoV infection.[67,79]

is negative, and the patient still shows clinical indication of suspected MERS-CoV infection, other serologic tests or nucleic acid sequencing are indicated. Positive result of either of these alternative tests confirm the diagnosis; otherwise, the patient has no indication of MERS-CoV infection (**Fig. 11**).[79]

Serology tests detect antibodies against MERS-CoV in patients who either have had an earlier infection or have been exposed to the virus. These tests are generally not for diagnostic purposes but for checking the development of immune response. The enzyme-linked immunosorbent assay (ELISA) was recommended as a screening test to detect the presence of antibodies against 2 viral targets including the nucleocapsid (N) and spike (S) proteins. When the ELISA result is positive, a microneutralization test is conducted to confirm the positive result. This microneutralization test detects the presence of antibodies that can neutralize the virus and inhibit viral entry. Although it is labor intensive and may take up to 5 days to turn around, this microneutralization test is considered as a gold standard for detecting antibodies in serum samples.[60] According to current data, the protein-based tests are less sensitive than nucleic acid-based tests and provide higher risk of false-positive results.[79] A decision algorithm similar to that used for the rRT-PCR test can be used for serology testing in patients with suspected MERS-CoV (see **Fig. 10**).

Pharmacologic Therapy

The treatment of MERS-CoV infection has been mostly supportive, which includes the administration of analgesics and antipyretics such as acetaminophen or nonsteroidal anti-inflammatory drugs (NSAIDs), as well as hydration and MV support. Other pharmacologic supportive therapies included chloroquine, nitazoxanide, silvestrol, steroids, and mycophenolate mofetil (MMF).[82] In addition, antiviral agents such as ribavirin, ritonavir/lopinavir, alisporivir, and interferons have shown inhibitory activity against MERS-CoV in vitro.[82] As of this writing, there is no highly effective therapeutic regimen that specifically treats MERS-CoV infection. However, various treatment strategies have been used with partial success. For example, immunotherapy from convalescent plasma and intravenous immunoglobulin (IVIG) has been exploited, whereas other combination therapies of antivirals together with an immunosuppressant such as cyclosporine, mycophenolic acid, or interferon-alpha have also been investigated.

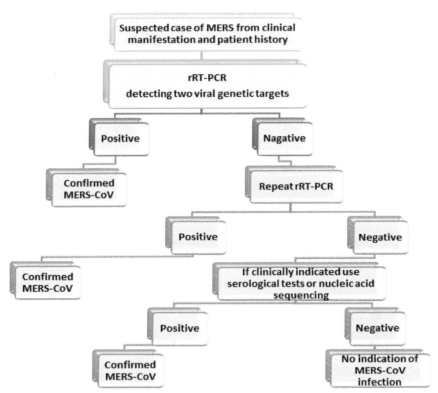

Fig. 11. Algorithm of suspected MERS-CoV infection using rRT-PCR for two viral genetic targets.[67,79]

Interestingly, ribavirin and interferon-alpha were reported to have synergistic effects during early infection,[76] whereas MMF showed synergistic effects with interferon-beta 1b.[82] The combination of interferon-alpha together with lopinavir, or ribavirin, or MMF has also been implemented.[82] Unfortunately, none of these studies has reduced the overall mortality rate in either human or animal models.[82,83] The role of antibiotics has been limited to patients who develop bacterial coinfection. Various antibiotic treatments may be considered; however, there are limited empiric data to support improved survival outcomes in this viral infection.[82] Until an effective prophylactic or therapeutic option becomes available, it is critically important to implement preventive measures by patient isolation, education, and supportive quarantine settings to prevent future outbreaks.

Vaccines
Despite several vaccine candidates under development, there is currently no vaccine licensed specifically for MERS.[84] MERS-CoV vaccine candidates are based mainly on the viral spike (S) protein (as the vital role in the viral infectivity), as well as other viral proteins including nucleocapsid (N) protein, envelope (E) protein, and NSP16.[85] There are currently 6 types of vaccines under investigation: viral vector-based vaccine, DNA vaccine, subunit vaccine, nanoparticle-based vaccine, inactivated-whole virus vaccine, and live-attenuated vaccine.[85] The first clinical study (phase 1b trial) of the ChAdOx1 MERS vaccine, conducted in Saudi Arabia, investigated the reactogenicity and immunogenicity of ChAdOx1 MERS in Middle Eastern adults.[84] Positive initial findings

led to a current phase 2 study, where a larger number of healthy adults, health-care workers, and occupationally exposed camel handlers will be recruited to explore vaccine safety and immunogenicity to prevent future MERS outbreaks. Limitations of this study were noted to include the small sample size and the open-label, nonrandomized, uncontrolled trial design.

SUMMARY

Although the development of MERS vaccines began with the emergence of MERS-CoV in 2012, vaccine developments have been slow, and most of the vaccine candidates have been evaluated in animal models.[85] The low occurrence of human-to-human transmission might be the reason for not prioritizing research in this area. However, the recent MERS outbreak in South Korea, which demonstrated virus emergence in second-generation and third-generation contacts, has reignited public awareness regarding the danger of MERS-CoV.[86] As no effective targeted treatment against MERS is currently available, the best solution is to develop a functional MERS vaccine to prevent MERS-CoV infection. More studies are focused on the viral vector-based and subunit vaccines. Even though many promising vaccine candidates have been proposed and reported, as of now, only 3 potential MERS-CoV vaccine candidates have progressed to phase I clinical trials: a DNA vaccine (GLS-5300) and 2 viral vector-based vaccines (MVA-MERS-S and MERS001).[85] It is likely that MERS vaccine for human use will not be available in the near future. Considerable efforts should be given to minimize delays in executing clinical trials, such as better understanding and coordination between sponsors, primary investigators, investigators, participants, and stakeholders.

CLINICS CARE POINTS

- Old age (ie, 80 years or older); gender (ie, male); and the presence of comorbid conditions, such as diabetes, chronic lung disease, cardiovascular disease, immunocompromising conditions, chronic kidney disease, and obesity, are risk factors for SARS-CoV2 with poor prognosis and death.
- The preferred method for detection of SARS-COV2 is the RT-PCR.
- The optimal days for RT-PCR testing via nasal or NP swab are days 3 to 4 after symptom onset.
- Asymptomatic testing can be expected to have a significantly high rate of false-negative results.
- Antigen tests can be used at point-of-care because they produce results in 15 to 30 minutes and may be useful as a biomarker to detect contagiousness.
- Vaccination is highly effective against COVID-19–associated hospitalization and death.
- Management of *nonhospitalized* patients included:
  - Nonpharmacological treatments such as drinking fluids, pulmonary hygiene, and resting in a prone position
  - Pharmacologic treatments such as ritonavir-boosted nirmatrelvir (Paxlovid) or remdesivir is recommended as the first-line therapy for patients who do not require supplemental oxygen.
  - Bebtelovimab and molnupiravir is reserved for cases where ritonavir-boosted nirmatrelvir and remdesivir are unavailable or their use is clinically inappropriate.
- Management of hospitalized patients may be subdivided into 3 treatment groups depending on the requirements of oxygen.
  - Patients who required minimal and conventional oxygen supplementation
    - May be treated with remdesivir or combination of remdesivir and dexamethasone. If remdesivir is not available, dexamethasone alone may be used.
    - If progressively increasing O_2 need, oral baricitinib or IV tocilizumab may be added.

○ Patients who required HFNC or NIV oxygen
  ■ Dexamethasone together with oral baricitinib (or alternatively tofacitinib) or IV tocilizumab (or alternatively sarilumab) are being considered first.
  ■ If baricitinib, tofacitinib, tocilizumab, or sarilumab is not available, dexamethasone alone may be given.
  ■ Remdesivir may be added in certain patients
○ Patients who required MV or ECMO
  ■ Dexamethasone plus oral baricitinib (or alternatively tofacitinib) or IV tocilizumab (or alternatively sarilumab) is given. Dexamethasone alone is considered, if baricitinib, tofacitinib, tocilizumab, or sarilumab is not available.

- The most effective primary prevention of COVID-19 infection is vaccination. COVID-19 vaccination schedule recommendations are published by the CDC and are determined by age, immune status, and the specific vaccine type (see **Figs. 8** and **9**).

- The MERS-CoV is caused by a single-stranded positive-sense RNA virus.

- This viral infection has been linked to dromedary camels, from which the virus has jumped to humans perhaps during calving season.

- There is one current rRT-PCR test available under EUA for the detection of MERS. When a suspected case of MERS-CoV presents, an rRT-PCR that detects at least 2 viral genetic targets should be ordered.

- The treatment of MERS-CoV infection has been mostly supportive, which includes the administration of analgesics and antipyretics such as acetaminophen or NSAIDs, as well as hydration and MV support.

- The IVIG has been used and other combination therapies of antivirals together with an immunosuppressant such as cyclosporine, mycophenolic acid, or interferon-alpha have also been investigated.

- Unfortunately, none of these studies has reduced the overall mortality rate in either human or animal models.

- Despite several vaccine candidates under development, there is currently no vaccine licensed specifically for MERS.

DISCLOSURE

The authors have nothing to disclose.

REFERENCES

1. GBD 2017 Influenza Collaborators. Mortality, morbidity, and hospitalisations due to influenza lower respiratory tract infections, 2017: an analysis for the Global Burden of Disease Study 2017. Lancet Respir Med 2019;7(1):69–89.
2. Abate SM, Checkol YA, Mantefardo B. Global prevalence and determinants of mortality among patients with COVID-19: A systematic review and meta-analysis. Ann Med Surg (Lond) 2021;64:102204 (In eng).
3. Disease Burden of Flu. Centers for Disease Control and Prevention website. Available at: https://www.cdc.gov/flu/about/burden/index.html. 2022. Accessed May 25, 2022.
4. Prevention CfDCa. Covid Data Tracker. Available at: https://covid.cdc.gov/covid-data-tracker/#prevention-measures-social-impact. Accessed September 6, 2022.
5. Prevention CfDCa. Covid Data Tracker. 2022. Available at: https://covid.cdc.gov/covid-data-tracker/#datatracker-home. Accessed July 16, 2022.
6. Dorjee K, Kim H, Bonomo E, et al. Prevalence and predictors of death and severe disease in patients hospitalized due to COVID-19: A comprehensive systematic

review and meta-analysis of 77 studies and 38,000 patients. PLoS One 2020; 15(12):e0243191 (In eng).

7. Hasoksuz M, Kilic S, Sarac F. Coronaviruses and SARS-COV-2. Turk J Med Sci 2020;50(Si-1):549–56 (In eng).

8. Chams N, Chams S, Badran R, et al. COVID-19: A Multidisciplinary Review. Front Public Health 2020;8:383 (In eng).

9. Singh SP, Pritam M, Pandey B, et al. Microstructure, pathophysiology, and potential therapeutics of COVID-19: A comprehensive review. J Med Virol 2021;93(1): 275–99 (In eng).

10. Ji YL, Wu Y, Qiu Z, et al. The Pathogenesis and Treatment of COVID-19: A System Review. Biomed Environ Sci 2021;34(1):50–60 (In eng).

11. Pascarella G, Strumia A, Piliego C, et al. COVID-19 diagnosis and management: a comprehensive review. J Intern Med 2020;288(2):192–206 (In eng).

12. Xiao F, Tang M, Zheng X, et al. Evidence for Gastrointestinal Infection of SARS-CoV-2. Gastroenterology 2020;158(6):1831–1833 e3.

13. Tan YK, Goh C, Leow AST, et al. COVID-19 and ischemic stroke: a systematic review and meta-summary of the literature. J Thromb Thrombolysis 2020;50(3): 587–95. In eng.

14. Pagali S, Parikh RS. Severe urticarial rash as the initial symptom of COVID-19 infection. BMJ Case Rep 2021;14(3):e241793.

15. Mir T, Almas T, Kaur J, et al. Coronavirus disease 2019 (COVID-19): Multisystem review of pathophysiology. Annals of Medicine and Surgery 2021;69:102745. Available at: https://www.ncbi.nlm.nih.gov/pmc/articles/PMC8381637/pdf/main.pdf. Accessed September 6, 2022.

16. Gomez-Mesa JE, Galindo-Coral S, Montes MC, et al. Thrombosis and Coagulopathy in COVID-19. Curr Probl Cardiol 2021;46(3):100742.

17. Prevention CfDCa. Guidance for Antigen Testing for SARS-CoV-2 for Healthcare Providers Testing Individuals in the Community. 2022. Available at: https://www.cdc.gov/coronavirus/2019-ncov/lab/resources/antigen-tests-guidelines.html. Accessed June 20, 2022.

18. Dinnes J, Deeks JJ, Berhane S, et al. Rapid, point-of-care antigen and molecular-based tests for diagnosis of SARS-CoV-2 infection. Cochrane Database Syst Rev 2021;3(3):Cd013705 (In eng).

19. Teymouri M, Mollazadeh S, Mortazavi H, et al. Recent advances and challenges of RT-PCR tests for the diagnosis of COVID-19. Pathol Res Pract 2021;221: 153443.

20. Lopera TJ, Alzate-Angel JC, Diaz FJ, et al. The Usefulness of Antigen Testing in Predicting Contagiousness in COVID-19. Microbiol Spectr 2022;10(2): e01962-21.

21. Prevention CfDCa. Interim Guidelines for COVID-19 Antibody Testing. 2022. Available at: https://www.cdc.gov/coronavirus/2019-ncov/lab/resources/antibody-tests-guidelines.html. Accessed July 21, 2022.

22. Mekonnen D, Mengist HM, Derbie A, et al. Diagnostic accuracy of serological tests and kinetics of severe acute respiratory syndrome coronavirus 2 antibody: A systematic review and meta-analysis. Rev Med Virol 2021;31(3):e2181.

23. Peeling RW, Heymann DL, Teo Y-Y, et al. Diagnostics for COVID-19: moving from pandemic response to control. Lancet 2022;399(10326):757–68.

24. Guan WJNZ, Hu Y, Liang WH, et al. Clinical characteristics of coronavirus disease 2019 in China. N Engl J Med 2020;382:1708–20.

25. Fu L, Wang B, Yuan T, et al. Clinical characteristics of coronavirus disease 2019 (COVID-19) in China: A systematic review and meta-analysis. J Infect 2020;80(6): 656–65 (In eng).

26. Kovacs A, Palasti P, Vereb D, et al. The sensitivity and specificity of chest CT in the diagnosis of COVID-19. Eur Radiol 2021;31(5):2819–24.

27. Radiology ACo. ACR Recommendations for the use of Chest Radiography and Computed Tomography (CT) for Suspected COVID-19 Infection. 2020. Available at: https://www.acr.org/Advocacy-and-Economics/ACR-Position-Statements/Re commendations-for-Chest-Radiography-and-CT-for-Suspected-COVID19-Infection. Accessed July 26, 2022.

28. Jacobi AC, BernheimA EC. Portable chest X-ray in coronavirus disease-19 (COVID-19): a pictorial review. Clin Imag 2020;(64):35–42. https://doi.org/10.1016/j.clinimag.2020.04.001.

29. Panel. C-TG. Coronavirus Disease 2019 (COVID-19) Treatment Guidelines. National Institutes of Health. . 2021 Available at: https://www.covid19treatmentguidelines.nih.gov/overview/clinical-spectrum/. Accessed July 27, 2022.

30. Yek C, Warner S, Wiltz JL, et al. Risk Factors for Severe COVID-19 Outcomes Among Persons Aged ≥18 Years Who Completed a Primary COVID-19 Vaccina-tion Series — 465 Health Care Facilities, United States, December 2020–October 2021. MMWR Morb Mortal Wkly Rep 2022;71:19–25.

31. Panel C-TG. Covid-19 Treatment Guidelines Clinical Management Summary. 2022 Available at: https://www.covid19treatmentguidelines.nih.gov/management/clinical-management/clinical-management-summary/. Accessed July 26, 2022.

32. Panel C-TG. Covid-19 Treatment Guidelines Therapeutic Management of Nonhospitalized Adults With COVID-19. 2022 Available at: https://www.covid19treatmentguidelines.nih.gov/management/clinical-management/nonhospitalized-adults–therapeutic-management/. Accessed July 26, 2022.

33. NIH. Antiviral Agents, Including Antibody Products. NIH. Available at: https://www.covid19treatmentguidelines.nih.gov/therapies/antivirals-including-antibody-products/summary-recommendations/. Accessed March 6, 2022.

34. Inc. P. Paxlovid (nirmatrelvir/ritonavir) (fact sheet). Available at: https://www.fda.gov/media/155050/download#:~:text=The%20dosage%20for%20PAXLOVID%20is,each%20active%20ingredient%20within%20PAXLOVID. Accessed June 28, 2022.

35. Veklury (remdesivir) (package insert). Foster City, CA: Gilead Sciences, Inc. Available at: https://www.gilead.com/-/media/files/pdfs/medicines/covid-19/veklury/veklury_pi.pdf. Revised June, 2022. Accessed June 20, 2022.

36. Merck and Co. Lagevrio (molnupiravir) (fact sheet). U.S. Food and Drug Admin-istration website. Available at: https://www.fda.gov/media/155054/download. Ac-cessed June 20, 2022.

37. Eli Lilly and Company. Bebtelovimab (fact sheet). U.S. Food and Drug Adminis-tration website. Available at: https://www.fda.gov/media/156152/download. Ac-cessed June 28, 2022.

38. LP AP. EVUSHELD (tixagevimab co-packaged with cilgavimab) (Fact sheet). US Food and Drug Administration website. 2022 Available at: https://www.fda.gov/media/154701/download. Accessed August 10, 2022.

39. Prevention CfDCa. COVID-19 Treatments and Medications. CDC. Available at: https://www.cdc.gov/coronavirus/2019-ncov/your-health/treatments-for-severe-illness.html. Accessed March 6, 2022.

40. Sanofi & Regeneron Pharmaceuticals I. KEVZARA (sarilumab) (Fact sheet). Sanofi & Regeneron Pharmaceuticals, Inc. 2018 Available at: https://products. sanofi.us/Kevzara/Kevzara.pdf. Accessed August 24, 2022.

41. Health Nlo. COVID-19 Treatment Guidelines: Interleukin-6 Inhibitors. 2021 https://www.covid19treatmentguidelines.nih.gov/therapies/immunomodulators/interleukin-6-inhibitors/. Accessed August 24, 2022.

42. Genentech, Inc. Actemra (tocilizumab). U.S. Food and Drug Administration website. Available at: https://www.fda.gov/media/150321/download. Accessed June 28, 2022.

43. Eli Lilly and Company. Baricitinib (fact sheet). U.S. Food and Drug Administration website. Available at: https://www.fda.gov/media/143823/download. Accessed June 28, 2022.

44. Health Nlo. COVID-19 Treatment Guidelines: Kinase Inhibitors: Janus Kinase Inhibitors and Bruton's Tyrosine Kinase Inhibitors. 2022 Available at: https://www.covid19treatmentguidelines.nih.gov/therapies/immunomodulators/kinase-inhibitors/. Accessed August 24, 2022.

45. Health Nlo. COVID-19 Treatment Guidelines: Corticosteroids. 2022 Available at: https://www.covid19treatmentguidelines.nih.gov/therapies/immunomodulators/corticosteroids/. Accessed August 24, 2022.

46. Panel. C-TG. Coronavirus Disease 2019 (COVID-19) Treatment Guidelines. National Institutes of Health. Therapeutic Management of Hospitalized Adults With COVID-19. 2022 Available at: https://www.covid19treatmentguidelines.nih.gov/management/clinical-management/hospitalized-adults–therapeutic-management/. Accessed July 27, 2022.

47. NIH. COVID-19 Treatment Guidelines. 2022 Available at: https://www.covid19treatmentguidelines.nih.gov/tables/management-of-hospitalized-adults-summary/. Accessed March 8, 2022.

48. Karampitsakos T, Papaioannou O, Tsiri P, et al. Tocilizumab versus baricitinib in hospitalized patients with severe COVID-19: an open label, randomized controlled trial. Clin Microbiol Infect 2023;29(3):372–8 (In eng).

49. Panel. C-TG. Coronavirus Disease 2019 (COVID-19) Treatment Guidelines. Special Populations. National Institutes of Health. 2022 Available at: https://www.covid19treatmentguidelines.nih.gov/special-populations/. Accessed August 3, 2022.

50. Panel. C-TG. Coronavirus Disease 2019 (COVID-19) Treatment Guidelines. Antithrombotic Therapy in Patients With COVID-19. National Institutes of Health. 2022 Available at: https://www.covid19treatmentguidelines.nih.gov/therapies/antithrombotic-therapy/. Accessed August 3, 2022.

51. NIH. COVID-19 Treatment Guidelines. 2022 Available at: https://www.covid19treatmentguidelines.nih.gov/tables/management-of-nonhospitalized-adults-summary/. Accessed March 7, 2022.

52. West E. China and India approve nasal COVID vaccines — are they a game changer? Nature 2022;609 (News) Available at: https://www.nature.com/articles/d41586-022-02851-0.pdf. Accessed August 3, 2022.

53. Sano K, Bhavsar D, Singh G, et al. SARS-CoV-2 vaccination induces mucosal antibody responses in previously infected individuals. Nat Commun 2022;13(1):5135.

54. Prevention CfDCa. Overview of COVID-19 Vaccines. 2022 Available at: https://www.cdc.gov/coronavirus/2019-ncov/vaccines/different-vaccines/overview-COVID-19-vaccines.html?s_cid=11758:different%20covid%20vaccines:sem.ga:p:RG:GM:gen:PTN:FY22. Accessed August 24, 2022.

55. Andrews N, Al E, Author Affiliations NA, et al. Covid-19 vaccine effectiveness against the Omicron (B.1.1.529) variant. N Engl J Med 2022;386(16):1532–46.
56. Prevention CfDCa. COVID Data Tracker. Atlanta, GA: US Department of Health and Human Services, CDC; 2022. Available at: https://covid.cdc.gov/covid-data-tracker. Accessed September 6, 2022.
57. Borobia AM, Carcas AJ, Perez-Olmeda M, et al. Immunogenicity and reactogenicity of BNT162b2 booster in ChAdOx1-S-primed participants (CombiVacS): a multicentre, open-label, randomised, controlled, phase 2 trial. Lancet 2021; 398(10295):121–30.
58. Benning L, Tollner M, Hidmark A, et al. Heterologous ChAdOx1 nCoV-19/ BNT162b2 prime-boost vaccination induces strong humoral responses among health care workers. Vaccines 2021;9(8):857. Available at: https://mdpi-res. com/d_attachment/vaccines/vaccines-09-00857/article_deploy/vaccines-09-00857.pdf?version=1628080404.
59. Rashedi R, Samieefar N, Masoumi N, et al. COVID-19 vaccines mix-and-match: The concept, the efficacy and the doubts. J Med Virol 2022;94(4):1294–9.
60. Schmidt T, Klemis V, Schub D, et al. Immunogenicity and reactogenicity of heterologous ChAdOx1 nCoV-19/mRNA vaccination. Nat med 2021;27(9):1530-1535. Available at: https://www.ncbi.nlm.nih.gov/pmc/articles/PMC8440177/pdf/41591_2021_Article_1464.pdf.
61. Prevention CfDCa. At-A-Glance COVID-19 Vaccination Schedules. Available at: https://www.cdc.gov/vaccines/covid-19/downloads/COVID-19-vacc-schedule-at-a-glance-508.pdf. Accessed August 31, 2022.
62. Prevention CfDCa. Interim Clinical Considerations for Use of COVID-19 Vaccines Currently Approved or Authorized in the United States. 2023 Available at: https://www.cdc.gov/vaccines/covid-19/clinical-considerations/interim-considerations-us.html. Accessed March 8, 2022.
63. Prevention CfDCa. Interim Clinical Considerations for Use of COVID-19 Vaccines Currently Approved or Authorized in the United States. 2022 Available at: https://www.cdc.gov/vaccines/covid-19/clinical-considerations/interim-considerations-us.html. Accessed March 8, 2022.
64. Administration UFD. COVID-19 Vaccines. Available at: https://www.fda.gov/emergency-preparedness-and-response/coronavirus-disease-2019-covid-19/covid-19-vaccines. Accessed August 31, 2022.
65. Novavax I. NOVAVAX COVID-19 VACCINE, ADJUVANTED (Fact Sheet). 2022 Available   at: https://www.fda.gov/media/159897/download.   Accessed September 6, 2022.
66. Astrazeneca I. COVID-19 Vaccine (ChAdOx1-S (recombinant)) (Package insert). 2021. Available at: https://www.fda.gov.ph/wp-content/uploads/2021/04/Package-insert-v3.0.pdf. Accessed August 31, 2022.
67. Yan Y, Chang L, Wang L. Laboratory testing of SARS-CoV, MERS-CoV, and SARS-CoV-2 (2019-nCoV): Current status, challenges, and countermeasures. Rev Med Virol 2020;30(3):e2106. https://doi.org/10.1002/rmv.2106 (In eng).
68. Prevention CfDCa. Middle East Respiratory Syndrome (MERS). 2019 Available at: https://www.cdc.gov/coronavirus/mers/about/index.html. Accessed April 20, 2022.
69. de Wit E, van Doremalen N, Falzarano D, et al. SARS and MERS: recent insights into emerging coronaviruses. Nat Rev Microbiol 2016;14(8):523–34 (In eng).
70. Dudas G, Carvalho LM, Rambaut A, et al. MERS-CoV spillover at the camel-human interface. Elife 2018;7. https://doi.org/10.7554/eLife.31257. In eng.

71. Bleibtreu A, Bertine M, Bertin C, et al. Focus on Middle East respiratory syndrome coronavirus (MERS-CoV). Med Mal Infect 2020;50(3):243–51 (In eng).
72. Organization WH. MERS Situation Update July 2022. World Health Organization Regional Office for the Eastern Mediterranean. 2022. Available at: https://applications.emro.who.int/docs/WHOEMCSR546E-eng.pdf?ua=1. Accessed September 6, 2022.
73. Heesoo Joo P, Brian A, Maskery PhD, et al. Economic Impact of the 2015 MERS Outbreak on the Republic of Korea's Tourism-Related Industries. Health Security 2019;17(2):100–8.
74. Widagdo W, Sooksawasdi Na Ayudhya S, Hundie GB, et al. Host Determinants of MERS-CoV Transmission and Pathogenesis. Viruses 2019;11(3). https://doi.org/10.3390/v11030280 (In eng).
75. Bosch BJ, Raj VS, Haagmans BL. Spiking the MERS-coronavirus receptor. Cell Res 2013;23(9):1069–70.
76. Al Mutair A, Ambani Z. Narrative review of Middle East respiratory syndrome coronavirus (MERS-CoV) infection: updates and implications for practice. J Int Med Res 2020;48(1). https://doi.org/10.1177/0300060519858030. 300060519858030.
77. Nam HS, Park JW, Ki M, et al. High fatality rates and associated factors in two hospital outbreaks of MERS in Daejeon, the Republic of Korea. Int J Infect Dis 2017;58:37–42. In eng.
78. Seys LJM, Widagdo W, Verhamme FM, et al. DPP4, the Middle East Respiratory Syndrome Coronavirus Receptor, is Upregulated in Lungs of Smokers and Chronic Obstructive Pulmonary Disease Patients. Clin Infect Dis 2017;66(1):45–53.
79. Chong ZX, Liew WPP, Ong HK, et al. Current diagnostic approaches to detect two important betacoronaviruses: Middle East respiratory syndrome coronavirus (MERS-CoV) and severe acute respiratory syndrome coronavirus 2 (SARS-CoV-2). Pathol Res Pract 2021;225:153565. https://doi.org/10.1016/j.prp.2021.153565 (In eng).
80. Shirato K, Nao N, Matsuyama S, et al. Ultra-Rapid Real-Time RT-PCR Method for Detecting Middle East Respiratory Syndrome Coronavirus Using a Mobile PCR Device, PCR1100. Japn J Infect Dis 2020;73(3):181–6.
81. Kim SY, Park SJ, Cho SY, et al. Viral RNA in Blood as Indicator of Severe Outcome in Middle East Respiratory Syndrome Coronavirus Infection. Emerg Infect Dis 2016;22(10):1813–6. In eng.
82. Rabaan AA, Al-Ahmed SH, Sah R, et al. MERS-CoV: epidemiology, molecular dynamics, therapeutics, and future challenges. Ann Clin Microbiol Antimicrob 2021;20(1):8. In eng.
83. Mo Y, Fisher D. A review of treatment modalities for Middle East Respiratory Syndrome. J Antimicrob Chemother 2016;71(12):3340–50.
84. Bosaeed M, Balkhy HH, Almaziad S, et al. Safety and immunogenicity of ChAdOx1 MERS vaccine candidate in healthy Middle Eastern adults (MERS002): an open-label, non-randomised, dose-escalation, phase 1b trial. Lancet Microbe 2022;3(1):e11-e20. (Available at: https://www.ncbi.nlm.nih.gov/pmc/articles/PMC8565931/pdf/main.pdf).
85. Yong CY, Ong HK, Yeap SK, et al. Recent advances in the vaccine development against Middle East respiratory syndrome-coronavirus. Front microb 2019;10:1781. (Available at: https://www.ncbi.nlm.nih.gov/pmc/articles/PMC6688523/pdf/fmicb-10-01781.pdf).
86. Organization WH. MERS Outbreak in the Republic of Korea, 2015. Available at: https://www.who.int/westernpacific/emergencies/2015-mers-outbreak. Accessed September 6, 2022.

Influenza Viruses

Brent Luu, PharmD, BCACP[a],*,
Virginia McCoy-Hass, DNP, MSN, RN, FNP-C, PA-C[a], Teuta Kadiu, RN, MSL[a],
Victoria Ngo, PhD[a], Sara Kadiu, PharmD[b], Jeffrey Lien, PharmD[c]

KEYWORDS

- Influenza viruses • Flu • Infection • *Orthomyxoviridae* • H1N1 • Hemagglutinin
- Neuraminidase

KEY POINTS

- The 3 genera of Influenza viruses that cause human disease are A, B, & C; however, influenza A & B are responsible for the annual epidemics with more than 500,000 deaths worldwide.
- Influenza associated with lower respiratory infections among adults older than 70 y.o has the highest mortality rate.
- High-risk patients such as obesity (BMI>30), pregnant women, smokers, infants (<6 months), and older adults (>65y.o) with influenza-like illness should be tested for influenza and treated appropriately to prevent mortality.
- Annual vaccination is the best means to prevent influenza infection; however, chemoprophylaxis with antiviral medication can be used for pre or postexposure prevention.

INTRODUCTION

Influenza viruses are RNA virus that belong to the *Orthomyxoviridae* family. Three genera of influenza viruses - A, B, and C - (IAV, IBV, ICV) cause human illness. A fourth genera, influenza D, does not cause human disease.[1] ICVs are endemic and typically cause mild illness. IAVs and IBVs are responsible for annual influenza epidemics, with an estimated 5 million infections and 500,000 excess deaths worldwide.[2] IBVs cause human disease only. They are currently classified in 2 lineages (B/Victoria and B/Yamagata) and cause localized epidemics.[2] IAVs cause both human and animal infection with zoonotic crossover. Because of the antigenic variability of IAVs, they are the cause of large epidemics and occasional pandemics. IAVs are further classified based on the antigenic properties of 2 surface glycoproteins. Currently, 18 hemagglutinin (H or HA) and 11 neuraminidase (N or NA) subtypes are identified. Viruses associated

[a] UC Davis Betty Irene Moore School of Nursing, 2450 48th Street, Sacramento, CA 95817, USA;
[b] Partners Pharmacy, 181 Cedar Hill Road Suite 1610, Marlborough, MA 01752, USA;
[c] Walgreens, 227 Shoreline Hwy, Mill Valley, CA 94941, USA
* Corresponding author.
E-mail address: brluu@ucdavis.edu

Physician Assist Clin 8 (2023) 531–553
https://doi.org/10.1016/j.cpha.2023.03.003
2405-7991/23/© 2023 Elsevier Inc. All rights reserved.
physicianassistant.theclinics.com

with all subtypes have not yet been isolated. The majority of IAV subtypes circulate in avian species, primarily wild birds.[1] Zoonotic IAV infection occurs in humans intermittently, often resulting in severe disease (eg, highly pathogenic H5N1 with a mortality rate of 60%). However, limited human-to-human transmission reduces the epidemic potential of these viruses. Only the H1, H2, and H3 subtypes have been associated with significant human-to-human transmission. Two IAV subtypes currently circulate in humans: A(H1N1) and A(H3N2).[1,3] There have been 5 IAV pandemics since the advent of the modern transportation age. The most severe was the 1918 H1N1 pandemic, in which an estimated 40 to 50 million people died. The most recent, the pH1N1/09 pandemic in 2009 to 2010, had an estimated mortality of 151,700 to 575,400.[3]

EPIDEMIOLOGY

Annual influenza A and B virus epidemics are associated with significant morbidity and mortality in the United States (US) and globally. The US Centers for Disease Control and Prevention (CDC) estimates that influenza caused "9 million–41 million illnesses, 140,000 to 710,000 hospitalizations and 12,000 to 52,000 deaths annually between 2010 and 2020."[4] Estimating the global burden of influenza is challenging due to the need for high-quality surveillance data. The 2017 Global Burden of Disease Study (GBD) estimated 11.5% of lower respiratory infection (LRI) episodes were due to influenza, resulting in an estimated 54.5 million episodes and 8.2 severe episodes, 9.46 million hospitalizations due to LRIs and 81.53 million hospital days globally. Influenza-associated LRI also resulted in 145,000 deaths of all ages in 2017. The influenza LRI mortality rate was highest among adults older than 70 years (16.4 deaths per 100,000), and the highest rate among all ages was in eastern Europe (5.2 per 100,000).[5] A 2018 statistical modeling study of data from 92 countries estimated that 291,243 to 645,832 seasonal influenza–associated respiratory deaths occur annually worldwide, with the majority (58%) among those age 65 years and over.[6] Global influenza activity was unusually low during the 2020 to 2021 season. From September 2020 to May 2021, the US incidence of positive influenza tests at clinical laboratories was 0.2% (1675 of 818,939 specimens). This can be compared with the prior 3 seasons (2017–2020), in which specimens testing positive for influenza peaked between 26.2% and 30.3%. As might be expected, the rates of influenza-associated hospitalization and death were also the lowest on record in recent decades.[7] CDC postulates that COVID-19 mitigation measures including the use of face masks, staying home, hand washing, school closures, reduced travel, increased ventilation of indoor spaces, and physical distancing, contributed to the decline in 2020 to 2021 flu incidence, hospitalizations, and deaths. Additionally, a record number of influenza vaccine doses were distributed in the US from 2020 to 2021, which also may have contributed to reduced flu illness.[7]

SCREENING AND DIAGNOSIS

Diagnostic tests available for the detection of influenza viruses in respiratory specimens include molecular assays (including rapid molecular assays, reverse transcription polymerase chain reaction (RT-PCR), and other nucleic acid amplification tests); and antigen detection tests (including rapid influenza diagnostic tests and immunofluorescence assays) and viral cultures.[8] Several rapid influenza diagnostic tests (RIDT) for antigen detection and rapid molecular assays (RMA) for influenza viral RNA or nucleic acid detection are CLIA-waived and available for outpatient clinic or home use (**Table 1**).

Table 1
Influenza virus testing methods

Testing Method[a]	Influenza Types Detected	Acceptable Specimens[b]	Sensitivity/Specificity[c]	Test Time	CLIA Waived[d]
Rapid Influenza Diagnostic Tests (RIDT)[e] (antigen detection)	A and B	NP swab, aspirate or wash, nasal swab, aspirate or wash, throat swab	Moderate to High/High	<15 min.	Yes/No
Rapid Molecular Assay [influenza viral RNA or nucleic acid detection]	A and B	NP swab, nasal swab	High/High	15–30 min	Yes/No
Immunofluorescence, Direct (DFA) or Indirect (IFA) Florescent Antibody Staining [antigen detection]	A and B	NP swab or wash, bronchial wash, nasal or endotracheal aspirate	Moderate/High	1–4 h	No
RT-PCR[f] (singleplex and multiplex; real-time and other RNA-based) and other molecular assays [influenza viral RNA or nucleic acid detection]	A and B	NP swab, throat swab, NP5 or bronchial wash, nasal or endotracheal aspirate, sputum	Very high/Very high	Varies (1–8 h, varies by assay)	No
Rapid cell culture (shell vials; cell mixtures; yields live virus)	A and B	NPswab, throat swab, NP5 or bronchial wash, nasal or endotracheal aspirate, sputum; (specimens placed in VTM8)		1–3 d	No
Viral tissue cell culture (conventional; yields live virus)	A and B	NP swab, throat swab, NP or bronchial wash, nasal or endotracheal aspirate, sputum (specimens placed in VTM)		3–10 d	No

[a] Serologic (antibody detection) testing is not recommended for routine patient diagnosis and cannot inform clinical management. A single acute serum specimen for seasonal influenza serology is uninterpretable and should not be collected. Serologic testing for the detection of antibodies to seasonal influenza viruses is useful for research studies and requires the collection of appropriately timed acute and convalescent serum specimens and testing of paired sera at specialized research or public health laboratories.

[b] Approved clinical specimens vary by influenza test. Approved respiratory specimens vary among FDA-cleared influenza assays. Consult the manufacturer's package insert for the approved clinical specimens for each test.

c General range provided, consult manufacturer's package insert for specific information.
d Clinical Laboratory Improvement Amendments (CLIA) of 1988. https://www.cms.gov/regulations-and-guidance/legislation/clia. CLIA waiver does not apply to all tests of this type; follow the manufacturer's directions.
e Chromatographic- and/or fluorescence-based lateral flow and membrane-based immunoassays. Some approved rapid influenza diagnostic assays utilize an analyzer reader device. The US Food & Drug Administration now requires RIDTs to achieve 80% sensitivity. Detection of viral antigen does not necessarily indicate the presence of viable infectious virus.
f Reverse transcription polymerase chain reaction, including FDA-approved test systems, reference laboratory testing using ASR or lab-developed reagents. Some approved molecular assays can produce results in approximately 60 to 80 min.
   Overview of Influenza Testing Methods. CDC. https://www.cdc.gov/flu/professionals/diagnosis/overview-testing-methods.htm.

During periods of influenza activity:

- Clinicians *should* test for influenza in high-risk patients[9–11] (**Table 2**) who present with influenza-like illness (ILI) if the test result will influence clinical management **Fig. 1**).[12]
- Clinicians *should* test for influenza in patients who present with acute respiratory symptoms (with or without fever) and either exacerbation of chronic medical conditions[10–12] (see **Table 2**) or known complication of influenza (eg, pneumonia) if the test result will influence clinical management **Fig. 1**).[13]
- Clinicians could consider influenza testing for patients not at high risk for influenza complications who present with ILI, pneumonia, or nonspecific respiratory illness (eg, cough without fever) and who are likely to be treated outpatient if the results might influence antiviral treatment decisions or reduce the use of unnecessary antibiotics, further diagnostic testing, time in the emergency department, or if the results might influence antiviral treatment or chemoprophylaxis decisions for high-risk household contacts (see **Fig. 1**).[13]
- Clinicians must also be able to appropriately interpret test results based on pretest probability. During periods of the influenza outbreak, the positive predictive value of RIDTs and RMAs for influenza is high and the negative predictive value is low.

Table 2
Patient-related risk factors for severe disease and complications in influenza infection

Risk Factor	Proposed Mechanisms
Obesity (BMI > 30)	• Diminished antibody response • Immune dysregulation due to adiposity • Deficit adaptive responses
Pregnancy or sex	• Increased immune tolerance during pregnancy to prevent fetal rejection • Sex steroid influence on immune response
Age	• Age < 6 mo: Lack of prior immunity; Immune immaturity (predominant Type 2 immunity, less effective response to viral infection) • Age > 65 y: Immunosenescence characterized by impaired humoral response and reduction in T cell receptor diversity and T cell function
Comorbid Conditions	Heart disease: systemic inflammatory response that increases the risk of acute cardiovascular event (heart failure, ischemic heart disease, and less commonly myocarditis, pericarditis) Lung disease (chronic obstructive pulmonary disease, asthma): impaired epithelial and immune cell function and altered fibroblast repair responses to viral infection Metabolic (obesity, metabolic syndrome): multifactorial, related to defective adaptive immune response, chronic dysfunction of inflammatory signaling related to adiposity, and insufficient responses to annual epidemic influenza virus vaccination Immunocompromise: Acquired or primary immunosuppressive states such as AIDS, immunosuppressive drug therapy, primary immunodeficiency syndromes
Tobacco Smoking	Impaired epithelial, immune, and fibroblast function

Sources: Flerlage T, Boyd DF, Meliopoulos V. et al. Nat Rev Microbiol. 2021;19:425–441.[9]; Rothberg MB, Haessler SD. Critical Care Medicine. April 2010;38(4suppl):e91-e97.[10]; Behrouzi, Bahar, and Jacob A. Udell. Current Atherosclerosis Reports. 2021;23(12):1-10.[11]

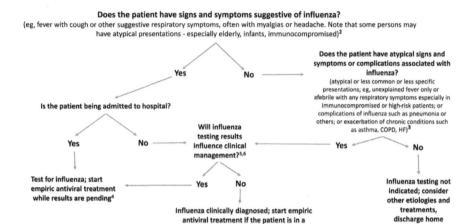

Fig. 1. Algorithm for influenza testing during periods of influenza activity. Timothy M Uyeki et al., Clinical Practice Guidelines by the Infectious Diseases Society of America: 2018 Update on Diagnosis, Treatment, Chemoprophylaxis, and Institutional Outbreak Management of Seasonal Influenza, Clinical Infectious Diseases, Volume 68, Issue 6, 15 March 2019, Pages e1–e47. https://doi.org/10.1093/cid/ciy866.

Fig. 2 outlines the interpretation of influenza testing results and clinical decision-making during periods when influenza viruses are circulating in the community.[9]

INFLUENZA PATHOGENESIS

Influenza belongs to the Orthomyxoviridae family of viruses, composed of 5 genera, 2 of which (influenza A and B) are medically relevant in humans. Influenza A virus subtypes are based on the antigenic properties of the 2 major viral surface glyco-proteins, hemagglutinin (HA) and neuraminidase (NA). Due to its antigenic vari-ability, type A is the cause of large epidemics and pandemics and associated with possible severe course of infection; type B causes localized epidemics, and type C causes mild infection, primarily in children. Because types A and B cause the majority of morbidity and mortality due to influenza, this section will focus on the pathogenesis of those types.[1,9,14] In humans, only viruses of the H1N1, H2N2, and H3N2 subtypes have circulated for extended periods. The H1–H16 HA and the N1–N9 NA subtypes are believed to be endemic to wild waterfowl. The ge-netic material of influenza viruses of the H17N10 and H18N11 subtypes has been detected only in bats. From their natural reservoirs, influenza A viruses can be transmitted across species, primarily poultry, pigs, and humans without becoming endemic. For example, avian influenza types A(H5N1) and A(H7N9) have caused serious illness in humans since 1997 and 2013, respectively, but have not spread efficiently among humans. In recent decades, studies have identified influenza HA protein as the major host restriction factor that limits interspecies transmission and the development of new virus lineages.[14] Influenza A has significant propensity for mutation, driven by viral mutation and genetic "reassortment" in which gene segments responsible for encoding HA or NA proteins are swapped between influ-enza viruses when two or more infect a host simultaneously. Small changes due to reassortment result in antigenic "drift" which is responsible for epidemic outbreaks of variable size every 1 to 4 years. Antigenic "shift" results when major changes in

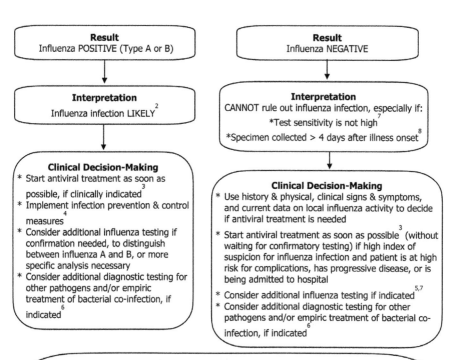

Fig. 2. Interpretation of influenza testing results and clinical decision-making during periods when influenza viruses are circulating in the community. Overview of Influenza Testing Methods. CDC. https://www.cdc.gov/flu/professionals/diagnosis/overview-testing-methods.htm.

gene sequences encoding HA and NA occur, creating novel strains capable of causing a pandemic.[1,9,15]

Influenza is spread primarily through large particle (>5μ) droplets and, to a lesser degree, by contact with fomites. Respiratory droplets containing influenza virus are exhaled when an infected person coughs, sneezes, or talks.[16] Once these droplets are inhaled by nearby people, the viral HA surface proteins bind to respiratory epithelial cell surface receptors that contain a sialosaccharide (sialic acid [SA]) linked to a galactose [Gal]). The influenza subtypes that cause human infection (A[H3N2], A [H1N1], and influenza B subtypes) bind preferentially to SA linked to Gal by α(2,6) linkage (SAα2,6Gal). SAα2,6Gal receptors are found predominantly in the upper respiratory tract (nasal mucosa, sinuses, pharynx, and larynx), to a lesser degree in the trachea and lower respiratory tract.[9,13] Sialosaccharides are present in cell types throughout the body. Thus, influenza virus-producing cells can be found in the mucous layer of the respiratory tract, the gastrointestinal tract, endothelial layers, myocardium, and brain. Influenza has also been shown to cause viremia in cases of severe disease.[16] Therefore, all respiratory secretions and bodily fluids, including diarrheal stools, of patients with influenza are considered to be potentially infectious, though the detection of influenza virus in blood or stool in influenza-infected patients is very uncommon.[17]

The influenza NA protein encodes a sialidase that cleaves sialic acids from sialyloligosaccharides, which permits the release of viruses from host cells.[13] Influenza matrix protein 2 (M2) is a transmembrane proton channel that facilitates efficient viral replication.[18,19] The influenza virus surface glycoproteins and M2 channel are illustrated in **Fig. 3**.[20]

Progression of Influenza Infection

The severity of human influenza infection ranges from asymptomatic to death. The development of symptoms or severe complications is mediated by adaptive immune memory from prior infection or immunization. Thus individuals such as young children without prior influenza virus exposure and those who are immunocompromised are at risk for severe disease.[9]

A meta-analysis of 56 human volunteer challenge studies evaluated viral shedding and clinical illness timelines in healthy adult subjects. After inoculation with influenza

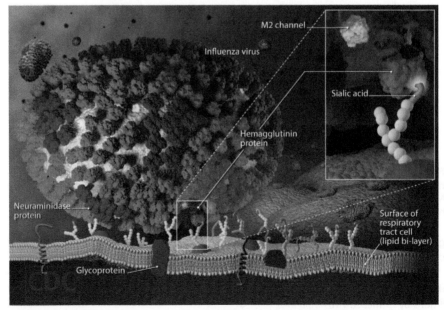

Fig. 3. Influenza Virus - surface glycoproteins and M2 Channels. Images of Influenza Viruses. CDC. https://www.cdc.gov/flu/resource-center/freeresources/graphics/images.htm.

virus, viral shedding increased rapidly within 24 hours, consistently peaked on day 2, and the average duration of viral shedding was 4 to 5 days and typically resolved by day 7. Symptomatic infection occurred in 66.9% of subjects. Importantly, viral shedding preceded symptom onset by 1 day. Symptom scores increased on day 1, with systemic symptom scores peaking on day 2 and total symptom scores on day 3. Symptoms resolved by day 8 to 9.[21]

Symptomatic influenza infection is characterized by abrupt onset of symptoms that include fever (typically 38o to 40o C), chills, headache, myalgias, anorexia, malaise, fatigue, upper respiratory symptoms (sore throat, nasal congestion, ear pain), and cough. While none of these is specific to influenza, the presence of respiratory and systemic symptoms during a period of confirmed local or epidemic influenza activity increases the likelihood of influenza infection.[9,22] Severe disease, resulting in hospitalization, pneumonia, acute respiratory distress syndrome, and death, is seen more frequently in high-risk populations (see **Table 2**).

Influenza Infection: Risk Factors and Complications

Several risk factors for severe disease and complications of influenza infection have been identified. Those at the extremes of age (>65 years or <6 months) are at particular risk. In the elderly, immunosenescence and increased prevalence of comorbid disease are hypothesized. In the very young, immature immune systems and absence of prior influenza exposure are thought to contribute.[9,10] Additional risk factors include obesity, pregnancy, sex (men have disproportionate hospitalization compared with nonpregnant women), chronic health conditions such as heart failure, chronic obstructive pulmonary disease, asthma, diabetes and metabolic syndrome, and environmental factors (eg, tobacco smoking) contribute to the severity of disease (see **Table 2**).

At-risk individuals are often less able to immunologically control infection, and because the infection itself can exacerbate the underlying condition (**Fig. 4**), complications of influenza are seen disproportionately among those with chronic medical

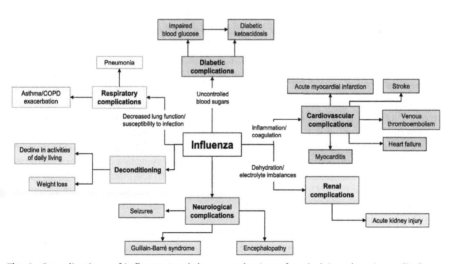

Fig. 4. Complications of influenza and the exacerbation of underlying chronic medical conditions by influenza virus infection. Alejandro E. Macias et al. The disease burden of influenza beyond respiratory illness, Vaccine, 39, Supplement 1, 2021, A6-A14, https://doi.org/10.1016/j.vaccine.2020.09.048.

conditions. Persons with chronic heart or respiratory disease are at highest risk of both severe influenza illness and exacerbated comorbidities, and this risk increases with age. This population accounts for up to 80% of hospital admissions with laboratory-confirmed influenza in adults, and 50% of those in children.[23]

GUIDELINES FOR TREATMENT AND CHEMOPROPHYLAXIS OF SEASONAL INFLUENZA
Treatment of Influenza

In the majority of cases, influenza is a self-limiting illness that can be treated on an outpatient basis with supportive care only. However, severe disease and complications may occur in high-risk populations. Current guidelines for the treatment of seasonal influenza recommend antiviral therapy for patients hospitalized with influenza, those with severe or progressive disease, and those at high-risk for complications from influenza (**Box 1**).[12]

Influenza chemoprophylaxis in community settings

Annual vaccination is the best means to prevent influenza infection. However, when vaccination is contraindicated or has not been administered, chemoprophylaxis with antiviral medication can be used for pre- or postexposure prevention and to control outbreaks in defined populations(see **Box 1**).[12]

Institutional or semiclosed settings include locations in which large groups of people live or congregate, including long-term care facilities, hospitals, schools, dormitories, correctional facilities, and cruise ships.[24] When a laboratory-confirmed influenza case is identified in such a setting, active surveillance for additional cases should begin as soon as possible. When 2 cases of laboratory-confirmed influenza are identified within 72 hours, outbreak control measures (**Table 3**),[13,17,25,26] including antiviral chemoprophylaxis should start as soon as possible. If same-day laboratory results are not available, chemoprophylaxis can be considered if influenza is suspected but not confirmed (see **Table 3**).[12,24]

Pharmacotherapy for Treatment and Chemoprophylaxis of Seasonal Influenza

Antiviral agents can shorten the duration of influenza illness and reduce the incidence of serious complications. Six prescription medications are currently approved by the US Food & Drug Administration (FDA) for the treatment or chemoprophylaxis of influenza. Four of these are recommended by the Centers for Disease Control for current use. Three chemically similar drugs—oseltamivir (oral), zanamivir (inhaled), and peramivir (intravenous)—are neuraminidase inhibitors (NAIs) that block the viral neuraminidase enzyme required for the release of the virus from the host cell. NAIs reduce the duration of symptoms and are effective against both influenza A and B viruses.[27–29] A new NAI, laninamivir (inhaled) is approved for use in Japan; it is not approved for use in the US. Baloxavir marboxil (oral) (hereafter baloxavir), a selective inhibitor of influenza cap-dependent endonuclease, blocks the proliferation of the influenza virus by inhibiting the initiation of mRNA synthesis.[30] The antiviral adamantanes (amantadine and rimantadine) target the M2 ion channel protein of influenza A viruses, though not influenza B. The adamantanes are not currently recommended for influenza treatment or chemoprophylaxis due to very high levels of resistance (>99%) among circulating influenza A viruses (A[H3N2] and A[H1N1]).[31] Antiviral resistance to the neuraminidases and baloxavir is currently low among circulating influenza viruses.[31] However, clinicians should monitor surveillance data on the susceptibility of circulating influenza viruses to the recommended antivirals each flu season. In the United States, these data are published by the CDC (https://www.cdc.gov/flu/weekly/index.htm).

Box 1
Summary of Guidelines for treatment and chemoprophylaxis of seasonal influenza

Treatment of Seasonal Influenza

- Initiate antiviral treatment as soon as possible for adults and children with documented or suspected influenza, regardless of vaccination history, who are:
  o Hospitalized with influenza.
  o Outpatients with severe or progressive disease, regardless of illness duration.
  o Outpatients at high risk of complications from influenza.
  o Younger than 2 years or ≥65 years.
  o Currently pregnant or within 2 weeks postpartum.
- Consider antiviral treatment for adults and children with documented or suspected influenza, who are *not* at high risk of influenza complications, regardless of vaccination history, who are:
  o Outpatients with illness onset ≤2 days before presentation.
  o Symptomatic outpatient who are household contacts of persons who are at high risk of influenza complications.
  o Symptomatic healthcare providers who care for patients who are at high risk of developing influenza complications.

Antiviral PRE-exposure Chemoprophylaxis to Prevent Influenza in the Absence of Institutional Outbreak
- Antiviral drugs should not be used for routine or widespread preexposure chemoprophylaxis outside of institutional outbreaks.
- *Consider* antiviral chemoprophylaxis for the duration of the influenza season for adults and children age ≥3 months who have the highest risk of influenza complications (eg, persons on immunosuppressant therapy).
- *Consider* short-term antiviral chemoprophylaxis for unvaccinated for adults and children age 3 months and over who have the highest risk of influenza complications in whom influenza vaccination is expected to be effective.
- *Consider* short-term antiviral chemoprophylaxis for unvaccinated for adults, including healthcare workers, and for children ≥3 months who have close contact with persons at high risk for influenza complications when vaccination is contraindicated or unavailable and these high-risk persons cannot take antiviral chemoprophylaxis.
- *Consider* educating patients and patients to arrange for early empiric antiviral treatment as an alternative to antiviral chemoprophylaxis

Antiviral POST-exposure Chemoprophylaxis to Prevent Influenza in Community Settings
- Consider postexposure antiviral chemoprophylaxis for asymptomatic adults and children aged ≥3 months who are at very high risk of developing complications from influenza and for whom influenza vaccination is contraindicated, unavailable, or expected to have low effectiveness, after household exposure to influenza.
- Consider postexposure antiviral chemoprophylaxis (AND influenza vaccination) for adults and children aged ≥3 months who are unvaccinated and are household contacts of a person at very high risk of complications from influenza, after exposure to influenza.
- Consider educating patients/parents and arranging for early empiric initiation of antiviral treatment as an alternative to postexposure antiviral chemoprophylaxis.
- IF chemoprophylaxis is given, administer postexposure antiviral chemoprophylaxis as soon as possible after exposure, ideally no later than 48 hours after exposure.
- Do not administer once-daily postexposure antiviral chemoprophylaxis if >48 hours have elapsed since exposure. Full-dose empiric antiviral treatment should be initiated as soon as symptoms occur, if treatment is indicated
- In nonoutbreak settings, administer postexposure antiviral chemoprophylaxis for 7 days after the most recent exposure to a close contact with influenza.
- Test for influenza and switch to antiviral treatment dosing in persons receiving postexposure antiviral chemoprophylaxis who become symptomatic, preferably with an antiviral drug with a different resistance profile if not contraindicated.

Implementation of Chemoprophylaxis for Control of Influenza in Institutional Settings

- Begin active surveillance for additional cases as soon as possible when one laboratory-confirmed influenza case is identified in an institutional setting.
- Begin outbreak control measures (see **Table 4**) as soon as possible, including antiviral chemoprophylaxis of residents/patients, when 2 cases of laboratory-confirmed influenza are identified within 72 hours of each other and continue active surveillance.
- Consider implementation of outbreak control measures as soon as possible if one or more residents/patients have suspected influenza and same-day results of influenza molecular testing are not available.
- When an influenza outbreak has been identified in an institutional setting, influenza testing should be done for any resident/patient with one or more acute respiratory symptoms, with or without fever, or any of the following without respiratory symptoms: temperature elevation or reduction, or behavioral change (delirium).
- Empiric antiviral treatment should be administered as soon as possible to any resident/patient with suspected influenza during an influenza outbreak without waiting for the results of influenza diagnostic testing.
- Antiviral chemoprophylaxis should be administered as soon as possible to all exposed residents/patients who do not have suspected or laboratory-confirmed influenza regardless of influenza vaccination history, in addition to the implementation of all other recommended influenza outbreak control measures, when an influenza outbreak has been identified in a long-term care facility or hospital.
- Antiviral chemoprophylaxis should be administered to residents on outbreak-affected units, in addition to implementing active daily surveillance for new influenza cases throughout the facility.
- Consider antiviral chemoprophylaxis for unvaccinated staff, including those for whom chemoprophylaxis may be indicated based upon underlying conditions of the staff or their household members (see recommendations 8–12) for the duration of the outbreak.
- Consider antiviral chemoprophylaxis for 14 days postvaccination for staff who receive inactivated influenza vaccine during an institutional influenza outbreak.
- Consider antiviral chemoprophylaxis for staff regardless of influenza vaccination status to reduce the risk of short staffing in facilities and wards whereby clinical staff are limited and to reduce staff reluctance to care for patients with suspected influenza.
- Administer antiviral chemoprophylaxis for 14 days and continue for at least 7 days after the onset of symptoms in the last case identified during an institutional influenza outbreak.

Adapted from Timothy M Uyeki et al., Clinical Practice Guidelines by the Infectious Diseases Society of America: 2018 Update on Diagnosis, Treatment, Chemoprophylaxis, and Institutional Outbreak Management of Seasonal Influenza, Clinical Infectious Diseases, Volume 68, Issue 6, 15 March 2019, Pages e1–e47, https://doi.org/10.1093/cid/ciy866.

The CDC recommends oral oseltamivir for patients with severe, complicated, or progressive influenza illness who are not hospitalized. For hospitalized influenza patients antiviral therapy with oral or enteric oseltamivir is recommended as soon as possible.[31] A comparison of the currently recommended influenza antiviral medications is in **Table 4**. The recommended dosage, duration, and adverse effects of influenza antiviral medications for treatment or chemoprophylaxis are detailed in **Table 5**.[32–35] Antiviral therapy has been demonstrated to reduce morbidity and oration in hospitalized influenza patient, even if started greater than 48 hours after onset of symptoms. There are insufficient data showing clinical benefit in hospitalized influenza patients to recommend inhaled zanamivir, oral baloxavir, or intravenous peramivir in this population.[31] Outpatients with suspected or confirmed influenza who have progressive disease or high risk for complications should also begin antiviral therapy as soon as possible, even if > 48 hours since illness onset. Non–high-risk outpatients with suspected or confirmed influenza can begin antiviral therapy if treatment can be started within 48 hours of symptom onset.[12,31] In a meta-analysis of 26 controlled trials including 11,987 subjects comparing the safety and

Table 3
Precautions to prevent the spread of influenza in community and institutional settings

Standard Precautions for all Patient Care[a]	Transmission-Based Precautions[a,b]
• Perform hand hygiene before and after each patient contact. • Use personal protective equipment (PPE) whenever there is an expectation of possible exposure to infectious material. • Follow respiratory hygiene/cough etiquette principles. • Proper handling and cleaning of patient care equipment and devices. • Clean and disinfect the environment appropriately. • Handle trash, textiles, and laundry carefully. • Follow safe injection practices, including proper handling and disposal of sharps. • Wear a surgical mask when performing lumbar punctures. • Ensure appropriate patient/resident placement.	• For patients in healthcare facilities or other institutional settings with suspected or confirmed influenza, implement droplet precautions[c] PLUS contact precautions[d] for 7 d after illness onset or until 24 h after fever and respiratory symptoms resolve, whichever is longer.[e,f] • Exercise caution when performing aerosol-generating procedures (eg, bronchoscopy, elective intubation, suctioning).[g] • Limit visitors for patients in isolation for influenza to persons necessary for the patient's care and emotional health. If consistent with facility policy, visitors can be advised to contact their healthcare provider (HCP) for information on influenza vaccination.

[a] Standard precautions are recommended by the CDC for inpatient and outpatient care settings, including care of ill residents in congregate residential settings (eg, dormitories, correctional facilities).
[b] .Implement all standard precautions AND transmission-based precautions specific to influenza.
[c] Droplet precautions include: Source control (put a mask on the patient); appropriate patient placement; use of PPE (face mask, or N95 respirator if indicated—see #7 below); limit transport and movement of patients (https://www.cdc.gov/infectioncontrol/basics/transmission-based-precautions.html).
[d] Contact precautions include: Appropriate patient placement; use of PPE, including gloves and gown; limit transport and movement of patient; use disposable or dedicated patient-care equipment; prioritized cleaning and disinfection of room (https://www.cdc.gov/infectioncontrol/basics/transmission-based-precautions.html).
[e] Influenza is spread primarily large (>5μ) droplets; and less commonly by direct contact with fomites. If coinfection with SARS-CoV2 (Covid19) is suspected, initiate airborne precautions plus contact precautions.
[f] Persons with influenza are most contagious in the first 3 to 4 d after the onset of symptoms. Viral shedding, and thus contagiousness, may span from 1 d before to 7 d after symptom onset. Young children and those with immunocompromise may shed viruses for longer periods.
[g] Avoid these procedures unless postponement will compromise care. Ensure that HCP present during the procedure are offered influenza vaccination. Conduct these procedures in and airborne infection isolation room if possible and consider the use of portable HEPA vibration units. Ensure the use of PPE (gown, gloves, and face shield or goggles). HCP should wear a fitted N95 respirator or equivalent (eg, powered air purifying respirator) during the procedure. Complete environmental surface cleaning after the procedure.
Sources: Neumann G, Kawaoka Y. Virology. 2015;479–480:234-246;[13] CDC. https://www.cdc.gov/flu/professionals/infectioncontrol/healthcaresettings.htm;[17] CDC. https://www.cdc.gov/infection control/basics/standard-precautions.html;[25] CDC.https://www.cdc.gov/infectioncontrol/guidelines/isolation/appendix/type-duration-precautions.html#I.[26]

efficacy of the four recommended influenza antivirals (the NAIs oseltamivir, zanamivir, peramivir, and the endonuclease inhibitor baloxavir), zanamivir was associated with the greatest reduction in symptom duration and baloxavir was associated with the lowest risk of influenza-related complications. Nausea and vomiting were the most common adverse effects.[28] One randomized, double-blind controlled trial (n = 1163) comparing baloxavir to placebo and to oseltamivir in high-risk adolescent

Table 4
Antiviral medications for treatment and chemoprophylaxis of influenza

Antiviral Agent	Activity Against	Indication	Recommended For	Not Recommended For
Oseltamivir (Oral)	Influenza A and B	Treatment	Any age[a]	Hypersensitivity to drug or ingredient
		Chemoprophylaxis	≥3 mo	Hypersensitivity to drug or ingredient
Zanamivir (Inhaled)	Influenza A and B	Treatment	≥7 y[b]	People with underlying respiratory disease (eg, asthma, COPD)[b]
		Chemoprophylaxis	≥5 y	
Peramivir (Intravenous)	Influenza A and B[c]	Treatment	≥6 mo[c]	Hypersensitivity to drug or ingredient
		Chemoprophylaxis[d]	Not recommended	Hypersensitivity to drug or ingredient
Baloxavir (Oral)	Influenza A and B[e]	Treatment	≥12 y[e]	Hypersensitivity to drug or ingredient and pregnancy or lactation
		Chemoprophylaxis	Postexposure prophylaxis in ages ≥12 y[f]	Hypersensitivity to drug or ingredient and pregnancy or lactation

Abbreviations: COPD, chronic obstructive pulmonary disease; N/A, not applicable.

[a] Oral oseltamivir is FDA-approved of acute uncomplicated influenza within 2 d of illness onset in people 14 d and older, and for chemoprophylaxis in people ≥1 y. Although not part of the FDA-approved indications, use of oral oseltamivir for the treatment of influenza in infants less than 14 day old, and for chemoprophylaxis in infants 3 mo to 1 y, is recommended by the CDC and the American Academy of Pediatrics. due to limited data, use of oseltamivir for chemoprophylaxis is not recommended in children younger than 3 month old, unless the situation is judged critical.

[b] Inhaled zanamivir is contraindicated in patients with underlying airway disease such as asthma or COPD, and those with a history of allergy to lactose or milk protein.

[c] Intravenous peramivir is FDA-approved of acute uncomplicated influenza within 2 d of illness onset in people ≥6 mo. Peramivir efficacy is based on clinical trials versus placebo for which the predominant influenza virus was type A; there is limited data on activity against influenza type B.

[d] There are no data for use of peramivir for chemoprophylaxis of influenza.

[e] Oral baloxavir marboxil is FDA-approved for the treatment of acute uncomplicated influenza within 2 d of illness onset in people aged ≥12 y who are otherwise healthy, or at high risk of developing influenza-related complications. The safety and efficacy of baloxavir for the treatment of influenza have been established in pediatric patients ≥12 y weighing at least 40 kg. For patients with influenza B virus infection, baloxavir significantly reduced the median time to the improvement of symptoms compared with oseltamivir by more than 24 h. However, there are no available data for baloxavir treatment of influenza in pregnant women, immunocompromised people, or in people with severe influenza who are not hospitalized.

[f] Baloxavir is FDA-approved postexposure prophylaxis of influenza in persons aged ≥12 y.

Influenza Antiviral Medications: Summary for Clinicians. CDC. https://www.cdc.gov/flu/professionals/antivirals/summary-clinicians.htm.

and adult outpatients found the efficacy of single-dose baloxavir was comparable to oseltamivir, with a lower adverse event profile (comparable to placebo).[36] A double-blind, placebo-controlled trial found that combination neuraminidase inhibitor and baloxavir for the treatment of hospitalized influenza patients aged ≥12 years did not result in superior clinical benefit compared with neuraminidase inhibitor monotherapy, though the combination of baloxavir and NAI did not significantly increase adverse events. Thus, the routine combination of antivirals is not recommended, even in hospitalized patients.[37]

Table 5

Antiviral medications for treatment or chemoprophylaxis of influenza: recommended dosage, duration, and adverse events

Antiviral Agent	Use	Children	Adults	Adverse Events	Drug Interactions
Oseltamivir (Oral)	Treatment (5 d)[a]	If < 1 year old[b]: 3 mg/kg/dose twice daily[c,d] If ≥1 y, dose varies by weight: >15–23 kg, dose is 45 mg twice daily >23–40 kg, dose is 60 mg twice daily >40 kg, dose is 75 mg twice daily	75 mg twice daily	Nausea, vomiting, headache. Postmarketing reports of serious skin reactions and sporadic, transient neuropsychiatric events[f]	intranasal LAIV[g]
	Chemo-prophylaxis (7 d)[e]	<3 mo, not recommended[e] ≥3 mo to <1 y[b]: 3 mg/kg/dose once daily[c] ≥1 y, dose varies by weight: >15–23 kg, dose is 45 mg once daily >23–40 kg, dose is 60 mg once daily >40 kg, dose is 75 mg once daily	75 mg once daily		
Zanamivir[h] (Inhaled)	Treatment (5 d)	Children ≥7 y: 10 mg (two 5-mg inhalations) twice daily	10 mg (two 5-mg inhalations) twice daily	Risk of bronchospasm, especially in the setting of underlying airway disease Sinusitis, and dizziness Post marketing reports of serious skin reactions and sporadic, transient neuropsychiatric events[f]	Intranasal LAIV[g]
	Chemo-prophylaxis (7 d)[e]	Children ≥5 y: 10 mg (two 5-mg inhalations) once daily	10 mg (two 5-mg inhalations) once daily		

(continued on next page)

Table 5
(continued)

Antiviral Agent	Use	Children	Adults	Adverse Events	Drug Interactions
Peramivir[i] (Intravenous [IV])	Treatment (1 d)[a]	Age 6 mo to 12 y: One 12 mg/kgdose, up to 600 mg maximum, by IV infusion over a minimum of 15 min	≥13 y: One 600 mg dose, via IV infusion over a minimum of 15 min	Diarrhea. Post marketing reports of serious skin reactions and sporadic, transient neuropsychiatric events[f]	Intranasal LAIV7
	Chemo-prophylaxis[i]	Not recommended	Not recommended		
Baloxavir[i] (Oral)	Treatment (1 d)[a]	≥5y.o: [<20kg] 2 mg/kg/dose orally x1 [20-79 kg] 40mg orally x 1 [≥80 kg] 80 mg orally x 1	≥12 y: Weight <80 kg: One 40 mg dose Weight ≥80 kg: One 80 mg dose[j]	None more common than placebo in clinical trials	Intranasal LAIV9 Polyvalent cation-containing products (eg, laxative, antacids, mineral supplements)[k]
	Chemo-prophylaxis[j]	≥5y.o: [<20kg] 2 mg/kg/dose orally x1; [20-79 kg] 40mg orally x 1; [≥80 kg] 80 mg orally x 1	≥12 y: Weight <80 kg: One 40 mg dose Weight ≥80 kg: One 80 mg dose[j]		

Abbreviations: LAIV, live attenuated influenza vaccine.

[a] Longer treatment duration may be needed for severely ill patients.

[b] Oral oseltamivir is approved by the FDA for the treatment of acute uncomplicated influenza within 2 d of illness onset with twice-daily dosing in people 14 d and older, and for chemoprophylaxis with once-daily dosing in people ≥1 y. Although not part of FDA-approved indications, the use of oral oseltamivir for the treatment of influenza in infants less than 14 day old, and for chemoprophylaxis in infants 3 mo to 1 y of age, is recommended by CDC and the American Academy of Pediatrics.[32]

[c] This FDA-approved oral oseltamivir treatment dose for infants 14 d and older and less than 1 year old provides oseltamivir exposure in children similar to that achieved by the approved dose of 75 mg orally twice daily for adults, as shown in 2 studies of oseltamivir pharmacokinetics in children.[33,34] The American Academy of Pediatrics recommended an oseltamivir treatment dose of 3.5 mg/kg orally twice daily for infants 9 to 11 month old, based on data that indicated the higher dose of 3.5 mg/kg was needed to achieve the protocol-defined targeted exposure for this cohort as defined in the CASG 114 study.[34]

[d] Current weight-based dosing recommendations are not appropriate for premature infants. Immature renal function in premature infants may result in slower clearance of oral oseltamivir leading to very high drug concentrations at doses recommended for full-term infants. CDC recommends dosing as also recommended by the American Academy of Pediatrics.[32]

[e] See Implementation of Chemoprophylaxis for Control of Influenza in Institutional Settings (see **Table 3**) for details regarding the duration of chemoprophy-laxis for outbreaks in institutional settings.

f Self-injury or delirium; mainly reported among Japanese pediatric patients.

g Concurrent administration of antiviral drugs with intranasal LAIV may inhibit viral replication of LAIV and thus decrease vaccine effectiveness. LAIV should not be given within: 48 h of oseltamivir or zanamivir administration within 48 h of planned vaccination; 5 d of peramivir administration; or 17 d of baloxavir administration. Persons who receive these antiviral medications within 2 weeks after receiving LAIV should be revaccinated with another appropriate influenza vaccine (eg, IIV or RIV4).

h Inhaled zanamivir is approved for the treatment of acute uncomplicated influenza within 2 d of illness onset with twice-daily dosing in people aged ≥7 y; and for chemoprophylaxis with once-daily dosing in people aged ≥5 y.

i Intravenous peramivir is approved for the treatment of acute uncomplicated influenza within 2 d of illness onset with a single dose in people aged ≥6 mo. There are no data for use of peramivir for chemoprophylaxis of influenza.

j Oral baloxavir is FDA-approved for the treatment and the post-exposure prophylaxis of uncomplicated influenza in adults and pediatric patients. These patients are at age ≥5 y and older, who are otherwise healthy with onset of symptoms no more than 48 hours.

k Coadministration of baloxavir with polyvalent cation-containing products can decrease plasma concentrations of baloxavir which may reduce efficacy. Baloxavir should not be administered with dairy products, calcium-fortified beverages, polyvalent cation-containing laxatives, antacids, or oral supplements (eg, calcium, iron, magnesium, selenium, or zinc).[35]

Influenza Antiviral Medications: Summary for Clinicians. CDC. https://www.cdc.gov/flu/professionals/antivirals/summary-clinicians.htm.

Vaccines

Annual vaccination is the best method for preventing or mitigating the impact of seasonal and pandemic influenza, which can prevent or reduce the severity of influenza infection. As previously discussed, the propensity of IAV for antigenic drift/shift allows influenza to evade the host adaptive immune response from prior infection or vaccination.[38]

The CDC Advisory Committee on Immunization Practices (ACIP) recommends that with rare exceptions, everyone age 6 months and older should get an influenza vaccine every season. This recommendation is particularly important for people who are at high risk of developing serious influenza complications (see **Table 2**).[12,39] Current available influenza vaccines include quadrivalent inactivated influenza vaccine [IIV4], recombinant influenza vaccine [RIV4], or live attenuated influenza vaccine (LAIV4). CDC updates specific recommendations for influenza vaccination by age group and based upon anticipated circulating influenza strains annually. For the 2022 to 2023 flu season, all influenza vaccines are quadrivalent and designed to protect against 4 flu strains, including 2 influenza A viruses and 2 influenza B viruses (**Table 6**). A smmary of these annual recommendations can be found at https://www.cdc.gov/flu/professionals/vaccination/vax-summary.htm.

DISCUSSION

Sixty percent of infectious diseases in people are zoonotic, and zoonotic influenza is among the top 8 zoonotic diseases of greatest concern in the US.[40] Therefore, a One Health approach is essential to strengthening the national and global capacity for preventing and responding to these diseases. One Health is a transdisciplinary approach that recognizes the interconnection between humans, animals, plants, and the shared environment in order to achieve optimal health outcomes for all. CDC and the World Health Organization (WHO) monitor mutations in influenza viruses in both humans and animals as part of their missions to protect the public from emerging health threats. An animal virus that crosses an unexpected species (eg, bat influenza in a bird) means that a particular virus has mutated in a way that may present a new public health threat. In particular, animal influenza viruses that achieve the ability to infect humans are of concern because the majority of people will not have existing immunity to a novel virus. If such a virus also achieves the ability to transmit easily between people, there is a risk of pandemic.[41–43]

Zoonotic influenza infection can occur primarily through direct contact with infected animals or contaminated environments. Humans can be infected with avian, swine, and less often, other zoonotic influenza viruses. Zoonotic influenza virus infections in humans may cause diseases ranging from mild upper respiratory tract infection (fever and cough, and early sputum production) to rapid progression to severe pneumonia, sepsis with shock, acute respiratory distress syndrome, and death. Nonrespiratory symptoms such as conjunctivitis, gastrointestinal symptoms, encephalitis, and encephalopathy have also been reported depending on subtype.[43] The majority of human cases of avian influenza (A(H5N1) and A(H7N9)) have been associated with contact with live or dead poultry or surfaces contaminated with avian influenza viruses. Human-to-human transmission has occurred in rare circumstances, but these viruses are not yet capable of efficient or sustained transmission among humans.[44] Migratory birds are a vast reservoir of avian influenza that is impossible to eradicate. Thus, vigilant surveillance in both animal and human populations and risk-based pandemic planning is essential.

A global influenza pandemic is among the most feared potential public health emergencies of international concern. Zoonotic infections are increasing in frequency

Table 6
Influenza vaccines for the 2022–2023 flu season[a]

Trade Name (Manufacturer)	Presentations	Age Indication	Mercury (From Thimerosal, if Present), μg/0.5 mL
IIV4 (Standard-dose, Egg-Based vaccines[b])			
Afluria Quadrivalent (Seqirus)	0.5-mL PFS[c]	≥3 y[c]	— (not applicable)
	5.0-mL MDV[c]	≥6 mo[c]	24.5
		18 through 64 y	
Fluarix Quadrivalent (GlaxoSmithKline)	0.5-mL PFS	≥6 mo	—
FluLaval Quadrivalent (GlaxoSmithKline)	0.5-mL PFS	≥6 mo	—
Fluzone Quadrivalent (Sanofi Pasteur)	0.5-mL PFS[d]	≥6 mo[d]	—
	0.5-mL SDV[d]	≥6 mo[d]	—
	5.0-mL MDV[d]	≥6 mo[d]	25
ccIIV4 (standard-dose, cell culture–based vaccine)			
Flucelvax Quadrivalent (Seqirus)	0.5-mL PFS	≥6 mo	—
	5.0-mL MDV	≥6 mo	25
HD-IIV4 (high-dose, egg-based vaccine[b])			
Fluzone High-Dose Quadrivalent (Sanofi Pasteur)	0.7-mL PFS	≥65 y	—
aIIV4 (standard-dose, egg-based†vaccine with MF59 adjuvant)			
Fluad Quadrivalent (Seqirus)	0.5-mL PFS	≥65 y	—
RIV4 (recombinant HA vaccine)			
Flublok Quadrivalent (Sanofi Pasteur)	0.5-mL PFS	≥18 y	—
LAIV4 (egg-based vaccine[b])			
FluMist Quadrivalent (AstraZeneca)	0.2-mL prefilled single-use intranasal sprayer	2 through 49 y	—

Abbreviations: ACIP, advisory committee on immunization practices; FDA, food and drug administration; HA, hemagglutinin; IIV4, inactivated influenza vaccine; quadrivalent, IM, intramuscular; LAIV4, live attenuated influenza vaccine, quadrivalent; MDV, multidose vial, NAS, intranasal; PFS, prefilled syringe, RIV4, recombinant influenza vaccine; quadrivalent, SDV, single-dose vial.

[a] Consult FDA-approved prescribing information for 2022 to 23 influenza vaccines for complete and updated information. Package inserts for U.S.-licensed vaccines are available at https://www.fda.gov/vaccines-blood-biologics/vaccines/vaccines-licensed-use-united-states.

[b] For persons with a history of severe egg allergy (eg, angioedema or swelling, respiratory distress, lightheadedness, or recurrent emesis) or who required epinephrine or another emergency medical intervention), cell-culture (ccIIV4) or recombinant (RIV4) influenza vaccine is preferred. However, ACIP recommends that persons with a history of egg allergy may receive egg-based vaccines (IIV4s and LAIV4). The setting for administration is determined by the severity of prior reaction. Those who report prior mild reactions to egg involving symptoms (eg, urticaria only) may receive vaccine in an outpatient setting such as a pharmacy or mass vaccination site. Those who report severe reactions to egg (as described above) should be vaccinated in a setting supervised by a health care provider who is able to recognize and manage severe allergic reactions.

[c] The approved dose volume for Afluria Quadrivalent is 0.25 mL for children aged 6 through 35 mo and 0.5 mL for persons aged $\geq$3 y. However, 0.25-mL prefilled syringes are not expected to be available for 2022 to 23 season. For children aged 6 through 35 mo, a 0.25-mL dose must be obtained from a multidose vial.

[d] Fluzone Quadrivalent is currently approved for ages 6 through 35 mo at either 0.25 mL or 0.5 mL per dose; however, 0.25-mL prefilled syringes are not expected to be available for the 2022 to 23 influenza season. If a prefilled syringe of Fluzone Quadrivalent is used for a child in this age group, the dose volume will be 0.5 mL per dose.

Influenza vaccines – United States, 2022 -23 influenza season*. CDC. https://www.cdc.gov/flu/professionals/acip/2022-2023/acip-table.htm.[45]

diversity, and global distribution. In the twenty-first century, there have been 3 novel zoonotic coronaviruses (SARS-CoV-1, MERS, and SARS-CoV2), an A(H1N1) swine influenza pandemic, Ebola epidemics, and global spread of Zika virus and other infectious diseases.[43] Based on the antigenic mutability of influenza and historic pattern of influenza, another pandemic is virtually inevitable.

The global experience of the SARS-CoV2 (Covid 19) epidemic exposed the vulnerabilities of the international public health system response to a novel, highly transmissible respiratory virus. Lessons learned and continuing to evolve from the Covid 19 pandemic can be used to strengthen the capacity of individual nations to respond to a crisis and improve coordination efforts at the international level. Continued surveillance for early detection of novel respiratory pathogens, including influenza, is essential to reducing the threat to human and animal populations. The One Health approach of collaborative, transdisciplinary partnerships is critical to responding to zoonotic disease and strengthening the US and global public health systems.

CLINICS CARE POINTS

- FDA-approved antiviral medications such as oseltamivir (PO), zanamivir (inhaled), and peramivir (IV) are neuraminidase inhibitors, which act against both influenza A & B viruses.

- Oral oseltamivir is indicated for acute uncomplicated influenza within 2 days of illness onset in people 14 days and older, and for chemoprophylaxis in people $\geq$1 year.

- Baloxavir is approved for uncomplicated influenza within 2 days of onset of illness in people with age $\geq$12 years.

- Do NOT administer once-daily postexposure antiviral chemoprophylaxis if more than 48 hours have lapsed since exposure. Full-dose empiric treatment should be implemented asap if treatment is indicated.

- Antiviral adamantanes such as amantadine and rimantadine are not recommended due to high levels of resistance (>99%) among influenza A viruses H3N2 and H1N1.

- Although resistance to neuraminidase inhibitors and baloxavir is currently low among the circulating influenza viruses, clinicians should monitor surveillance data on the susceptibility of circulating influenza viruses during each flu season.

- Annual flu vaccination is the best method for preventing and mitigating the impact of seasonal and pandemic flu.

DISCLOSURE

The authors have nothing to disclose.

REFERENCES

1. Types of Influenza Viruses. Centers for Disease Control and Prevention website. Available at: http://www.cdc.gov/flu/about/viruses/types.htm. 2021. Accessed 25 May, 2022.
2. Influenza (Seasonal). World Health Organization website. Available at:. https://www.who.int/news-room/fact-sheets/detail/influenza-(seasonal). 2018. Accessed 25 May, 2022.
3. Saunders-Hastings PR, Krewski D. Reviewing the history of pandemic influenza: Understanding patterns of emergence and transmission. Pathogens 2016; 5(4):66.
4. Disease Burden of Flu. Centers for Disease Control and Prevention website. Available at: https://www.cdc.gov/flu/about/burden/index.html. 2022. Accessed 25 May, 2022.
5. GBD 2017 Influenza Collaborators. Mortality, morbidity, and hospitalisations due to influenza lower respiratory tract infections, 2017: an analysis for the Global Burden of Disease Study 2017. Lancet Respir Med 2019;7(1):69–89.
6. Iuliano AD, Roguski KM, Chang HH, et al. Global Seasonal Influenza-associated Mortality Collaborator Network. Estimates of global seasonal influenza-associated respiratory mortality: a modelling study. Lancet 2018;391(10127): 1285–300.
7. 2020-2021 Flu Season Summary. Centers for Disease Control and Prevention website. Available at: https://www.cdc.gov/flu/season/faq-flu-season-2020-2021.htm. 2021. Accessed 22 May, 2022.
8. Influenza Virus Testing Methods. Centers for Disease Control and Prevention website. Available at: https://www.cdc.gov/flu/professionals/diagnosis/overview-testing-methods.htm. 2020. Accessed 25 May, 2022.
9. Flerlage T, Boyd DF, Meliopoulos V, et al. Influenza virus and SARS-CoV-2: pathogenesis and host responses in the respiratory tract. Nat Rev Microbiol 2021;19: 425–41.
10. Rothberg MB, Haessler SD. Complications of seasonal and pandemic influenza. Critical Care Medicine. April 2010;38(4suppl):e91–7.
11. Behrouzi B, Udell JA. Moving the needle on atherosclerotic cardiovascular disease and heart failure with influenza vaccination. Curr Atherosclerosis Rep 2021;23(12):1–10.
12. Uyeki TM, Bernstein HH, Bradley JS, et al. Clinical practice guidelines by the Infectious Diseases Society of America: 2018 update on diagnosis, treatment, chemoprophylaxis, and institutional outbreak management of seasonal influenza. Clin Infect Dis 2019;68(6):e1–47.
13. Neumann G, Kawaoka Y. Transmission of influenza A viruses. Virology 2015; 479–480:234–46.
14. Bouvier NM, Palese P. The biology of influenza viruses. Vaccine 2008 Sep 12; 26(Suppl 4):D49–53.
15. Infection Control - Transmission-Based Precautions. Centers for Disease Control and Prevention website. Available at: https://www.cdc.gov/infectioncontrol/basics/transmission-based-precautions.html. 2016. Accessed 17 June, 2022.
16. Tse H, To KK, Wen X, et al. Clinical and virological factors associated with viremia in pandemic influenza A/H1N1/2009 virus infection. PLoS One 2011;6(9):e22534.
17. Prevention Strategies for Seasonal Influenza in Healthcare Settings-Guidelines and Recommendations. Centers for Disease Control and Prevention website.

Available at: https://www.cdc.gov/flu/professionals/infectioncontrol/healthcaresettings.htm. 2021. Accessed 17 June, 2022.

18. Cady SD, Luo W, Hu F, et al. Structure and function of the influenza A M2 proton channel. Biochemistry 2009;48(31):7356–64.

19. Schnell JR, Chou JJ. Structure and mechanism of the M2 proton channel of influenza A virus. Nature 2008;451(7178):591–5.

20. Images of Influenza Viruses. Centers for Disease Control and Prevention website. Available at: https://www.cdc.gov/flu/resource-center/freeresources/graphics/images.htm. 2019. Accessed 15 May, 2022.

21. Carrat F, Vergu E, Ferguson NM, et al. Time lines of infection and disease in human influenza: A review of volunteer challenge studies. Am J Epidemiol 2008; 167(7):775–85.

22. Zambon MC. Epidemiology and pathogenesis of influenza. J Antimicrob Chemother 1999;44(suppl_2):3–9.

23. Macias AE, McElhaney JE, Chaves SS, et al. The disease burden of influenza beyond respiratory illness. Vaccine 2021;39(Suppl 1):A6–14.

24. Influenza virus testing in investigational outbreaks in institutional or other closed settings. Centers for Disease Control and Prevention website. Available at: https://www.cdc.gov/flu/professionals/diagnosis/guide-virus-diagnostic-tests.htm. 2019. Accessed 25 May, 2022.

25. Infection Control - Standard Precautions for

26. Infection Control - Type ansite. https://www.cdc.gov/infectioncontrol/guidelines/isolation/appendix/type-duration-precautions.html#I. 2019. Accessed 17 June, 2022.

27. Hayden FG, Treanor JJ, Fritz RS, et al. Use of the oral neuraminidase inhibitor oseltamivir in experimental human influenza: randomized controlled trials for prevention and treatment. JAMA 1999;282(13):1240–6.

28. Liu J, Lin S, Wang L, et al. Comparison of antiviral agents for seasonal influenza outcomes in healthy adults and children: A systematic review and network meta-analysis. JAMA Netw Open 2021;4(8):e2119151.

29. Su H, Feng I, Tang H, et al. Comparative effectiveness of neuraminidase inhibitors in patients with influenza: A systematic review and network meta-analysis. J Infect Chemother 2022;28(2):158–69.

30. Heo YA. Baloxavir: First global approval. Drugs 2018;78(6):693–7.

31. Influenza Antiviral Medications: Summary for Clinicians. Centers for Disease Control and Prevention website. Available at: https://www.cdc.gov/flu/professionals/antivirals/summary-clinicians.htm. 2022. Accessed 15 June, 2022.

32. Committee on Infectious Diseases. Recommendations for prevention and control of influenza in children. Pediatrics 2018;142(4):e20182367.

33. Gibiansky L, Ravva P, Parrott NJ, et al. Mechanistic population pharmacokinetic model of oseltamivir and oseltamivir carboxylate accounting for physiological changes to predict exposures in neonates and infants. Clinical Pharmacology & Therapeutics 2020;108(1):126–35.

34. Kimberlin DW, Acosta EP, Prichard MN, et al. Oseltamivir pharmacokinetics, dosing, and resistance among children aged <2 years with influenza. J Infect Dis 2013;207(5):709–20.

35. Baloxavir marboxil package insert. Food and Drug Administration website. Available at: https://www.accessdata.fda.gov/drugsatfda_docs/label/2019/210854s001lbl.pdf. Revised October 20, 2019. Accessed 16 June, 2022.

36. Ison MG, Portsmouth S, Yoshida Y, et al. Early treatment with baloxavir marboxil in high-risk adolescent and adult outpatients with uncomplicated influenza

(CAPSTONE-2): a randomised, placebo-controlled, phase 3 trial. Lancet Infect Dis 2020;20(10):204–1214.
37. Kumar D, Ison MG, Mira JP, et al. Combining baloxavir marboxil with standard-of-care neuraminidase inhibitor in patients hospitalised with severe influenza (FLAGSTONE): a randomised, parallel-group, double-blind, placebo-controlled, superiority trial. Lancet Infect Dis 2022;22(5):718–30.
38. Houser K, Subbarao K. Influenza vaccines: Challenges and solutions. Cell Host Microbe 2015;17(3):295–300.
39. What are the benefits of flu vaccination? Centers for Disease Control and Prevention website. Available at: https://www.cdc.gov/flu/prevent/vaccine-benefits.htm. 2021. Accessed 17 June, 2022.
40. Zoonotic Diseases Shared Between Animals and People of Most Concern in the U.S. Centers for Disease Control and Prevention website. Available at: https://www.cdc.gov/media/releases/2019/s0506-zoonotic-diseases-shared.html. 2019. Accessed 24 June, 2022.
41. CDC's One Health Office: What We Do. Centers for Disease Control and Prevention website. https://www.cdc.gov/onehealth/what-we-do/index.html 2022. Accessed 24 June, 2022.
42. Influenza (Avian and other zoonotic). World Health Organization website. Available at: https://www.who.int/news-room/fact-sheets/detail/influenza-(avian-and-other-zoonotic). 2018. Accessed 24 June, 2022.
43. National Association of State Public Health Veterinarians, Council of State and Territorial Epidemiologiest. Zoonotic Influenza Detection, Response, Prevention, and Control Reference Guide. Baltimore, MD: National Association of State Public Health Veterinarians; June 2022. Available at: http://nasphv.org/Documents/Zoonotic%20Influenza%20Reference%20Guide%20-%20June%202022.pdf. Accessed 23 June, 2022.
44. Bird Flu Virus Infections in Human. Centers for Disease Control and Prevention website. Available at: https://www.cdc.gov/flu/avianflu/avian-in-humans.htm. 2022. Accessed 24 June, 2022.
45. Influenza vaccines — United States, 2022–23 influenza season*. 2022. (Accessed 22 September, 2022, Available at: https://www.cdc.gov/flu/professionals/acip/2022-2023/acip-table.htm.)

Emerging Perinatal Infections

Jennifer Comini, MSPAS, PA-C[a],*, Greta Vines-Douglas, MSHS, PA-C[a],
Margarita Loeza, MD[b]

KEYWORDS

- Perinatal • Pregnancy • TORCH • Syphilis • COVID • Prevention • Screening
- Infection

KEY POINTS

- COVID-19 infection in pregnancy raises the risk of severe infection, preterm birth, cesarean section, and low birth weigh compared to nonpregnant individuals.
- Because of increasing syphilis case rates, thorough syphilis screening is required throughout pregnancy to prevent stillbirth, neonatal death, and congenital syphilis infections.
- Screening for group B streptococcus infections should be performed between 36 and 38 weeks of gestation.
- Increasing antibiotic resistance among common perinatal infections requires appropriate adherence to evidence-based treatment guidelines.

INTRODUCTION

Pregnant individuals are at risk for a variety of infections during the perinatal period. Although TORCH infections (toxoplasmosis, others, rubella, cytomegalovirus, herpes simplex virus) and group B streptococcus (GBS) are frequently referenced, there is an assortment of other pathogens that are important to note during pregnancy (**Table 1**). These infections can occur before conception, during pregnancy, or during the post-partum period with implications on maternal health, the development of congenital syndromes, and newborn complications (**Table 2**). Many of these infections are preventable, with appropriate transmission avoidance and vaccination, whereas others are manageable with proper screening and prompt treatment.

The prevention, screening, and management of perinatal infections requires comprehensive care, including laboratory surveillance, health education, and immunizations to

[a] Charles R. Drew University of Medicine and Science Physician Assistant Program, 1731 East 120th Street, Los Angeles, CA 90059, USA; [b] Charles R. Drew University of Medicine and Science Physician Assistant Program, Venice Family Clinic, 1731 East 120th Street, Los Angeles, CA 90059, USA
* Corresponding author. Charles R. Drew University of Medicine and Science, 1731 East 120th Street, Los Angeles, CA 90059.
E-mail address: jennifercomini@cdrewu.edu

Physician Assist Clin 8 (2023) 555–573
https://doi.org/10.1016/j.cpha.2023.02.003
2405-7991/23/© 2023 Elsevier Inc. All rights reserved.

physicianassistant.theclinics.com

Table 1
Perinatal infections

Viruses	
Influenza	Influenza A and B
COVID-19	SARS-CoV-2
Cytomegalovirus (CMV)	Human CMV
Hepatitis B	Hepatitis B virus
Hepatitis C	Hepatitis C virus
Herpes simplex virus (HSV)	HSV 1, HSV 2
HIV	HIV 1, HIV 2
Parvovirus B19 (fifth disease)	Human parvovirus B19
Rubella (German measles)	Rubella virus
Varicella (chickenpox)	Varicella-zoster virus
Human papilloma virus (HPV)	HPV
Zika	Zika virus
Bacteria and Mycobacteria	
Listeriosis	*Listeria monocytogenes*
Chlamydia	*Chlamydia trachomatis*
Bacteriuria from *Escherichia coli*	*E coli*
Gonorrhea	*Neisseria gonorrhoeae*
Maternal GBS	*Streptococcus agalactiae* or GBS
Pertussis (whooping cough)	*Bordetella pertussis*
Syphilis	*Treponema pallidum*
Tuberculosis	*Mycobacterium tuberculosis*
Bacterial vaginosis	*Gardnerella vaginalis*
Parasites and Protozoan	
Trichomoniasis	*Trichomonas vaginalis*
Malaria	*Plasmodium falciparum, Plasmodium vivax*
Chagas disease	*Trypanosoma cruzi*
Toxoplasmosis	*Toxoplasmosis gondii*

reduce morbidity and mortality and avoid vertical transmission to the newborn. Ree-merging infections, such as syphilis, have led to the transmission of infection during pregnancy or after birth resulting in an increase in congenital syphilis cases. COVID-19 is the most notable emerging infection affecting pregnancy.

Routine preconception counseling and timely access to prenatal care can reduce the morbidity and mortality caused by perinatal infections. Appropriate laboratory screening should be performed during each trimester at prenatal visits as guided by current evidence (**Table 3**). Early identification of perinatal infections can reduce newborn complications.

DISCUSSION
COVID-19

Epidemiology

First identified in Wuhan, China at the end of 2019, SARS-CoV-2 is a single-stranded RNA virus responsible for causing COVID-19, which was declared a global pandemic by World Health Organization in March 2020 (discussed elsewhere in this issue).[16,17]

Table 2
Congenital syndromes and newborn complications

Disease	Pathogen	Syndrome	Complications
Viruses			
Corona virus disease (COVID-19)	SARS-CoV-2		Pneumonia, preterm birth,[1,2] stillbirth[3]
Zika	Zika virus	Congenital Zika syndrome	Microcephaly, brain abnormalities, intracranial calcifications, congenital contractures[4]
Varicella (chickenpox)	Varicella-zoster virus	Congenital varicella syndrome	High neonatal death rate[4]
Parvovirus B19 (fifth disease)	Human parvovirus B19		Hydrops fetalis, severe neonatal anemia[4]
Cytomegalovirus	Human cytomegalovirus	Congenital cytomegalovirus	Jaundice, petechiae, thrombocytopenia, hepatosplenomegaly, growth restriction, myocarditis, nonimmune hydrops[4]
Genital herpes	Herpes simplex virus HSV 1, HSV 2	Neonatal herpes simplex	Symptomatic neonatal disease may be limited to surface lesions of the skin, eyes, or mouth, meningoencephalitis, or disseminated disease with symptoms of sepsis[4]
HIV	HIV 1, HIV 2	Neonatal HIV	Recurrent bacteremia, increased opportunistic infections, frequent diarrhea, cardiomyopathy, hepatitis, generalized lymphadenopathy, splenomegaly, hepatomegaly, oral candidiasis[5]
Hepatitis B	Hepatitis B virus	Neonatal hepatitis B	No signs or symptoms

(continued on next page)

Table 2
(continued)

Disease	Pathogen	Syndrome	Complications
Hepatitis C	Hepatitis C virus	Congenital hepatitis C	Newborn infants appear healthy[4]
Rubella (German measles)	Rubella virus	Congenital rubella syndrome	Congenital defects[4]
Bacteria and Mycobacteria			
Listeriosis	*Listeria monocytogenes*		Fetal loss, preterm labor,[6] neonatal sepsis, meningitis[4]
Maternal GBS	*Streptococcus agalactiae* or GBS	GBS early onset GBS late onset	Neonatal sepsis, low birth weight,[4] urinary tract infection[7]
Asymptomatic bacteriuria *Escherichia coli*	*E coli*	Early onset sepsis[8] Late-onset sepsis[8]	Early onset neonatal sepsis, low birth weight[4]
Chlamydia	*Chlamydia trachomatis*		Preterm birth, spontaneous abortion, stillbirth,[8] purulent conjunctivitis, pneumonia[4]
Gonorrhea	*Neisseria gonorrhoeae*	Ophthalmia neonatorum Disseminated infection	Conjunctivitis, systemic disease[4]
Tuberculosis	*Mycobacterium tuberculosis*	Congenital tuberculosis	Poor appetite, fever, irritability, hypoplasia, weight loss, cough, respiratory distress, hepatosplenomegaly, lymphadenopathy, abdominal distention[9]
Syphilis	*Treponema pallidum*	Congenital syphilis	Rhinitis, hepatosplenomegaly, skin rash with desquamation, chorioretinitis and pigmentary chorioretinopathy, glaucoma, cataracts, interstitial keratitis, optic neuritis, periostitis, and cortical demineralization of the bone[10]
Parasites and Protozoan			

Malaria	*Plasmodium falciparum, Plasmodium vivax*	Congenital malaria syndrome	Neonatal sepsis[4]
Chagas disease	*Trypanosoma cruzi*	Congenital trypanosoma	Low birth weight, hepatosplenomegaly, anemia, jaundice, edema, thrombocytopenia, petechiae, tremors, seizure disorders[11]
Toxoplasmosis	*Toxoplasmosis gondii*	Congenital toxoplasmosis	Prematurity, intrauterine growth restriction, jaundice, hepatosplenomegaly, myocarditis, pneumonitis, rash, chorioretinitis, hydrocephalus, intracranial calcifications, microcephaly, seizures

Table 3
Indications screening for prenatal infections in the United States

Disease	Organism/Pathogen	Prenatal Screening
Viruses		
Coronavirus disease (COVID-19)	SARS-CoV-2	Test all pregnant patients in labor and on admission[12]
Zika virus	Zika virus	Test symptomatic or at-risk patients[4]
Varicella (chickenpox)	Varicella-zoster virus	Check titer for immunity at first prenatal visit[4]
Parvovirus B19 (fifth disease)	Human parvovirus B19	No support for routine screening[4]
Cytomegalovirus (CMV)	Human CMV	No support for routine screening[13]
Herpes simplex virus (HSV)	HSV 1, HSV 2	No support for routine screening[4]
HIV	HIV 1, HIV 2	First prenatal visit and third trimester for high risk[4,14]
Hepatitis B	Hepatitis B virus	First prenatal visit and third trimester for high risk[14]
Hepatitis C	Hepatitis C virus	First prenatal visit[14]
Rubella (German measles)	Rubella virus	Check titer for immunity at first prenatal visit[4]
Bacteria and Mycobacteria		
Listeriosis	Listeria monocytogenes	No support for routine screening[4]
Maternal GBS	Streptococcus agalactiae or GBS	Screen all at 35–37 wk[4]
Asymptomatic bacteriuria caused by Escherichia coli	E coli	Screen with urine culture at first prenatal visit[15]
Chlamydia	Chlamydia trachomatis	All pregnant individuals younger than 25 y or with other risk factors at first prenatal visit and third trimester if high risk[4,14]
Gonorrhea	Neisseria gonorrhoeae	All pregnant individuals younger than 25 y or with other risk factors at first prenatal visit and third trimester if high risk[4,14]
Tuberculosis	Mycobacterium tuberculosis	First prenatal visit[4]

Syphilis	*Treponema pallidum*	First prenatal visit and third trimester and delivery[4,14]
Bacterial vaginosis	*Gardnerella vaginalis*	No support for routine screening[4]
Parasites and Protozoan		
Malaria	*Plasmodium falciparum, Plasmodium vivax*	No support for routine screening[4]
Chagas disease	*Trypanosoma cruzi*	No routine screening, screen pregnant individuals who have lived in Mexico, Central America, and South America[11]
Toxoplasmosis	*Toxoplasmosis gondii*	No support for routine serologic screening[4]

COVID-19 has a spectrum of disease severity. Asymptomatic disease is prevalent. Symptomatic disease can range from mild to fatal. Clinical manifestations include pulmonary disease consisting of fever, fatigue, anosmia, cough, and shortness of breath leading to pneumonia, respiratory failure, extrapulmonary complications, and death.[16] As of June 2022, there have been 84.9 million cases of COVID-19 in the United States causing more than 1 million deaths and affecting approximately 215,000 pregnant individuals.[18] Evaluation regarding severe maternal illness, pregnancy outcomes, and fetal impact is ongoing.

Clinical relevance
SARS-CoV-2 is transmitted via respiratory droplets, person-to-person contact, and fomites (**Table 4**).[16,17] Vertical transmission seems rare.[16] Infection in early pregnancy (first trimester) seems unlikely to impact the developing fetus because fetal immunoglobulin development does not occur until later in gestation.[20]

Assessment
There has been concern regarding pregnant individuals' risk for severe COVID-19 infection because of the physiologic changes occurring within the immune system, respiratory system (eg, decrease in total lung capacity), cardiovascular system, and hypercoagulability risk during gestation.[21] Pregnant individuals should be tested for COVID-19 on admission to labor and delivery wards (see **Table 3**). Asymptomatic and mild disease seem to predominate with positivity rates similar to the general population.[2,22] In symptomatic pregnant individuals, fever, cough, and mild respiratory symptoms are the most commonly reported symptoms.[2,22] Pregnant patients who are asymptomatic or with mild infection can be managed in the outpatient setting with close follow-up.

Published case studies and reviews since the start of the pandemic have demonstrated an increased risk for severe SARS-CoV-2 infection in pregnant individuals compared with their nonpregnant counterparts.[22,23] Severe disease appears most frequently in the second half of pregnancy.[22] Risk factors for severe infection include older maternal age, comorbidities (asthma, diabetes, hypertension), and obesity.[22] Hospitalization with multidisciplinary management and supplemental oxygen are needed for more severe COVID disease. Additional maternal outcomes with severe infection include an increased risk of intensive care unit (ICU) admission, mechanical ventilation, intubation, and extracorporeal membrane oxygenation compared with nonpregnant individuals.[2,20,22–24] Antiviral treatment should be offered in pregnancy as indicated (discussed elsewhere in this issue).

Complications
The most frequently recorded adverse pregnancy outcome is preterm birth.[1,2] Preterm birth rates were higher than the general pregnant population and additionally higher in symptomatic COVID-19-infected pregnant patients than those with asymptomatic infections.[25] Preterm delivery occurred most often because of worsening maternal status, rather than fetal condition.[22] Premature rupture of membranes and spontaneous deliveries were also reported.[26] The use of antenatal steroids (dexamethasone) can benefit the preterm neonate by enhancing fetal lung maturation. Additionally, there is an increased incidence of cesarean section among SARS-CoV-2-positive pregnant patients.[24]

Death among pregnant individuals with severe COVID-19 who are admitted to ICUs seemed to be slightly higher than nonpregnant counterparts, with Black women disproportionately affected.[2,23] Maternal death has been associated with preexisting comorbid conditions.[24]

Table 4
Prevention of vertical and horizontal infections during pregnancy

Immunizations		
Seasonal influenza	Influenza A and B	Immunize before, during, or after pregnancy
Coronavirus disease (COVID-19)	SARS-CoV-2	Immunize before, during, or after pregnancy
Varicella (chickenpox)	Varicella-zoster virus	Immunize before or after pregnancy[4]
Hepatitis B	Hepatitis B virus	Immunize before or after pregnancy[4]
Rubella (German measles)	Rubella virus	Immunize before or after pregnancy[4]
Pertussis (whooping cough)	*Bordetella pertussis*	Immunize with Tdap at 27–36 wk[4]
Condoms and Safe Sex During Pregnancy/Abstinence		
(HIV	HIV 1, HIV 2	
Herpes	HSV 1, HSV 2	
Hepatitis B virus	Hepatitis B virus	
Chlamydia infection	*Chlamydia trachomatis*	Treat patient and partners[4]
Gonorrhea infection	*Neisseria gonorrhoeae*	Treat patient and partners[4]
Syphilis	*Treponema pallidum*	
Zika virus	Zika virus	
Hepatitis C	Hepatitis C virus	
Cytomegalovirus (CMV)	Human CMV	
Chagas disease	*Trypanosoma cruzi*	
Insecticides		
Malaria	*Plasmodium falciparum, Plasmodium vivax*	Chemoprophylaxis, avoid mosquitoes, insecticide-treated bed nets[4]
Chagas disease	*T cruzi*	Insecticide to eliminate bugs, screen blood before transfusion[4]
Zika virus	Zika virus	Insecticide, avoid mosquitoes and travel to endemic areas[4]
Hand Washing		

(continued on next page)

Table 4
(continued)

Toxoplasmosis	*Toxoplasmosis gondii*	Avoid cat litter[19]
Escherichia coli	*E coli*	
Listeriosis	*Listeria monocytogenes*	
Parvovirus B19 (fifth disease)	Human parvovirus B19	
CMV	Human CMV	Personal hygiene[13]
Proper Handling and Avoidance of Certain Foods		
Toxoplasmosis		Cook meat at least 145°F[19]
E coli		Avoid raw milk, soft cheese, wash fruit, and vegetables
Listeriosis		Avoid raw milk, soft cheese, wash fruit, and vegetables, undercooked meat[4]

Other notable complications included an increased hypercoagulability risk in those infected, which is already elevated in pregnant individuals, further predisposing patients to venous thromboembolism. A low threshold for thromboprophylaxis should be used.[21]

There are rare serious adverse outcomes in neonates. Complications of maternal infection in the neonate include preterm birth, low birth weight, and fetal growth restriction.[24] No congenital malformations have been reported thus far, but more research is needed on the impact of first trimester infection on the developing fetus.[27] APGAR scores have been encouraging.[2,26] Neonates infected with SARS-CoV-2 were primarily asymptomatic, followed by symptoms of fever and mild respiratory manifestations.[28] Newborn ICU (NICU) admission rates were higher among newborns delivered to SARS-CoV-2-positive individuals, which may be related to low birth rates and premature delivery.[28,29]

Additional impacts of COVID-19 on maternal health include the cessation of in-office visits (replaced with telemedicine) and increased susceptibility to intimate partner violence, which is associated with adverse pregnancy outcomes.[21]

Recommendations

All pregnant individuals presenting to the hospital for admission should be screened for COVID-19.[12] Patients should be encouraged to breastfeed to pass on antibodies to the newborn.[21,22] The COVID-19 vaccine, granted Emergency Use Authorization by the Food and Drug Administration, should be offered to all pregnant and lactating individuals, consistent with recommendations in nonpregnant patients (**Table 5**). There is no safety concern regarding the vaccine's impact on pregnancy or fertility.[22,31] Titers do not seem to differ by trimester of vaccination. Maternal vaccination can provide protective immunity to the newborn without adverse effect on the developing fetus or postnatal development.[31] The incidence of pregnancy loss and preterm birth in vaccinated individuals is similar to prepandemic rates according to vaccine surveillance and reporting systems.[31]

Syphilis

Clinical relevance

Syphilis is a sexually transmitted infection caused by *Treponema pallidum*, a spirochetal bacterium (discussed elsewhere in this issue). It is spread by direct sexual contact with an infected partner or through vertical transmission from mother to fetus (see **Table 4**).[32] Vertical transmission can occur during delivery, but most frequently occurs in utero.

Preliminary 2021 data from the Centers for Disease Control and Prevention (CDC) show increasing rates of primary and secondary syphilis in men and women, with congenital syphilis on the rise.[32] Congenital syphilis has increased every year since 2013 with a 291.1% case increase occurring between 2015 and 2019.[33] With increased case rates, an increase in stillbirths and congenital syphilis–related deaths have also been observed.[33] Pregnant individuals lacking prenatal care are at increased risk. CDC data from 2019 cited an increase in congenital cases related to missed opportunity for treatment, lack of prenatal care, and lack of syphilis testing.[33] The influence of the COVID-19 pandemic on prenatal care delivery and screening of syphilis will be important to evaluate as congenital syphilis rates are monitored further.

Assessment

Syphilis has three stages: primary, secondary, and tertiary. The primary stage is distinguished by a chancre, a painless, round sore at the area of initial infection, and lymphadenopathy. Because of the location and absence of pain, the sore can go unnoticed by the individual, ultimately delaying detection and treatment, resulting in progression to the

Table 5
Transmission of perinatal infections

Disease	Transmission to Mother	Maternal-Fetal Transmission
Viruses		
Influenza	Person to person via respiratory droplets[4]	Contact with infected mother after delivery[4]
COVID-19	Person to person	Vertical,[3] postnatal contact with infected mother
Zika	Sex, arthropods	Vertical, breastfeeding
Varicella (chickenpox)	Person-to-person via respiratory droplets or close contact[4]	Vertical
Parvovirus B19 (fifth disease)	Respiratory secretions and hand to mouth contact[4]	Vertical, viral placental transport[4]
Cytomegalovirus	Person-to-person	Intrauterine, perinatal, postnatal, breast milk
Herpes simplex virus	Sex[4]	Vertical, ascending infection, or postnatal during vaginal delivery[4]
HIV	Transmitted by sexual contact with body fluids, such as saliva, urine, and breastmilk; and by blood transfusion and organ transplantation[4]	Vertical, breastfeeding[4]
Hepatitis B	Sex[4]	Vertical, exposure to maternal blood during labor and delivery[4]
Hepatitis C	Sex, arthropods	Vertical, breastfeeding
Rubella (German measles)	Person-to-person	Placental or vertical
Human papilloma virus	Sex[30]	Vertical[30]
Bacteria and Mycobacteria		
Listeriosis	Contaminated food or fluids	Transplacental, ascending intrauterine infection, exposure during delivery, vertical[4]
Maternal GBS	Person-to-person, maternal colonization[4]	Vertical[4]
Asymptomatic bacteriuria (*Escherichia Coli*)	Consumption of contaminated food or fluids	Vertical
Chlamydia	Sex[4]	Vertical[4]

Gonorrhea	Sex[4]	Vertical[4]
Tuberculosis	Person-to-person	At time of delivery because of aspiration, hematogenous dissemination, aspiration of infected amniotic fluid, vertical, breastfeeding[4]
Syphilis	Sex[4]	Hematogenous transplacental infection of the fetus in utero, direct contact lesions during delivery[4]
Parasites and Protozoan		
Malaria	Arthropod	Vertical
Chagas disease	Arthropod vector, blood or organ recipients, food, fluid	Vertical
Toxoplasmosis	Contaminated food, ingest oocytes after contact with cat feces[19]	Transplacentally (vertical)[4]

secondary stage (discussed elsewhere in this issue).[32] Latent syphilis occurs when the bacteria remain hidden in the body but there are no overt signs or symptoms of infection. This aspect of syphilis can last for years during which the patient remains infectious.[32,34]

Complications

Complications of syphilis specific to pregnancy include stillborn delivery, neonatal death, and congenital syphilis.[32,34] It is the second leading cause of stillbirths worldwide.[35] Additionally, neonates born to syphilis-positive individuals are more often preterm and of low birth weight.[34] In addition to a variety of symptoms, congenital syphilis can lead to developmental delay, seizures, and death (see **Table 2**).

Recommendations

Screening for syphilis should occur in all pregnant individuals, regardless of risk, at the first prenatal visit during the first trimester (see **Table 3**).[32] Repeat screening should occur twice during the third trimester, at 28 weeks gestation and delivery.[32] Testing should occur with each subsequent pregnancy, regardless of a prior negative result in a previous pregnancy. Testing begins with a nontreponemal test, such as rapid plasma reagin or venereal disease research laboratory test, with reflex to a confirmatory treponemal test, such as *T pallidum* particle agglutination.[34]

A positive syphilis test necessitates treatment with intramuscular benzathine penicillin G. Penicillin (PCN)-allergic patients should undergo desensitization. Early treatment is imperative to prevent complications. All sexual partners who may be exposed to the virus should also be treated to prevent reinfection.

Newborns born to syphilis-positive patients should receive screening for congenital syphilis.[32,36] Those with congenital syphilis should receive PCN as treatment.[34,36]

Other Notable Trends in Perinatal Infections

Listeriosis

In 2017, the largest outbreak of listeriosis to date occurred in South Africa, with more than 1000 documented cases.[37] The significance of this outbreak sparked renewed interest and research. Common foods associated with *Listeria monocytogenes* infection include unpasteurized dairy products and ready-to-eat processed meats. Within the last decade, nontraditional foods, such as sprouts, celery, melons, fruits, potatoes, caramel apples, and packaged salads, have been increasingly implicated as sources of infection.[6] Researchers found that outbreaks from novel foods increased 366% from 1998 to 2018.[6] Listeriosis is associated with a 20% fatality rate, which is higher than many other foodborne diseases.[6]

According to the CDC, listeriosis is the third leading cause of death from food poisoning in the United States, resulting in about 1600 infections per year, and around 260 deaths.[38] Although rare in the general population, pregnant individuals are 13 to 17 times more likely to become infected and can transmit this infection to their unborn babies.[38] Neonatal complications include meningitis, respiratory disease, and bacteremia, with a case fatality of 20% to 30% (see **Table 2**).[39]

Common symptoms of listeriosis include fever, body aches, abdominal pain, flulike symptoms, nausea, vomiting, and diarrhea. Pregnant individuals, however, often lack typical gastrointestinal symptoms, such as vomiting and diarrhea, making this diagnosis challenging during pregnancy.[39] The most common symptoms during pregnancy include fever, leukocytosis, and premature contractions.[39] Listeria should be considered a potential diagnosis in pregnant individuals presenting with these atypical symptoms. Inquiring about food exposures may prove beneficial when interviewing pregnant patients because of the rise in nontraditional contaminated food sources (see **Tables 4** and **5**).

Group B streptococcus

Approximately 25% of pregnant individuals have GBS infection.[40] GBS is the most common cause of neonatal infection and clindamycin-resistant GBS strains now cause more than 40% of cases.[40,41] Maternal colonization in the gastrointestinal and genitourinary tracts is associated with a 50% transmission rate, and 1% to 2% of infected newborns develop an infection within the first week of life.[41] Newborn complications include sepsis, pneumonia, and meningitis (see **Table 2**). Preterm infants are at highest risk when compared with term newborns, with a morbidity and mortality risk of 19.2% versus 2.1%, respectively.[42]

The American College of Obstetrics and Gynecology Committee provided an updated opinion about preventing early onset GBS infection in 2020, replacing the CDC 2010 guidelines.[41] This update addresses screening recommendations for pregnant patients and antibiotic stewardship.

Important updates for the prevention and treatment of early neonatal sepsis from GBS include the following[41]:

- Screen all pregnant individuals at 36 and 0/7 weeks to 37 and 6/7 weeks. This updated screening guideline reflects the goal of collecting specimens within 5 weeks of birth and covers a longer gestational period (up to 41 and 0/7 weeks). The prior screening recommendation was 35 and 0/7 weeks.
- Perform PCN allergy testing for all pregnant individuals who report a history of PCN allergy. This recommendation may decrease the need for alternative antibiotic use to eradicate infection. The guideline recommends that a PCN allergy be noted on all laboratory requisitions, so that susceptibility for clindamycin is performed when testing the specimen.
- Prophylactic intravenous (IV) intrapartum PCN is preferred for pregnant individuals with positive cultures or other risk factors for GBS. Risk factors include previous neonate with severe GBS infection, history of GBS bacteriuria during current pregnancy, increased risk for preterm delivery, prelabor premature rupture of membranes or rupture of membranes for 18-plus hours at term, and pregnant patients with fever at or above 100.4°F. IV prophylaxis excludes pregnant individuals planning for cesarean birth in the absence of labor and rupture of membranes. Alternatives to PCN are recommended based on low- versus high-risk classification for patients who have PCN allergy. These include:
  - Low risk: IV cefazolin
  - High risk: IV clindamycin or vancomycin (if clindamycin resistant)
  - Unknown risk: PCN allergy testing, IV cefazolin; clindamycin or vancomycin (based on susceptibility)

These updates aim to decrease GBS infection in neonates by addressing significant factors that contribute to neonatal morbidity and mortality.

Escherichia coli

Escherichia coli is a leading cause of severe infection (sepsis and pneumonia) in term and preterm neonates.[7] For term infants, E coli is second only to GBS in causing early onset sepsis.[7] Additional research indicates that the E coli–associated early onset sepsis is increasing and may surpass GBS as the most common cause of neonatal sepsis. Incidence rates can vary based on geographic region and population demographics. The estimated global incidence rate is 22 infections per 1000 births, with a mortality rate of 11% to 19%.[43]

There are high resistance rates to medications commonly used to treat E coli and GBS (eg, ampicillin and gentamicin).[7,44] The impact of this disease on vulnerable populations is concerning, and perinatal antibiotics to prevent GBS in 50% of pregnant individuals may drive resistance patterns.[7] Health care providers should be aware of resistance to commonly used medications to eradicate E coli. Ampicillin and a third-generation cephalosporin, or ampicillin plus amikacin (after ruling out central nervous system involvement) may be considered to eradicate resistant strains.[44]

Gonorrhea and chlamydia

During the last decade, the prevalence of sexually transmitted infection increased in most countries.[45] In the United States, chlamydia and gonorrhea increased by 19% and 56%, respectively, from 2014 to 2019.[46] Serious sequelae, such as ectopic pregnancy, infertility, and pelvic inflammatory disease, can result from untreated gonococcal and chlamydial infections.[47,48] Preterm birth, stillbirth, spontaneous abortion, neonatal conjunctivitis, or disseminated neonatal infection are additional consequences associated with infection during pregnancy (see **Table 2**).[8] Effective screening and treatment can help prevent pregnancy complications and vertical transmission of chlamydia and gonorrhea (see **Table 3**).

The CDC updated the sexually transmitted infection treatment guidelines in 2021. In pregnant females, 1 g of oral azithromycin is still the preferred treatment option for chlamydial infection, whereas amoxicillin is an alternative for those who are unable to tolerate azithromycin. Frequent use of azithromycin has resulted in increasing resistance to standard treatment regimens for chlamydial and gonococcal infections.[14] The preferred treatment of nonpregnant patients is now doxycycline rather than azithromycin.[49] However, the use of doxycycline is not recommended during pregnancy.[14] In addition to azithromycin, pregnant patients positive for Chlamydia trachomatis should also, (1) receive a test of cure 4 weeks after treatment, (2) be retested after 3 months, and (3) be retested during the third trimester or at time of delivery.[14] For gonococcal infections, a single 500-mg intramuscular dose of ceftriaxone is recommended, and cotreatment for chlamydia should also be given.[14] Consultation with an infectious disease specialist is recommended if a significant allergy to PCN precludes the use of ceftriaxone.[14]

SUMMARY

The management of perinatal infections requires a delicate balance between addressing maternal status and potential complications in the developing fetus. Fetal complications of perinatal infections can range from mild to fatal. COVID-19 infection remains the most significant emerging infection among pregnant individuals with an increased risk of preterm birth, cesarean section, NICU admission, and low birth weight. Additionally, increased risk of severe infection and a slight increase in morality is observed in pregnant patients with COVID-19 infection compared with nonpregnant patients. Vaccination against COVID-19 is strongly recommended. Drastically rising syphilis rates across the country requires attention to appropriate prenatal screening guidelines to prevent stillbirth, neonatal death, and congenital syphilis. Meaningful trends among established perinatal bacterial infections need to be acknowledged to allow for early detection, proper treatment, and the prevention of neonatal complications (eg, listeriosis, E coli, gonorrhea, chlamydia). There are additionally concerning trends regarding increased antibiotic resistance to clindamycin in GBS and azithromycin in chlamydia.

PAs in obstetrics and gynecology and related fields should be acutely aware of these current trends to deliver suitable screening, prompt diagnosis, and evidence-based treatment to provide the greatest reduction in maternal and neonatal morbidity and mortality. The importance of thorough prenatal care and infection prevention through vaccination and pathogen avoidance should be emphasized to the pregnant patient.

CLINICS CARE POINTS

- Test all pregnant individuals admitted to labor and delivery for SARS-CoV-2.
- Pregnant individuals should be tested for syphilis three times during pregnancy (first trimester, third trimester, and delivery).
- Despite a change in antibiotic selection for nonpregnant individuals, those who are pregnant and test positive for *Chlamydia trachomatis* should continue to receive azithromycin with amoxicillin as an alternative.
- Group B streptococcus testing should be performed between 36 weeks and 37 and 6/7 weeks.

DISCLOSURE

None of the authors have any disclosures to report.

REFERENCES

1. Dubey P, Reddy SY, Manuel S, et al. Maternal and neonatal characteristics and outcomes among COVID-19 infected women: an updated systematic review and meta-analysis. Eur J Obstet Gynecol Reprod Biol 2020;252:490–501.
2. Overton EE, Goffman D, Friedman AM. The epidemiology of COVID-19 in pregnancy. Clin Obstet Gynecol 2022;65(1):110–22.
3. Pashaei Z, SeyedAlinaghi S, Qaderi K, et al. Prenatal and neonatal complications of COVID-19: a systematic review. Health Sci Rep 2022;5(2):e510.
4. ACOG. Guidelines for perinatal care. 8th edition. Elk Grove Village IL, Washington, DC: American Academy of Pediatrics; The American college of Obstetricians and Gynecologists. 2017.
5. Abbas M., Bakhtyar A., Bazzi R., Neonatal HIV. [Updated 2022 Sep 20]. In: StatPearls [Internet]. Treasure Island (FL): StatPearls Publishing; 2022. Available from: https://www.ncbi.nlm.nih.gov/books/NBK565879/. Accessed June 19, 2022.
6. Desai AN, Anyoha A, Madoff LC, et al. Changing epidemiology of *Listeria monocytogenes* outbreaks, sporadic cases, and recalls globally: a review of ProMED reports from 1996 to 2018. Int J Infect Dis 2019;84:48–53.
7. Flannery DD, Akinboyo IC, Mukhopadhyay S, et al. Antibiotic susceptibility of *Escherichia coli* among infants admitted to neonatal intensive care units across the US from 2009 to 2017. JAMA Pediatr 2021;175(2):168.
8. Olaleye AO, Babah OA, Osuagwu CS, et al. Sexually transmitted infections in pregnancy: an update on *Chlamydia trachomatis* and *Neisseria gonorrhoeae*. Eur J Obstet Gynecol Reprod Biol 2020;255:1–12.
9. Li C, Liu L, Tao Y. Diagnosis and treatment of congenital tuberculosis: a systematic review of 92 cases. Orphanet J Rare Dis 2019;14(1):131.
10. Birth defects surveillance: quick reference handbook of selected congenital anomalies and infections. Geneva: World Health Organization; 2020.
11. Centers for Disease Control and Prevention. Congenital Chagas disease. US Department of Health and Human Services, CDC. Available at: https://www.cdc.gov/parasites/chagas/health_professionals/congenital_chagas.html.
12. Hashim NAF, Mahdy ZA, Abdul Rahman R, et al. Universal testing policy for COVID-19 in pregnancy: a systematic review. Front Public Health 2022;10:588269.
13. Hughes BL, Gyamfi-Bannerman C. Diagnosis and antenatal management of congenital cytomegalovirus infection. Am J Obstet Gynecol 2016;214(6):B5–11.

14. Workowski K, Bachmann L, Chan P, et al. Sexually transmitted infections treatment guidelines. 2021. Available at: https://www.cdc.gov/mmwr/volumes/70/rr/pdfs/rr7004a1-H.pdf. Published 2021. Accessed June 10, 2022.

15. US Preventive Services Task Force. Screening for asymptomatic bacteriuria in adults: US Preventive Services Task Force Recommendation Statement. JAMA 2019;322(12):1188–94.

16. Moore KM, Suthar MS. Comprehensive analysis of COVID-19 during pregnancy. Biochem Biophys Res Commun 2021;538:180–6.

17. Centers for Disease Control and Prevention. Basics of COVID-19. US Department of Health and Human Services, CDC. Available at: https://www.cdc.gov/coronavirus/2019-ncov/your-health/about-covid-19/basics-covid-19.html. Published 2021. Updated November 4, 2021. Accessed June, 2022.

18. Centers for Disease Control and Prevention. COVID Data Tracker. US Department of Health and Human Services, CDC. Available at: https://covid.cdc.gov/covid-data-tracker. Published 2022. Accessed June 9, 2022.

19. Jones J, Lopez A, Wilson M. Congenital toxoplasmosis. Am Fam Physician 2003; 67(10):2131–8.

20. Kazemi SN, Hajikhani B, Didar H, et al. COVID-19 and cause of pregnancy loss during the pandemic: a systematic review. PLoS One 2021;16(8):e0255994.

21. Wastnedge EAN, Reynolds RM, van Boeckel SR, et al. Pregnancy and COVID-19. Physiol Rev 2021;101(1):303–18.

22. Nana M, Nelson-Piercy C. COVID-19 in pregnancy. Clin Med 2021;21(5):e446–50.

23. Zambrano LD, Ellington S, Strid P, et al. Update: characteristics of symptomatic women of reproductive age with laboratory-confirmed SARS-CoV-2 infection by pregnancy status—United States, January 22–October 3, 2020. MMWR Morb Mortal Wkly Rep 2020;69:1641–7.

24. Thompson JL, Nguyen LM, Noble KN, et al. COVID-19-related disease severity in pregnancy. Am J Reprod Immunol 2020;84(5):e13339.

25. Delahoy MJ, Whitaker M, O'Halloran A, et al. Characteristics and maternal and birth outcomes of hospitalized pregnant women with laboratory-confirmed COVID-19 - COVID-NET, 13 states, March 1-August 22, 2020. MMWR Morb Mortal Wkly Rep 2020;69(38):1347–54.

26. Di Toro F, Gjoka M, Di Lorenzo G, et al. Impact of COVID-19 on maternal and neonatal outcomes: a systematic review and meta-analysis. Clin Microbiol Infect 2021;27(1):36–46.

27. Rodrigues C, Baía I, Domingues R, et al. Pregnancy and breastfeeding during COVID-19 pandemic: a systematic review of published pregnancy cases. Front Public Health 2020;8:558144.

28. Ciapponi A, Bardach A, Comandé D, et al. COVID-19 and pregnancy: an umbrella review of clinical presentation, vertical transmission, and maternal and perinatal outcomes. PLoS One 2021;16(6):e0253974.

29. Lassi ZS, Ana A, Das JK, et al. A systematic review and meta-analysis of data on pregnant women with confirmed COVID-19: clinical presentation, and pregnancy and perinatal outcomes based on COVID-19 severity. J Glob Health 2021;11:5018.

30. Sarr EHM, Mayrand MH, Coutlée F, et al. Exploration of the effect of human papillomavirus (HPV) vaccination in a cohort of pregnant women in Montreal, 2010-2016. Heliyon 2019;5(8):e02150.

31. Shook LL, Fallah PN, Silberman JN, et al. COVID-19 vaccination in pregnancy and lactation: current research and gaps in understanding. Front Cell Infect Microbiol 2021;11:735394.

32. Centers for Disease Control and Prevention. Preliminary 2021 data: syphilis. Available at: https://www.cdc.gov/std/statistics/2020/preliminary2021.htm?CDC_AA_refVal=https%3A%2F%2Fwww.cdc.gov%2Fstd%2Fstatistics%2F2020%2FCongenital-Syphilis-preliminaryData.htm. Published 2022. Accessed June 9, 2022.

33. Centers for Disease Control and Prevention. National overview: sexually transmitted disease surveillance. 2019. Available at: https://www.cdc.gov/std/statistics/2019/overview.htm#CongenitalSyphilis. Published 2021. Accessed.

34. Peeling RW, Mabey D, Kamb ML, et al. Syphilis. Nat Rev Dis Primers 2017;3:17073.

35. Lawn JE, Blencowe H, Waiswa P, et al. Stillbirths: rates, risk factors, and acceleration towards 2030. Lancet 2016;387(10018):587–603.

36. Centers for Disease Control and Prevention. Congenital syphilis. US Department of Health and Human Services, CDC. Available at: https://www.cdc.gov/std/treatment-guidelines/congenital-syphilis.htm. Published 2021. Accessed.

37. National Institute for Communicable Diseases (NICD) South Africa. Situation Report, 26. 2018. Available at: https://www.nicd.ac.za/wp-content/uploads/2018/07/Listeriosis-outbreak-situation-report-_26July2018_fordistribution.pdf. Published 2018. Accessed June 7, 2022.

38. Center for Disease Control and Prevention. Listeria (listeriosis), people at risk. Available at: https://www.cdc.gov/listeria/risk-groups/pregnant-women.html. Published 2016. Accessed June 7, 2022.

39. Fouks Y, Amit S, Many A, et al. Listeriosis in pregnancy: under-diagnosis despite over-treatment. J Perinatol 2018;38(1):26–30.

40. Center for Disease Control and Prevention. Clindamycin-resistant group B streptococcus. Available at: https://www.cdc.gov/drugresistance/pdf/threats-report/gbs-508.pdf. Published 2019. Accessed June 9, 2022.

41. Prevention of Group B. Streptococcal early-onset disease in newborns: ACOG Committee Opinion, Number 797. Obstet Gynecol 2020;135(2):e51–72.

42. Puopolo KM, Lynfield R, Cummings JJ, et al. Management of infants at risk for group B streptococcal disease. Pediatrics 2019;144(2):e20191881.

43. Fleischmann-Struzek C, Goldfarb DM, Schlattmann P, et al. The global burden of paediatric and neonatal sepsis: a systematic review. Lancet Respir Med 2018; 6(3):223–30.

44. Mendoza-Palomar N, Balasch-Carulla M, González-Di Lauro S, et al. *Escherichia coli* early-onset sepsis: trends over two decades. Eur J Pediatr 2017;176(9): 1227–34.

45. Peyriere H, Makinson A, Marchandin H, et al. Doxycycline in the management of sexually transmitted infections. J Antimicrob Chemother 2018;73(3):553–63.

46. Dalby J, Stoner BP. Sexually transmitted infections: updates from the 2021 CDC guidelines. Am Fam Physician 2022;105(5):514–20.

47. Cyr S, Barbee L, Workowski K, et al. Update to CDC's treatment guidelines for gonococcal infection. 2020. Available at: https://www.cdc.gov/mmwr/volumes/69/wr/pdfs/mm6950a6-H.pdf. Published 2020. Accessed June 10, 2022.

48. Center for Disease Control and Prevention Sexually Transmitted Infections Treatment Guidelines 2021. Chlamydial infections. Available at: https://www.cdc.gov/std/treatment-guidelines/chlamydia.htm. Published 2021. Accessed June 10, 2022.

49. Wind CM, De Vries E, Schim Van Der Loeff MF, et al. Decreased azithromycin susceptibility of *Neisseria gonorrhoeae* isolates in patients recently treated with azithromycin. Clin Infect Dis 2017;65(1):37–45.

Emerging Infectious Diseases and Bioterrorism

Samuel Paik, PA-C

KEYWORDS

- Infectious disease • Terrorism • Bioterrorism • Emerging infection

KEY POINTS

- Emerging infections globally and their use in bioterrorism
- Examples of bioterrorism
- Historical timeline
- Lessons from COVID
- Defense again future Bioterrorism

INTRODUCTION

The Enlightenment Period brought us the theory that globalization will bring peace as all sovereign nations would become interdependent and interconnected. After WWII, we saw that Kantian supposition expressed as the world became more and more woven together. It is all the more intriguing that the same globalization that brought relative peace helped spread COVID-19 with devastating international consequences. Shakespearean is how this pandemic is ending, the start of an international war in Ukraine.

Warfare has traditionally been thought of as material objects from swords to nuclear weapons to dominate an opposing group. There are many aspects of warfare such as killing your target or possibly even more effective, harnessing the threat of it. Warfare advances have developed over centuries to where there are now cyber-attacks, chemical warfare, and for the last few centuries, biological warfare. We have seen infectious diseases and bioterrorism play out for centuries. The first recorded use being the Tartars catapulting infested corpses into the port city of Caffa (now Ukraine) in 1347 to much more systematic horrors committed during WWI, to our current situation, mainly terrorism that is motivated by political reasons or more sinister aspirations.[1]

This particular class of war, bioterrorism, is incredibly frightening in its magnitude because unlike a nuclear warhead which would destroy indiscriminately but has been used very rarely in the history of humankind, biological warfare may be used discreetly and has the potential to cripple nations. It is also much easier to produce

Charles Drew University PA Program, 1731 East 120th Street, Los Angeles, CA 90059, USA
E-mail address: samuelpaik@cdrewu.edu

Physician Assist Clin 8 (2023) 575–581
https://doi.org/10.1016/j.cpha.2023.03.004
2405-7991/23/© 2023 Elsevier Inc. All rights reserved.

than a nuclear missile and easier to obtain. So dangerous is its very existence, the international world has largely agreed to prohibit the use of biological weapons. Alas, there are still individuals, terrorist organizations, and nations that have used them and are currently developing biological terrorism as a weapon.

What Is Bioterrorism?

Bioterrorism is defined as "the intentional release or threat of release of biologic agents (ie, viruses, bacteria, fungi or their toxins) to cause disease or death among human population or food crops and livestock to terrorize a civilian population or manipulate the government and in the present scenario of increased terrorist activity has become a real possibility."[2]

Like any other technology, bioterrorism has evolved and gone are the days of catapulting rotting corpses to strike fear into an enemy. Terrorists now are using advances in medicine and science to create agents that are becoming effectively deadly. There are countless bacteria, viruses, chemical agents, fungi, and other pathogens you could choose from, but we will narrow it down. The Center for Disease Control and Prevention (CDC) breaks down agents and diseases into three main categories (**Box 1**).[3]

What We Learned from COVID

We found out how unprepared the US government and the US health care system were during the COVID pandemic, which at the time of this writing is up ticking again. The challenges posed by bioterrorism are very similar to the COVID epidemic with variables such as incubation periods, mortality rates, geographically strategic hubs for travel, infrastructure, public health preparedness, treatment options, testing options, routes of entry (airborne, droplet, GI, etc. ...), national and international epidemiology communication, and many more. COVID -19 is an example of a near-perfect pathogen that could be used as a bioterrorism weapon. It was perfect in that it was incredibly virulent, there was initially very ineffective treatment of it, testing was not developed nor distributed well, there was not enough personal protective equipment (PPE) distributed to protect vulnerable health care workers, and symptoms varied greatly, killing some people whereas others remained asymptomatic, thereby, spreading the virus easier.[4]

One could argue that bioterrorism has been in its adolescent stage up to this point. It was largely curtailed after the international community witnessed the horrors of WWI and WWII. Governments and militaries have long used bioterrorism, but in modern times, most have converted the research to a more defensive approach. Bioterrorism is now more associated with selected attacks. One of the most infamous unsolved murder cases involved cyanide in Tylenol capsules in the Chicago suburbs 50 years ago, for which we still have no motive and many unanswered questions to this day. We also saw the anthrax attacks after September 11 that killed very few but created mass chaos and panic throughout the country.[5] But imagine a totalitarian government watching this COVID pandemic playing out the past few years. It can readily be argued that a robust biological warfare program would be much more effective than a nuclear arsenal if the goal is destruction. It would not be farfetched to imagine a government or terrorist organization creating another coronavirus or another virulent pathogen. The health care system of the United States was decimated by COVID-19 and the thought of another pandemic-related attack could possibly break an already fragile system.

Future Threats

As technology progresses in medicine and bioscience, so does the threat of a complicated genetically modified pathogen. Smallpox has been essentially wiped out with

Box 1
Categorical assignments of agents and pathogens by the CDC

Category A—The US public health system and primary health care providers must be prepared to address various biological agents, including pathogens that are rarely seen in the United States. High-priority agents include organisms that pose a risk to national security because they
1. Can be easily disseminated or transmitted from person to person;
2. Result in high mortality rates and have the potential for major public health impact;
3. Might cause public panic and social disruption; and
4. Require special action for public health preparedness.

Agents/Disease

Anthrax (*Bacillus anthracis*)

Botulism (*Clostridium* botulinum toxin)

Plague (*Yersinia pestis*)

Smallpox (variola major)

Tularemia (*Francisella tularensis*)

Viral hemorrhagic fevers, including
   Filoviruses (Ebola, Marburg)
   Arenaviruses (Lassa, Machupo)

Category B—Second highest priority agents include those that
• Are moderately easy to disseminate;
• Result in moderate morbidity rates and low mortality rates; and
• Require specific enhancements of CDC's diagnostic capacity and enhanced disease surveillance.

Agents/Disease

Brucellosis (*Brucella* species)

Epsilon toxin of *Clostridium perfringens.*

Food safety threats (*Salmonella* species, *Escherichia coli* O157:H7, *Shigella*)

Glanders (*Burkholderia mallei*)

Melioidosis (*Burkholderia pseudomallei*)

Psittacosis (*Chlamydia psittaci*)

Q fever (*Coxiella burnetii*)

Ricin toxin from *Ricinus communis* (castor beans)

Staphylococcal enterotoxin B

Typhus fever (*Rickettsia prowazekii*)

Viral encephalitis (alphaviruses, such as eastern equine encephalitis, Venezuelan equine encephalitis, and western equine encephalitis])

Water safety threats (*Vibrio cholerae, Cryptosporidium parvum*)

Category C

The third highest priority agents include emerging pathogens that could be engineered for mass dissemination in the future because of
• Availability;
• Ease of production and dissemination; and
• Potential for high morbidity and mortality rates and major health impact.

Agents/Disease
• Emerging infectious diseases such as the Nipah virus and hantavirus

There are also categorizations of chemical agents by the CDC. See **Figs. 1–4**.

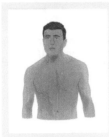
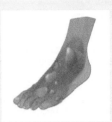

Chemicals causing severe blisters in the eyes, skin, and lining of the nose, sinuses, mouth, throat, and lungs (respiratory tract).

- Lewisite (L, L-1, L-2, L-3)
- Nitrogen mustard (HN-1, HN-2, HN-3)
- Phosgene oxime (CX)
- Sulfur mustard (H) (mustard gas)

More Information about Blister Agents

Fig. 1. Chemical Emergencies - Blister Agents (Vesicants). CDC. https://www.cdc.gov/chemicale mergencies/hcp/chemicals-by-category.html.

mass vaccinations that took a herculean effort last century. The caveat is that there are still different strains of the virus such as its cousin monkey pox which is spiking at the time of this writing. We are removed enough from smallpox that it is no longer a required vaccination which leaves this country vulnerable. The United States had stores of smallpox and even monkeypox vaccinations just in case of an outbreak of biological attack but a recent article has pointed out that before the monkeypox outbreak, 20 million doses of the vaccine expired.[6] This speaks volumes to the unpreparedness of our public health infrastructure.

Technology that gave us the mRNA COVID vaccines, CRISPR gene editing, AI, and other advances are like any other tool in the history of mankind. It can be used for good or evil. These advances may lead to malevolent breakthroughs in developing

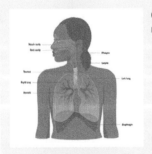

Chemicals causing severe irritation or swelling the lining of the respiratory tract.

- Ammonia
- Bromine (CA)
- Chlorine (CL)
- Hydrogen chloride
- Methyl bromide
- Methyl isocyanate

- Osmium tetroxide
- Phosgene (CG)
- Phosphine
- Phosphorus, elemental, white or yellow
- Sulfuryl fluoride

More Information about Pulmonary Agents

Fig. 2. Chemical Emergencies - Choking/Lung Agents (Pulmonary). CDC. https://www.cdc.gov/chemicalemergencies/hcp/chemicals-by-category.html.

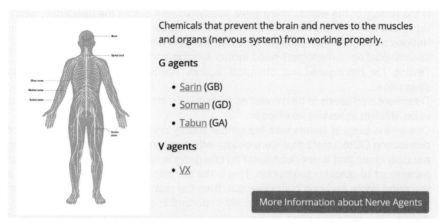

Chemicals that prevent the brain and nerves to the muscles and organs (nervous system) from working properly.

G agents

- Sarin (GB)
- Soman (GD)
- Tabun (GA)

V agents

- VX

More Information about Nerve Agents

Fig. 3. Chemical Emergencies - Nerve Agents. CDC. https://www.cdc.gov/chemicalemergencies/hcp/chemicals-by-category.html

previous pathogens that have the ominous history of the near extinction of humanity such as the Spanish flu, the plague, or smallpox. Nefarious groups could even make those previous pathogens even more deadly. They could, for example, create a strain with a longer incubation period allowing for further infection through asymptomatic carriers or make those pathogens even more virulent or create a more mutagenic version of the pathogen thereby decreasing the likelihood of an effective vaccine or testing.

How to Defend Against Such Attacks

COVID was a travesty on a scale we have not seen in a century. It disrupted the world but because of our firsthand experience with this disease, it has shown our vulnerabilities. We unequivocally must do better to prepare for the next pandemic, epidemic, or bioterrorist attack. The following is a list of steps that need to be addressed to prepare for the said attack.

1. International governments need to work for the betterment of humanity and not just for self-preservation. We saw those countries rich in resources did not readily distribute surplus vaccines to countries without vaccines. That allowed the virus to mutate and then prolong the pandemic. The world is not cleanly divided into borders. International organizations must invest in the public health and health care infrastructure of all nations for the preservation of all people.
2. Only through massive funding did scientists create the first mRNA vaccines. Never has a completely new technology been created and distributed in such a short time

- Biotoxins
- Blood Agents
- Caustics (Acids)
- Incapacitating Agents
- Metals
- Riot Control Agents/Tear Gas
- Toxic Alcohols

Fig. 4. Chemical Emergencies - Additional Chemicals by Category. CDC. https://www.cdc.gov/chemicalemergencies/hcp/chemicals-by-category.html.

in the history of the world. There were whistleblowers before the pandemic, warning of not only the possibility of a pandemic or epidemic but the inevitability of it. Nations must continue funding to prevent the next disaster.

3. International epidemiologists need further funding and support.
4. Testing for pathogens and chemical agents needs to be fast, reliable, and streamlined.
5. Treatment also needs to be developed fairly quickly and evidence-based data need to be efficient in testing its efficacy.
6. One of the biggest issues was the global supply chain that limited the speed of distributing COVID tests that were cheap, effective, and readily available. Creating a supply chain that is not dependent on one geographic area or one item would be paramount to quicker distribution. This is the Christmas light theory. If there are a thousand lights and one bulb goes out, then the rest go out. This cannot happen when testing and treatment are gravely important in containing pathogens. Companies have already turned to automation and AI, which would negate some of the vulnerabilities of manpower. The global supply chain is out of this author's and many health care professionals' area of expertise but nonetheless, if a physician associate (PA) does not have the tools to treat, they are made ineffective.
7. Politicization of health care has rooted deep distrust in the health care system. This will not be easily solved but is an incredibly important topic to tackle. Misinformation, disinformation, and political posturing almost became worse than the virus itself and it can be argued that the anti-vaccine movement sputtered our defense against COVID and weakened our health care system. This is a complicated topic beyond the scope of this section but again, nonetheless incredibly important to note in our defense against bioterrorism.
8. The health care system is deeply troubled. Caregiver burnout is rampant and the COVID pandemic broke a system that was already stressed. Many experienced health care workers have quit and without their experience and expertise, our health care system is incredibly vulnerable at the moment. Providing staffing, providing PPE, and decreasing the root causes of burnout are essential. This virus was particularly harmful because inadequate PPE allowed front line health care workers to contract COVID which created staffing shortages, and there might not be clear data yet, but anecdotally, the deaths related to the failure of the health care system were a difficult pill to swallow.
9. There needs to be further training of health care professionals including PAs, especially in hospital and inpatient settings to look out for evidence of bioterrorism.[7]

It is said that before the eruption of Mt. Vesuvius, there were ample warning signs that the volcano would erupt. Ash, seismic activity, and gas emissions all progressively increased months before the eruption, but were largely ignored by the population.[8] Our human tendency to believe that "everything will be all right" inhibits our ability to prepare and take seriously the red flags waving before us. As PAs, we are but a small chain in the link that is this country, but we must do our part to educate ourselves, our patients, and our health care systems, to be proactive in our pursuit of safety and security.

CLINICS CARE POINTS

- When considering differential diagnoses in odd settings or out-of-place signs and symptoms, one should include biochemical agents.
- If an agent is suspected, poison control is an excellent resource.

- Know your local resources and local public health guidelines. If working in a large metropolitan area, there may be disaster scenarios related to bioterrorism.
- The CDC has preparation and planning information for bioterrorism emergencies for health care workers on their Web site.
- Consider working with your hospital management on emergency plans for the next pandemic or any bioterrorism attack that includes supply chain vulnerabilities and medication allocation.

DISCLOSURE

No disclosures have been identified.

REFERENCES

1. Schneider BR. Biological weapons in history. In: Britannica EoE, editor. Britannica. "Weapon of Mass Destruction." *Encyclopædia Britannica*, Encyclopædia Britannica, Inc., 2023, Available at: https://www.britannica.com/technology/weapon-of-mass-destruction. Accessed March 23, 2023.
2. Das S, Kataria VK. Bioterrorism : A Public Health Perspective. Med J Armed Forces India 2010;66(3):255–60.
3. Bioterrorism Agents/Diseases. 2022. Available at: https://emergency.cdc.gov/agent/agentlist-category.asp. Accessed August 13, 2022.
4. Michalski A, Knap J, Bielawska-Drózd A, et al. Lessons learned from 2001-2021 - from the bioterrorism to the pandemic era. Ann Agric Environ Med 2022; 29(1):1–11.
5. Gostin LO, Nuzzo JB. Twenty Years After the Anthrax Terrorist Attacks of 2001: Lessons Learned and Unlearned for the COVID-19 Response. JAMA 2021;326(20): 2009–10.
6. Goldstein J. How the U.S. Let 20 Million Doses of Monkeypox Vaccine Expire. New York Times. 2022. Available at: https://www.nytimes.com/2022/08/01/nyregion/monkeypox-vaccine-jynneos-us.html. Accessed August 13, 2022.
7. Nofal A, AlFayyad I, AlJerian N, et al. Knowledge and preparedness of healthcare providers towards bioterrorism. BMC Health Serv Res 2021;21(1):426.
8. Bertagnini A, Cioni R, Guidoboni E, et al. Eruption early warning at Vesuvius: The A.D. 1631 lesson. Geophys Res Lett 2006;33(18). https://doi.org/10.1029/2006GL027297.

The Antivaccination Movement and Vaccine Hesitancy

James F. Cawley, MPH, PA-C[a,b]

KEYWORDS

- Vaccine hesitancy • Antivaccine • Immunization • COVID-19 vaccine

KEY POINTS

- Vaccination is a highly effective method to prevent infectious diseases. However, progress in the control of vaccine-preventable disease has stagnated in recent years due to vaccine hesitancy.
- Vaccine uptake is also hampered by socioeconomic factors, political viewpoints, or access to care barriers or structural barriers.
- Vaccine hesitancy is observed among all strata of society and includes health care workers.
- National surveys steadily report greater degrees of COVID-19 vaccine hesitancy in BIPOC (black, indigenous, and people of color) communities.
- Misinformation on social media platforms has a significant effect on citizen willingness to be vaccinated.

INTRODUCTION

Immunization against disease is among the most successful global public health efforts of the modern era, and substantial gains in vaccination coverage rates have been achieved worldwide. Vaccination is a highly effective method to prevent a number of infectious (communicable) diseases. Immunization has led to significant improvements in child, traveler, and adult health over the past 60 years. Many infectious diseases common in prior generations, like polio and measles, are less common today due to immunization. Common vaccine-preventable diseases also include diphtheria, *Haemophilus influenzae* type b, hepatitis A and B, human papillomavirus, influenza (flu), meningococcal infections, mumps, pertussis (whooping cough), pneumococcal infections, rotavirus, rubella, tetanus, and varicella (chickenpox).[1]

[a] Physician Assistant Leadership and Learning Academy, University of Maryland Baltimore, Baltimore, MD, USA; [b] Professor Emeritus of Prevention and Community Health, Milkin Institute School of Public Health, The George Washington University
E-mail address: jcawley@umaryland.edu

Physician Assist Clin 8 (2023) 583–591
https://doi.org/10.1016/j.cpha.2023.02.004
2405-7991/23/© 2023 Elsevier Inc. All rights reserved.

However, progress in the control of vaccine-preventable disease has stagnated in recent years due to vaccine hesitancy. Vaccine hesitancy is defined as a "delay in acceptance or refusal of vaccines despite availability of vaccination services" and has become a key driver in the control of vaccine-preventable diseases.[2] We now know that in society there are a vocal minority of people who are sternly opposed to vaccination, and most vaccine-hesitant individuals fall on a spectrum from vaccine acceptance to vaccine denial. Vaccine uptake is also hampered by socioeconomic factors, political viewpoints, or access to care barriers or structural barriers to access.[3] Vaccine hesitancy is observed among all strata of society and includes health care workers. This article describes the phenomena of vaccine hesitancy, certain groups affected by hesitancy, the barriers to acceptance of vaccines as an important public health primary prevention intervention, and some thoughts on the future of the control of infectious disease through the use of immunizations.

Historical Perspectives

To gain an understanding of modern-day fear of vaccines and the serious diseases that they prevent, we must first focus on smallpox (*Variola vera*). The earliest written description of a disease like smallpox appeared in China in the fourth century. Historians trace the global spread of smallpox to the growth of civilizations and exploration. Expanding trade routes over many centuries led to the spread of the disease. In 1796, the English doctor Edward Jenner noticed that milkmaids who had gotten cowpox were protected from smallpox. Jenner also knew about variolation and guessed that exposure to cowpox could be used to protect against smallpox. Vaccination became widely accepted and gradually replaced the practice of variolation. At some point in the 1800s, the virus used to make the smallpox vaccine changed from cowpox to vaccinia virus. Almost 2 centuries after Jenner hoped that vaccination could annihilate smallpox, the World Health Organization (WHO) in the late 1960s embarked on a global campaign to eradicate smallpox. Shortly after the last known case of the disease was documented in Somalia in 1977, the WHO declared the world free of this disease in 1980. Many people consider smallpox eradication to be the biggest achievement in international public health and one of the most impressive scientific achievements of the twentieth century.[4]

In the last 100 years, science has produced vaccines that prevent or modify more than 30 human infectious diseases. Smallpox was eradicated globally in 1980. Three diseases (polio, measles, and congenital rubella syndrome) have been effectively eliminated from many developed countries (although outbreaks of measles have recently been observed in the United States), and morbidity from six other diseases has been reduced by more than 97% in the United States. Approximately 95% of children are now protected against diphtheria, tetanus, pertussis, measles, mumps, rubella, and varicella by age 6 years in most US jurisdictions with few racial or socioeconomic disparities, in part due to successful administration of required school immunizations.[5] Estimates project that vaccines recommended for children in the United States and territories will prevent 21 million hospitalizations and avert 730,000 deaths in the 10-year cohort of children born between 1994 and 2013, while saving $295 billion in direct costs and US$1.38 trillion in societal costs (both net cost of vaccination).[6]

The root of the modern era of antivaccine attitudes began in 1998 when British gastroenterologist Andrew Wakefield[7] published a case series in the *Lancet* that suggested that the measles, mumps, and rubella (MMR) vaccine seemed to predispose children to behavioral regression and autism. Despite a small sample size (n = 12), an uncontrolled design, and the speculative nature of the conclusions, the paper received wide publicity and MMR vaccination rates began to drop due to parental concern about the risk of autism.[7] Soon after, scientists, epidemiologists, and public health organizations began to criticize the speculative association asserted by Wakefield, but evidence and informed opinion that refuted this assertion received much less attention.[8] It took more than 10 years before the *Lancet* issued a retraction of Wakefield's paper admitting that several elements in the paper were incorrect, contrary to the findings of the earlier investigation.[9] By this time, Britain's General Medical Council had stripped Wakefield of his medical license, and he and his colleagues were held guilty of ethical violations (they had conducted invasive investigations on the children without obtaining the necessary ethical clearances) and scientific misrepresentation. In 2004, after an extensive review of vaccine safety, the Institute of Medicine of the National Academy of Science issued a report stating flatly that "that the evidence favors rejection of a causal relationship between thimerosal containing vaccines and autism."[10]

Vaccine Hesitancy

Vaccine hesitancy is pervasive, perhaps affecting as much as a quarter of US parents. Clinicians report that they routinely receive requests to delay vaccines and that they routinely acquiesce. Vaccine rates vary by state and locale and by specific vaccine, and vaccine hesitancy results in personal risk and in the failure to achieve or sustain herd immunity to protect others who have contraindications to the vaccine or fail to generate immunity to the vaccine. It has been recommended that clinicians should adopt a variety of practices to combat vaccine hesitancy, including a variety of population health management approaches that go beyond the usual call to educate patients, clinicians, and the public. Strategies include using every visit to vaccinate, and the creation of standing orders for immunization or practice protocols to provide vaccination, and adopting the practice of stating clear recommendations. Up-to-date, trusted resources exist to support clinicians' efforts in adopting these approaches to reduce vaccine hesitancy and its impact.[11]

Although there are medical, religious, and philosophic considerations that contribute to vaccine hesitancy, the data continuously show that coronavirus disease (COVID) vaccines are safe and effective and reduce the number of hospitalizations and deaths. Yet a growing number of Americans including frontline health care workers remain incredulous about the COVID vaccine campaign. According to the Kaiser Family Foundation survey, 16% of respondents will "definitely not" get the vaccine. Frontline health care workers understand their duty to protect patients but are not immune from antivaccination views and may harbor similar distrust as some in the public concerning the COVID vaccine campaign.[12] This distrust may be in part due to the rapid development and availability of COVID vaccines in under 1 year, whereas nearly all other prior vaccines have taken years to complete the regulatory approval process before public distribution. This difference may give the impression that the vaccines were rushed and not scientifically vetted for potential side effects and downstream risks, which is underscored by a 2021 community survey, which showed 71% of respondents citing concerns about side effects.[13]

Furthermore, vaccine distrust may have been fueled by the imposition of mandates, which some have pontificated violated their constitutional freedom. Moreover, changing guidance from the Centers for Disease Control and Prevention (CDC) and contradictory statements by officials have led to confusion and criticism sparking antivirus sentiment in many segments of society. Some would argue that the constant mixed messaging and polarization of the virus by authorities is undermining public trust and calling into question, whether there is alignment between public health experts and elected officials. This has often played out in the courts, where rolling vaccine mandates issued by the federal government have been blocked, perhaps exacerbating the confusion around the importance of vaccines.

Another factor contributing to vaccine hesitancy is misinformation on social media platforms. A great deal of misinformation, propagated largely on social media, has a significant effect on citizen willingness to be hesitant regarding COVID-19 vaccines. A disturbing myth held by more than a third of unvaccinated persons and 40% of blacks is that the vaccine itself causes COVID-19. Another myth is that the vaccines cause infertility. About 29% of unvaccinated adults believe that or do not know, as do 31% of Republicans and the same percentage of unvaccinated adults believe that vaccines changed a person's DNA. Two-thirds of unvaccinated adults believe at least one of these vaccine myths.[12] Detoxifying malicious content about vaccines is no easy task and requires concerted efforts between public health officials and social media administrators to help disarm the proliferation of COVID-19 vaccine conspiracy theories. As was seen in the COVID-19 pandemic, not only were unvaccinated individuals a threat to public health but also there was a substantial economic burden that resulted from that segment of the US population (**Fig. 1**).

Vaccine Hesitancy Among Vulnerable Populations

National surveys steadily report greater degrees of COVID-19 vaccine hesitancy in BIPOC (black, indigenous, and people of color) communities, and there are multiple historical reasons to justify skepticism about vaccines among this group. A long list historical experiences with medical research abuses, most notably the US Public Health Service Syphilis Study at Tuskegee. The goal of this inhuman research study was to observe the natural history of untreated syphilis in black sharecroppers in Alabama, but the subjects were completely unaware of the researchers' true intentions and were told they were receiving treatment of bad blood (assessed from https://www.cdc.gov/tuskegee/timeline.htm). Unfortunately, the sharecroppers never received any treatment and succumbed to latent syphilis. This incident led to greater mistrust of the American health care system among the black population who were already subject to profound racial injustice, inequity, and marginalization.

The Tuskegee experiment remains a stain on American history, and decades later, blacks continue to experience worse health care outcomes when compared with their white counterparts.[14] Consequently, blacks have been disproportionately affected by

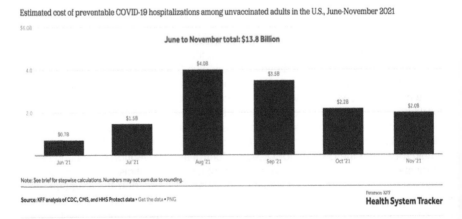

Estimated cost of preventable COVID-19 hospitalizations among unvaccinated adults in the U.S., June-November 2021

June to November total: $13.8 Billion

Note: See brief for stepwise calculations. Numbers may not sum due to rounding.

Source: KFF analysis of CDC, CMS, and HHS Protect data • Get the data • PNG

Peterson-KFF
Health System Tracker

Fig. 1. Cost of the unvaccinated.

COVID-19 and vaccination rates remain uneven in people of color.[15] One way the health care community can build trust with black Americans is through culturally appropriate communication coupled with an understanding and acknowledgment of black Americans' negative experiences within the US health care system.

One recent study compared vaccine uptake and hesitancy among minority populations in the United States and the United Kingdom. In the United States ($n = 87,250$) compared with white participants, vaccine hesitancy was greater for black and Hispanic participants and those reporting more than one or the other race. In the United Kingdom ($n = 1,254,294$), racial and ethnic minority participants showed similar levels of vaccine hesitancy to the United States. However, associations between participant race and ethnicity and levels of vaccine uptake were observed to be different in the US and the UK studies. Among US participants, vaccine uptake was significantly lower among black participants, which persisted among participants who self-reported being vaccine willing. In contrast, statistically significant racial and ethnic disparities in vaccine uptake were not observed in the UK sample. In this study of self-reported vaccine hesitancy and uptake, lower levels of vaccine uptake in black participants in the United Sates during the initial vaccine rollout may be attributable to both hesitancy and disparities in access.[16]

Polarization of Vaccines

Over the past decade, antivaccine groups and leaders have begun to organize politically founded state political action committees, formed coalitions with other constituencies, and built a vast network that is now the foundation of vaccination opposition by conservative groups and legislators across the country.[17] These groups and leaders use common-sense concepts, for example, that parents should be able to raise their children as they see fit, and that medical decisions should be autonomous, private, and not government paternalism. Undoubtedly, polarization has opened political rifts in vaccination rates and vaccine efficacy. The antivaccine movement is expanding and so is its alliances and influence among those skeptical of government overreach. This discourse has plagued every facet of society and instilled uncertainty in a fluid situation. Owing to the evolving nature of COVID-19, public health experts despite their best efforts have struggled to combat polarization. Subsequently, some Americans leery of the polarized American political climate have turned to other sources of information, which may be inaccurate, anecdotal, and perpetuate the spread of fake news. The Director General of the WHO mentioned "We're not just fighting an epidemic; we're fighting an infodemic. Fake news spreads faster and more easily than this virus, and is just as dangerous."[18] Thus, the term "infodemic" rose from relative obscurity to international prominence. The WHO went on to note that the 2019-novel coronavirus outbreak and response "has been accompanied by a massive 'infodemic'–an over-abundance of information–some accurate and some not–that makes it hard for people to find trustworthy sources and reliable guidance when they need it."[18] Observers from the University of Oxford have commented on the technical inaccuracy of this epidemiologic metaphone but admit that, when it comes to COVID-19 vaccine information, we are in an era of increasing misinformation.[19]

Given the number of news, social media outlets, and partisan divide, it is impossible to stop the flow of disinformation or debunk every piece of fake news or Internet thread. Consequently, politicians need to rally behind the public health infrastructure and promote the inherent and historical benefits of vaccination programs throughout modern history that have made a fundamental contribution to the American health care system and life expectancy. In addition, Facebook, Twitter, and other social media platforms need greater safeguards and restrictions to stem the flow of vaccine misinformation and strategies to address antivaccine accounts that frequently overstep the companies' terms of service.

Evidence-Based Strategies to Help Clinicians Address Vaccine Hesitancy

An effective evidence-based strategy must be comprehensive in scope to address vaccine hesitancy. Given the average American does not understand the intricacies of vaccine development, a recommended strategy is to reassure patients that COVID vaccines were created without compromising safety. Patients who are on the fence about COVID vaccines may be more inclined to get inoculated if they are assured that vaccines manufacturers did not cut corners and the vaccines are as safe as the required traditional immunizations.

Vaccine Hesitancy: Health Care Workers

Health care providers (HCPs) hold considerable influence in the decision of their patients to be vaccinated.[20] In one review it was shown that HCPs who were vaccinated themselves (or who intended to be vaccinated) were more likely to recommend vaccination to their patients. Older individuals, males, and those with past flu vaccination history or compliance with other vaccines were more likely to accept COVID-19 vaccination. Some vaccinated HCPs believed that by getting vaccinated themselves they could provide a reassuring example to patients, particularly those who have concerns.[21]

Recently vaccine hesitancy has been observed among health care workers globally. In many respects, there are curious incongruities regarding vaccines that are evident among health care workers who have risked their employment over the COVID-19 vaccine. As part of their employment on-boarding, most new hires are required to take a series of immunizations including shots against hepatitis B. The CDC recommends that all health care workers, emergency personnel, and other individuals who are exposed to blood or bodily fluids should be vaccinated against hepatitis B.[22] Most medical students, physician assistants (PA) students, and other health professional schools require students to be immunized against hepatitis before serving on clinical training rotations. Yet, despite the apparent familiarity of most health care workers with commonly required vaccines, the expression of vaccine hesitancy and outright refusal among health care workers during the COVID-19 pandemic was widespread.

A scoping review of the published literature was conducted, and a final pool of 51 studies ($n = 41,098$ nurses) from 36 countries was included in this review. The overall pooled prevalence rate of COVID-19 vaccine refusal among 41,098 nurses worldwide was 20.7% (95% CI = 16.5%–27%). The rates of vaccination refusal were higher from March 2020 to December 2020 compared with the rates from January 2021 to May 2021. The major reasons for COVID-19 vaccine refusal were concerns about vaccine safety, side effects, and efficacy; misinformation and lack of knowledge; and mistrust in experts, authorities, or pharmaceutical companies. It should be noted that most of the studies included in this review were conducted when the vaccines were approved under emergency use authorization.[23]

Vaccine Hesitancy and Vaccine Refusal

Vaccine hesitancy is closely related to outright vaccine refusal. Of late there has been an uptick in the occurrence of common vaccine-preventable infectious diseases like measles and pertussis. Vaccine refusal has been associated with an increased risk for measles among people who refuse vaccines and among fully vaccinated individuals. Most of the US measles cases in the era after measles elimination represent cases of higher risk due to intentionally unvaccinated children. Although pertussis resurgence has been attributed to waning immunity and other factors, vaccine refusal was still associated with an increased risk for pertussis in some populations.[11]

The Role of Vaccine Inequity as a Risk Factor for Vaccine Hesitancy

Strategies to improve vaccine compliance in the wake of case decisions by the judiciary. New approaches are needed to mitigate barriers to accessing routine and pandemic-related vaccination services, build trust between patients and providers to encourage effective communication about vaccines, and dispel the myths and misinformation that erode public confidence in vaccines.

SUMMARY

There is concern that the antivaccine movement has now become assimilated into the wider political world under the flag of infringement on individual freedom.[24] America exists in an era of anti-intellectualism and antiscience.[25] Notable experts in medicine and public health, particularly during the COVID-19 pandemic, have repeatedly been subjected to harsh and unfair criticism. Thus, it is not surprising that the antivaccine movement in the United States has emerged and thrived in society and more recently has assumed a stance that federal and/or state imposition of vaccine requirements constitutes a denial of a civil right.

Antivaccine attitudes have changed and expanded in the last several years. The "Disneyland" measles outbreak drew vaccine opposition into the political mainstream, followed by promotional campaigns conducted in pages framing vaccine refusal as a civil right. Political mobilization in state-focused campaigns followed in 2019. The dynamics of health misinformation on Facebook pose a threat to vaccination programs. Social media exposure is theorized to amplify vaccine skepticism.[26] As a result, public health officials, political leaders, and health researchers should expect more attempts to amend state-legislated regulations associated with vaccine exemptions, potentially accompanied by fiercer lobbying from specific celebrities.[26]

The benefit of immunization as a public health measure has had an immense, unassailable impact on the health of children and adults due to highly effective vaccines. Newer vaccines, such as the coronavirus vaccine, have also been proved to be safe and effective. Despite these unquestioned successes, all vaccines face continuing obstacles bred of ignorance and mistrust in the quest to achieve sufficient levels of public acceptance.[27]

CLINICS CARE POINTS

- Vaccine hesitancy is prevalent and presents challenges to public health as well as indivual clinicians.

DISCLOSURE

The authors have nothing to disclose.

REFERENCES

1. Association of Professionals in Infection Control and Epidemiology. Vaccination saves lives. Available at: https://apic.org/monthly_alerts/vaccination-saves-lives/.

2. National Academies of Sciences, Engineering, and Medicine. The critical public health value of vaccines: tackling issues of access and hesitancy: proceedings of a workshop. Washington, DC: The National Academies Press; 2021.

3. Centers for Disease Control and Prevention National Center for Immunization and Respiratory Diseases. Vaccinate with confidence. Atlanta, GA: CDC NCIRD; 2019.

4. Centers for Disease Control and Prevention. History of Smallpox. Available at: https://www.cdc.gov/smallpox/history/history.html.

5. Centers for Disease Control and Prevention. Diseases you almost forgot about (thanks to vaccines). 2020. Available at: https://www.cdc.gov/vaccines/parents/diseases/forgot-14-diseases.html.

6. Whitney CG, Zhou F, Singlreton J, et al, Centers for Disease Control and Prevention. Benefits from immunization during the vaccines for children program era—United States, 1994–2013. Morb Mortal Wkly Rep 2014;63:352–5.

7. Wakefield AJ, Murch SH, Anthony A, et al. Ileal-lymphoid-nodular hyperplasia, non-specific colitis, and pervasive developmental disorder in children. Lancet 1998;351:637–41.

8. Taylor B, Miller E, Farrington CP, et al. Autism and measles, mumps, and rubella vaccine: No epidemiologic evidence for a causal association. Lancet 1999;353:2026–9.

9. Eggertson L. Lancet retracts 12-year-old article linking autism to MMR vaccines. CMAJ (Can Med Assoc J) 2010;182:E199–200.

10. National Academy of Sciences. Institute of Medicine. Immunization safety review: vaccines and autism. Washington, D.C.: National Academy Press; 2004.

11. Mayo Clinic Proceedings. Vaccine Hesitancy. Available at: https://www.mayoclinicproceedings.org/article/S0025-6196(15)00719-3/fulltext.

12. Altman D. Persistent Vaccine Myths. Available at: https://www.kff.org/coronavirus-covid-19/perspective/persistent-vaccine-myths/.

13. SteelFisher G, Blendon R, Caporello H. An Uncertain Public – Encouraging Acceptance of Covid-19 Vaccines. N Engl J Med 2021;384:1483–8.

14. Commonwealth Fund. Achieving racial and ethnic equity in U.S. health care. Scorecard. 2021. November 18, 2021). Available at: https://www.commonwealthfund.org/publications/scorecard/2021/nov/achieving-racial-ethnic-equity-us-health-care-state-performance.

15. Centers for Disease Control and Prevention. Risk for COVID-19 infection, hospitalization, and death by Race/Ethnicity. Centers for Disease Control and Prevention. Retrieved May 23, 2022, Available at: https://www.cdc.gov/coronavirus/2019-ncov/covid-data/investigations-discovery/hospitalization-death-by-race-ethnicity.html.

16. Nguyen LH, Joshi AD, Drew DA, et al. Self-reported COVID-19 vaccine hesitancy and uptake among participants from different racial and ethnic groups in the United States and United Kingdom. Nat Commun 2022;13:636.

17. Mnookin S. The panic virus: fear, myth, and the vaccination debate. New York: Simon & Schuster; 2011.

18. World Health Organization, Novel Coronavirus (2019 = n19), *Situation Report*, 13, 2020, 1-2.

19. Oxford Internet Institute, University of Oxford. Are We Really Living in and 'Infodemic'? Science Suggests a Different Story. 2021. Available at: https://www.oii.ox.ac.uk/news-events/news/are-we-really-living-in-an-infodemic-science-suggests-a-different-story/.

20. Heyerdahl L, Dielen S, Nguyen T, et al. Doubt at the Core: Unspoken Vaccine Hesitancy Among Healthcare Workers. Lancet Regional Health-Europe 2021. https://doi.org/10.1016/j.lanepe.2021.100289.
21. Centers for Disease Control and Prevention (CDC). Hepatitis B Vaccination. Available at: https://www.cdc.gov/vaccines/vpd/hepb/index.html#:~:text=The%20hepatitis%20B%20vaccine%20is,factors%20for%20hepatitis%20B%20infection.
22. Paterson P, Meurice F, Stanbury L, et al. Vaccine Hesitancy and Healthcare Providers. Vaccine 2016;6700–6.
23. Khubchandani J, Bustos E, Chowdhury S, et al. COVID-19 Vaccine Refusal Among Nurses Worldwide: Review of Trends and Predictors. Vaccines(Basel) 2022;10:230.
24. Velasquez-Manaff M. The Anti-Vaccine Movement's New Frontier. New York Times, Sunday 2022.
25. Hotez P. The antiscience movement is escalating, going global and killing thousands. Scientific American 2021;21:45–51.
26. Broniawtoski DA, Jamison A, Johnson N, et al. Facebook Pages, The Disneyland Measles Outbreak, and Promotion of Vaccines as a Civil Right, 2009-2019. Am J Public Health 2020;110:S312–8.
27. Modlim JF, Schaffner W, Orenstein W, et al. Journal of Infectious Disease 2021; 224(Issue Supplement):S307–8.

Intersection of Emerging Infectious Diseases and Substance Use Disorder
Emerging Trends, Epidemiology, Human Immunodeficiency Virus, Hepatitis

Sampath Wijesinghe, DHSc, AAHIVS, PA-C[a],*,
Anne Walsh, MMSc, PA-C, DFAAPA[b], Jenn Stauffer, MHS, PA-C, AAHIVS[c],
Nancy Hamler, DMSc, MPA, RDN, PA-C[d,e], Olivia Sawh, MS, PA-C[f]

KEYWORDS

- Substance use disorder • Infectious disease • HIV • Hepatitis
- Emerging infectious disease

KEY POINTS

- There is a strong correlation between emerging infections and substance use disorder.
- Understanding the correlation between SUD and HIV.
- Understanding the correlation between SUD and Hepatitis.

INTRODUCTION

Infectious diseases (IDs) and substance use disorders (SUD) are accountable for numerous alarming health conditions in the world. Individuals with high-risk behaviors associated with drug use put themselves at risk for contracting or transmitting viral infections, such as human immunodeficiency virus (HIV) or hepatitis. Indisputably, HIV,

[a] Stanford School of Medicine – MSPA Education, 1265 Welch Road, Suite 100, Stanford, CA 94305, USA; [b] Chapman University – MMS-PA Studies Program, 9401 Jeronimo Road, Irvine, CA 92618, USA; [c] Oklahoma State University Center for Health Sciences Physician Assistant Program, 1111 West 17th Street, Tulsa, OK 74107, USA; [d] Department of MS Physician Assistant Science, University of the Pacific | School Health Sciences, 3200 Fifth Avenue, Sacramento, CA 95817, USA; [e] Department of MS Clinical Nutrition, University of the Pacific | School Health Sciences, 3200 Fifth Avenue, Sacramento, CA 95817, USA; [f] Instructional Faculty and Stanford Educators4Care (E4C)-PA, Stanford School of Medicine, 1265 Welch Road, Suite 100, Stanford, CA 94305, USA
* Corresponding author.
E-mail address: samwije@stanford.edu

Physician Assist Clin 8 (2023) 593–612
https://doi.org/10.1016/j.cpha.2023.02.009
2405-7991/23/© 2023 Elsevier Inc. All rights reserved.

viral hepatitis, and SUD continue to be a threat not only in the United States but also globally. The following facts demonstrate the significance of this threat.

In 2018, 7.2 million medical visits were related to infectious and parasitic diseases. Of those, 3.4 million occurred in the emergency department. Out of these 3.4 million people, 523,000 were admitted to the hospital with a principal hospital discharge diagnosis of infectious and parasitic diseases.[1]

Since 1999, drug overdose has killed approximately 932,000 people. In 2020, approximately 75% of drug overdose mortalities involved an opioid. Overdose deaths have increased more than eight-fold since 1999.[2] In 2020, opioids killed almost 69,000 people, and more than 82% of those deaths were from synthetic opioids.[3]

In 2019, there were 36,801 newly diagnosed HIV cases in the United States and dependent areas. Of those, people who inject drugs accounted for 7% (2,508). The same year, there were 15,815 deaths among people with diagnosed HIV in the United States and dependent areas.[4]

In 2018, although 12,474 cases of hepatitis A were reported in the United States, the actual number of cases is estimated to be 24,900 largely due to underreporting. The current evidence suggests that there has been an increase of hepatitis A infections since 2016.[5]

In 2018, a total of 3,322 hepatitis B cases were reported. After adjusting for case underascertainment and underreporting, the actual number of cases were estimated to be 21,600.[5]

In 2019, a total of 4,136 cases of acute hepatitis C were reported. After adjusting for underascertainment and underreporting, the total was estimated as 57,500. Injection-drug use caused many infections and was the most common mode of hepatitis C virus (HCV) transmission in the United States.[6]

In general, clinicians may appreciate that patients with SUD frequently suffer from other mental health conditions, such as depression, anxiety disorders, and personality disorders. Furthermore, individuals with SUD are susceptible to ID. This chapter focuses on emerging trends and epidemiology between SUD and HIV/hepatitis as well as screening and treatments for these diseases. Finally, calls for action are discussed to provide some helpful information to all clinicians about the implications of this investigation on clinical practice.

Hepatitis D and Hepatitis E

Hepatitis D virus (HDV) and hepatitis E virus (HEV) are uncommon in the United States. Most HDV occurs among people who migrate or travel to the United States from countries with high HDV endemicity. HDV is not a nationally notifiable condition in the United States; therefore, the actual number of HDV cases is unknown.[7] Most of the symptomatic HEV in the United States occurs among people who have traveled to a developing country where HEV is endemic. Random, non-travel-related cases of HEV have been reported in the United States.[8] No clear exposure was identified for these domestically acquired cases. Given the rarity of HDV and HEV infections in the United States, they are not discussed in this chapter.

DISCUSSION
Substance Use Disorder and Infectious Disease

SUD is defined as a problematic pattern of substance use that has caused significant impairment and/or distress to a person in a 12-month period. Specifically, it is defined by the *Diagnostic and Statistical Manual of Mental Disorders* (fifth edition) (*DSM-5*), by the 11 criteria listed, and the condition is named more specifically depending on the substance or substances involved (for example, alcohol use disorder or opioid use disorder). The severity of the SUD is determined by the number of criteria met. Two to 3 criteria indicate mild SUD; 4 or 5 criteria indicate moderate SUD, and 6 or more criteria indicate severe SUD.

The 11 *DSM-5* criteria for a substance use disorder are as follows[9]:

	Criteria
1	The substance is often taken in larger amounts or over a longer period than was intended.
2	There is a persistent desire or unsuccessful efforts to cut down or control use.
3	A great deal of time is spent in activities necessary to obtain the substance, use the substance, or recover from its effects.
4	There is a craving or a strong desire or urge to use the substance.
5	There is recurrent use resulting in a failure to fulfill major role obligations at work, school, or home.
6	There is continued use despite having persistent or recurrent social or interpersonal problems caused or exacerbated by its effects.
7	Important social, occupational, or recreational activities are given up or reduced because of use.
8	There is recurrent use in situations in which it is physically hazardous.
9	Use is continued despite knowledge of having a persistent or recurrent physical or psychological problem that is likely to have been caused or exacerbated by the substance.
10	Tolerance (there is a need for markedly increased amounts of the substance to achieve intoxication or the desired effected, or markedly diminished effect with continued use of the same amount of the substance).
11	Withdrawal (there are withdrawal symptoms that occur when substance use is cut back or stopped following a period of prolonged use).

Of note, it is important to distinguish SUD from substance dependence. In substance dependence, a patient shows signs of physiologic tolerance and/or withdrawal (ie, to opioids or benzodiazepines) but takes the substance as prescribed and does not show signs of impaired control, social impairment, or risky use.

Among people aged 12 years and older in the United States in 2020, 14.5% of people qualified for a diagnosis of SUD. Within that group, 10.2% met criteria for alcohol use disorder (the most common from of SUD), and 6.6% of people met criteria for illicit drug use disorder (illicit drugs were defined as marijuana, cocaine, heroin, hallucinogens, inhalants, methamphetamine, or misused prescription psychotherapeutic drugs). Of note, SUDs are not mutually exclusive.[10] More broadly, 13.5% of people reported using an illicit drug within the past month.[10] Of note, this survey by the US Substance Abuse and Mental Health Services Administration excludes people who are homeless and not in shelters, residents of institutional group living (jails, nursing homes, mental institutions, and long-term care hospitals), and military personnel on active duty, so the real numbers are likely higher.[10] Furthermore, the impact of the COVID-19 pandemic on these numbers is not fully known yet, but it is likely that the pandemic brought increases in substance use, increases in associated morbidity and mortality, and decreases in access to SUD treatment services.

Substance use and SUDs are risk factors for the transmission and progression of ID because people may engage in risky behaviors to become intoxicated and/or while intoxicated. In addition, chronic use of some substances may be associated a less robust immune system over time.[11]

First, ID may result from behaviors performed to become intoxicated. Routes of substance administration include oral, inhalation, intranasal ("snorting"), intravenous ("shooting up"), subcutaneous ("skin popping"), or intramuscular ("muscling"). More invasive routes are associated with increased risk of bacterial, viral, and fungal infections, and the use of invasive routes often points toward a more severe SUD.[12] For example, if a person is injecting a substance, they at higher risk for developing ID and is more likely to meet criteria for a more severe SUD (injection drug use aligns with SUD criteria 8 and/or 9). These risks are further increased by use of needles and supplies that are not sterile, repeatedly used, and/or shared. Infectious conditions that can result from these administration routes include, but are not limited to, cellulitis, localized abscesses, HIV, hepatitis, infectious endocarditis, bacteremia, and osteomyelitis.[11] As an example, one study suggested that the US opioid epidemic and the resulting increased injection drug use could likely explain the national increase in hepatitis C infection.[13] Therefore, while taking a substance use history, it is important to note the route or routes of administration for each substance. While completing a physical examination, it is important to look for signs of drug use (ie, injection sites or "track marks") and physical signs and sequelae of ID.

In addition to risky behaviors performed to become intoxicated, people who use substances are also at higher risk for ID because of behaviors performed while intoxicated. For example, people under the influence are more likely to engage in high-risk sexual activity, such as inconsistent use of barrier protection, engaging with multiple partners, or performing sexual acts in exchange for substances.[11] This increases the risk of sexually transmitted infections (STIs), such as gonorrhea, chlamydia, syphilis, herpes, HIV, or hepatitis.

Third, chronic substance use has been shown to decrease immunity over time, further contributing to the likelihood of contracting an ID.[11] Finally, it is important to note that substance use and ID are often compounded by other factors, such as poverty, housing instability, and decreased health care access and utilization.

Highlights for Clinicians

Given that substance use and SUDs are modifiable risk factors for the transmission and progression of ID, more training on the diagnosis and treatment of SUDs should be given to health care providers and trainees. Historically, SUD education has been minimal in medical schools, physician associate (PA), nurse practitioner (NP) programs, and other training programs, which leads to practicing providers with limited knowledge about SUDs. Increased training would allow providers to feel more confident in treating SUDs and would likely decrease the stigma surrounding SUDs.

Also, when appropriate, the treatment of the ID should include treatment of the underlying SUD. Therefore, the treatment of comorbid ID and SUD should be interdisciplinary and multimodal. It should also include harm reduction education and strategies (ie, clean needles and supplies, safe injecting sites), vaccines for the prevention of other ID, medications if available (ie, pre-exposure prophylaxis [PrEP] for HIV), barrier contraception for STI prevention, and access to psychosocial support.[11]

Finally, there is a lesson to be learned by focusing on the data provided in. According to the figure, 39% of physicians and 38% of patients are responsible for the opioid crisis. Therefore, it is reasonable to state that more physicians are responsible for the opioid crisis than patients. Besides, 9% of pharmacists are also responsible for the opioid crisis. An intervention to alleviate physician (including PAs an NPs) and pharmacist responsibility for the opioid crisis would alleviate some of the problems related to SUDs. Therefore, it is critical to study this problem thoroughly and come up with possible solutions to lessen this crisis. All health care team members should be aware that almost half of the opioid crisis was originated by them.

Hepatitis and Substance Use Disorder

Viral hepatitis

The prevalence of viral hepatitis has increased exponentially over the past 3 decades, despite the most common infections, hepatitis A virus (HAV), hepatitis B virus (HBV), and HCV, being preventable, treatable, or curable. The primary factor driving this increase is the opioid crisis.[14] Substance use disorder, particularly injection drug use, has fueled a wave of new viral hepatitis infections that challenge the health care system's ability to diagnose and manage chronic liver disease and oblige clinicians to address the associated high-risk behaviors. Clinicians caring for patients with SUD must be aware of the ongoing risk for both acute and chronic viral hepatitis and remain up-to-date, as new knowledge informs changes in clinical practice guidelines.

In patients without underlying liver disease, acute infection with HAV or HBV results in fulminant hepatic failure in 1% and 10% of cases, respectively. In patients with SUD, coinfections are common however, and patients with underlying chronic HBV or HCV who contract acute HAV are at much higher risk of fatal fulminant hepatic failure, approximately 33%, with a fatality rate more than 50%.[15] It is important to screen all patients diagnosed with viral hepatitis for coinfection with other hepatotropic viruses (HAV, HBV, HCV).

Chronic viral hepatitis owing to HBV or HCV is complicated by end-stage liver failure with or without hepatocellular carcinoma (HCC) in up to one-third of cases, necessitating liver transplant for survival. The presence of other chronic liver disease, including alcoholic and nonalcoholic fatty liver, increases the rate of disease progression and risk of complications, such as variceal bleeding and hepatic encephalopathy. Thousands of patients die each year waiting for a liver transplant. In the United States, liver transplant may cost approximately $875,000.[16] Liver transplant success varies based on many factors but continues to improve, with up to 90% of patients alive at 1 year and more than 75% alive at five years.[17]

Recommendations for two critical preventive measures, viral hepatitis screening and vaccination, have evolved in recent years based on changing patient demographics and novel drug development.

Hepatitis A

Characteristically transmitted through the fecal-oral route, HAV infections are typically related to contaminated food exposures, for example, via fecal contamination of fresh produce or infected food service workers. In an investigation of recent outbreaks, parenteral exposures have also been implicated, placing persons who use or inject illicit drugs at high risk.

HAV, which causes potentially severe acute hepatitis, is vaccine-preventable through a 2-dose series that provides close to 100% protection for a minimum of 25 years and is likely life-long. Although vaccination was first recommended for high-risk populations in 1996, the US Advisory Committee on Immunization Practices did not begin recommending routine childhood vaccination for HAV until 2006. In 2007, infection rates were the lowest ever recorded, and a 95% drop in cases occurred through 2011.[18] Since 2016, however, there has been an exponential increase in HAV infections (**Fig. 1**). Notable outbreaks have occurred among unhoused patients, most of whom also share SUD as a risk factor. The Centers for Disease Control and Prevention (CDC) now recommends all persons who use or inject illicit drugs be vaccinated against HAV.

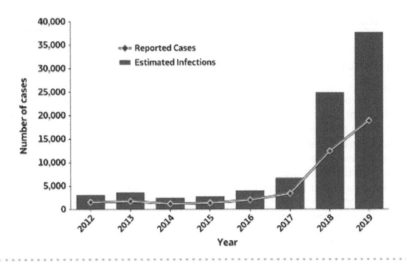

Fig. 1. Number of reported HAV infection cases and estimated infections, United States 2012 to 2019. Viral Hepatitis Surveillance Report 2018 — Hepatitis C. https://www.cdc.gov/hepatitis/statistics/2018surveillance/HepC.htm. Accessed 5/16/2022.

Hepatitis B and C

HBV and HCV infections are transmitted parenterally by infected blood and body fluids, including semen and vaginal secretions. Like other blood-borne pathogens such as HIV, the following 4 general categories of transmission and high-risk patient demographics are recognized.

- Iatrogenic: Blood- and organ-donor screening in the United States was not mandated for HBV until 1972, and for HCV until 1991; thus, anyone that received transfusions before these dates is at-risk. National health programs that used reusable needles, for example, in Egypt during the 1950s to 1980s to treat schistosomiasis, also transmitted millions of infections; Egypt is reported to have the highest prevalence of HCV in the world.
- Vertical: Prenatal screening and treatment of HBV, along with the vaccination of newborn infants which began in 1991, reduces vertical transmission rates. Unvaccinated infants born to HBV-positive mothers have up to a 90% chance of acquiring the infection (during pregnancy or through breastfeeding), and up to a 90% chance that the infection becomes chronic.[19] Vertical transmission is the primary risk factor for patients born in HBV-endemic nations (carrier rates >8%), including those in southeast and central Asia, sub-Saharan Africa, and the Amazon basin.
- Sexual: High-risk sexual behaviors involve any exposure to blood and body fluids without barrier protection. The presence of HIV infection confers an increased risk of both HBV and HCV upon exposure.
- Intravenous drug use (IVDU): Injection drug use was popularized in the United States in the early twentieth century when heroin was widely prescribed in place of opium to treat respiratory and other conditions. After addiction risk was noted, medical use ceased. However, the market for drug trafficking was created, and the use of reusable glass syringes and needles facilitated viral spread. Single-use plastic syringes invented in the 1950s potentially reduced this risk; however, users still share their "works." The US "war on drugs" began in 1971 and

escalated in 1986, as cases of viral hepatitis were increasingly recognized. Widespread promotion of the long-acting oral opioid Oxycontin, beginning in 1996, led to a sharp increase in the prevalence of opiate addiction and overdose. Crackdowns on drug diversion and pill mills made oral opioids too difficult or expensive to obtain, relegating addicts back to injecting heroin. The reemergence of blood-borne infections (HCV, HBV, and HIV) in the United States has hit the rural south the hardest, where heroin use is at an all-time high in young adults.

The incidence of new acute and chronic HCV infections continues to increase across all ages (**Fig. 2**). Over the last decade, young adults have caught up to "Baby Boomers" as the highest prevalence age group (**Fig. 3**). Regions hardest hit by the opioid epidemic report the highest number of cases (**Fig. 4**).

Hepatitis B Virus Screening Recommendations

Although chronic HBV is preventable with vaccination and effectively managed with viral suppressive medications in specific patients, it is not curable. Therefore, the CDC screening guidelines have remained unchanged and support screening with hepatitis B surface antigen (HBsAg) in the following populations.

- People born in countries with greater than 2% HBsAg prevalence
- People born in the United States not vaccinated as infants whose parents were born in regions with high rates of HBV infection (HBsAg prevalence $\geq$8%)
- Men who have sex with men
- People who inject drugs
- People with HIV
- Household and sexual contacts of people with HBV infection
- People requiring immunosuppressive therapy

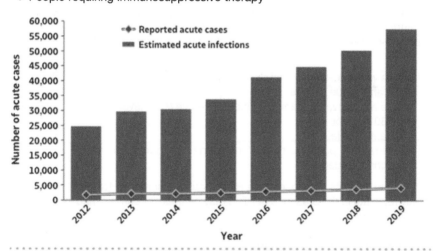

Acute Hepatitis C	2012	2013	2014	2015	2016	2017	2018	2019
Reported acute cases	1,778	2,138	2,194	2,436	2,967	3,216	3,621	4,136
Estimated acute infections	24,700	29,700	30,500	33,900	41,200	44,700	50,300	57,500

Fig. 2. Number of reported acute HCV infection cases and estimated infections, United States 2012 to 2019. Viral Hepatitis Surveillance Report 2018 — Hepatitis C. https://www.cdc.gov/hepatitis/statistics/2018surveillance/HepC.htm. Accessed 5/16/2022.

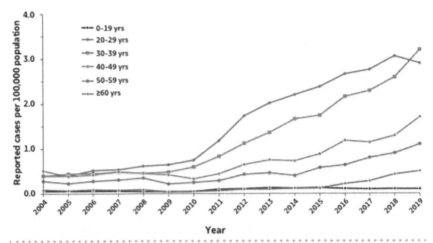

Age (years)	2004	2005	2006	2007	2008	2009	2010	2011	2012	2013	2014	2015	2016	2017	2018	2019
0–19	0.1	0.1	0.1	0.1	0.0	0.0	0.1	0.1	0.1	0.1	0.1	0.1	0.1	0.1	0.1	0.1
20–29	0.4	0.4	0.5	0.5	0.7	0.7	0.7	1.2	1.7	2.0	2.2	2.4	2.7	2.7	3.0	2.9
30–39	0.4	0.4	0.4	0.5	0.5	0.5	0.6	0.8	1.1	1.4	1.7	1.7	2.2	2.3	2.6	3.2
40–49	0.5	0.4	0.4	0.5	0.5	0.4	0.3	0.4	0.6	0.7	0.7	0.9	1.2	1.1	1.3	1.7
50–59	0.3	0.2	0.3	0.3	0.4	0.2	0.3	0.3	0.4	0.5	0.4	0.6	0.6	0.8	0.9	1.1
≥60	0.1	0.1	0.1	0.1	0.1	0.0	0.1	0.1	0.1	0.1	0.1	0.1	0.2	0.3	0.4	0.5

Source: CDC, National Notifiable Diseases Surveillance System.

Fig. 3. Over the last decade, young adults have caught up to "Baby Boomers" as the highest prevalence age group. Viral Hepatitis Surveillance Report 2018 — Hepatitis C. https://www.cdc.gov/hepatitis/statistics/2018surveillance/HepC.htm. Accessed 5/16/2022.

- People with end-stage renal disease (including those on hemodialysis)
- Blood and tissue donors
- People with elevated alanine aminotransferase (ALT) levels (>19 IU/L for women and >30 IU/L for men)
- Pregnant people
- Infants born to people with HBV infection (HBsAg and antibody to HBsAg only are recommended)

In addition, patients diagnosed with HBV should be screened for HDV. HDV, which can only replicate in the presence of HBV, may be acute or chronic, and increases the risk of liver failure.

Hepatitis B Virus Serologic Diagnosis

Fig. 5 illustrates how to interpret HBV and vaccination status. This is a very useful illustration for clinicians as they order and review HBV-related laboratory tests.

Hepatitis B Virus Vaccination

Vaccination for HBV is available for all ages and is given in a 3-dose series: 0, 1, to 2 months, and 4 to 6 months, with the minimum interval of 4 weeks between doses 1 and 2. The recommendation for routine vaccination of infants began in

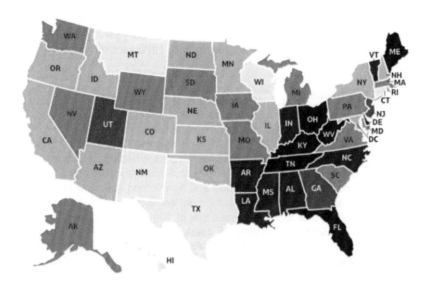

Color Key	Cases/100,000 Population	State or Jurisdiction
	0.0–0.2	CT, HI, MT, NM, TX, WI
	0.3–0.4	AZ, CA, CO, ID, IL, KS, MN, NH, NY, OK, OR
	0.5–0.8	AK, IA, MA, MD, MI, MO, NV, PA, SC, SD, VA, WA, WY
	0.9–1.1	GA, NJ, UT
	1.2–2.5	AL, AR, DE, IN, LA, MS, NC, VT
	2.6–4.3	FL, KY, ME, OH, TN, WV
	Data not available	DC, ND, NE, RI

Source: CDC. National Notifiable Diseases Surveillance System

Fig. 4. Acute HBV by state or jurisdiction—United States, 2019. Viral Hepatitis Surveillance Report 2018 — Hepatitis C. https://www.cdc.gov/hepatitis/statistics/2018surveillance/HepC.htm. Accessed 5/16/2022.

	Acute HBV	Chronic HBV	Cleared HBV	Vaccination
HBcAb IgM	+	-	-	-
HBcAb IgG	+	+	+	-
HBsAg	+	+	-	-
Anti-HBs	-	-	+	+
HBeAg	+	+/-	-	-
Anti-HBe	-	+/-	+/-	-
HBV DNA	High/Low	Low/High	-	-

Fig. 5. Helpful illustration to interpret HBV and vaccination status. IgG, immunoglobulin G; IgM, immunoglobulin M. Hepatitis B Serology Test Result Interpretation, by Acharya Tankeshwarin, Virology-Microbeonline.com, July 21, 2022. https://microbeonline.com/interpretation-of-hepatitis-b-serologic-test-results. Accessed 7/15/2022.

1991, and vaccination is now recommended for all adults through age 60 years regardless of risk factors. Adults over the age of 60 years with risk factors, including those with SUD, should be vaccinated. HBV vaccination also prevents HDV infection.

Hepatitis B Virus Treatment

The American Association for the Study of Liver Diseases (AASLD) provides guidelines for the treatment of chronic HBV. Approximately 0.5% of patients with chronic HBV per year will either spontaneously, or while on treatment, clear HBsAg, which is considered an immunologic "cure." HBV DNA remains in hepatocyte nuclei however, and the infection may reactivate. The goal of medical treatment, therefore, is to reduce morbidity and mortality; reducing viral load and normalizing ALT slow progression to end-stage liver disease and decrease (but do not eliminate) risk of HCC. In pregnant patients, reduction of viral load decreases risk of vertical transmission to the fetus. Treatment decisions are based on disease phase, which is determined by the patient's laboratory test values (ALT, viral load, and e-Antigen status): *immune tolerant phase*, *immune active phase*, *inactive phase*, or *reactivation phase*. The phase of chronic HBV evolves over time; when to start and stop medical treatment is beyond the scope of this article but is described by AASLD.[20]

Whether the patient is actively being treated, chronic HBV requires close laboratory monitoring and follow-up for life. Patients on medical treatment may develop drug resistance, particularly with low adherence, and all patients with chronic HBV need lifelong screening for HCC. Referral to a gastroenterologist, hepatologist, and/or ID specialist is recommended for optimal patient management.

Medications Approved for the Treatment of Hepatitis B Virus

Fig. 6 lists medications approved for the treatment of HBV, including the name of the medication, dose, pregnancy category, and adverse effects.

Medication	Dose	Pregnancy Category	Adverse Effects
Peg-Interferon alpha 2a – adults 2b – children	180 mcg injected SQ weekly (adults)	C	Flu-like symptoms, depression, cytopenias, autoimmune disorders in adults
Lamivudine	100 mg po daily	C	Pancreatitis, lactic acidosis
Telbivudine	600 mg po daily	B	Myopathy, neuropathy, Lactic acidosis. Not used in children.
Entecavir	0.5 – 1 mg po daily	C	Lactic acidosis
Adefovir	10 mg po daily	C	Acute renal failure, nephrogenic diabetes insipidus, lactic acidosis
Tenofovir	300 mg po daily	B	Nephropathy, osteomalacia, lactic acidosis

Fig. 6. Medications approved for the treatment of HBV. (Source: https://www.ncbi.nlm.nih.gov/pmc/articles/PMC5975958/.)

Medication	Dose	Pregnancy Category	Adverse Effects
Peg-Interferon alpha 2a, adults 2b, children	180 μg injected SQ weekly (adults)	C	Flulike symptoms, depression, cytopenias, autoimmune disorders in adults
Lamivudine	100 mg po daily	C	Pancreatitis, lactic acidosis
Telbivudine	600 mg po daily	B	Myopathy, neuropathy, lactic acidosis Not used in children
Entecavir	0.5–1 mg po daily	C	Lactic acidosis
Adefovir	10 mg po daily	C	Acute renal failure, nephrogenic diabetes insipidus, lactic acidosis
Tenofovir	300 mg po daily	B	Nephropathy, osteomalacia, lactic acidosis

Although medications used for chronic HBV may be also used for acute HBV, the vast majority of patients with acute HBV do not require medication and recover over several weeks to months with supportive care.

Hepatitis C Virus Screening Recommendations

Hepatitis C is the most commonly reported blood-borne infection in the United States. Although there is no vaccine for HCV, this infection is now curable with the advent of direct-acting antiviral agents (DAAs). Before development of these novel agents, interferon-based therapies were poorly tolerated and achieved cure rates of less than 50%; thus, routine screening was not recommended and remained risk-based. The recognition of "Baby Boomers" as a high-risk population began in 2016; birth cohort–based screening was recommended, for the first time including those with no identifiable risk factors nor ALT elevation. At that time, people born between 1945 and 1965 carried the highest infection rate, attributed in part to widespread drug use during the 1970s to 1980s.[21] New HCV infections have skyrocketed over the last decade in the young adult population, primarily because of the opioid epidemic. This shift in demographic, coupled with access to curative medications, forms the basis for new screening guidelines. The USPSTF now recommends that all persons aged 18 to 79 years be screened at least once with anti-HCV antibody testing.[22] The CDC also recommends screening for all adults over 18 years and pregnant patients with each pregnancy, in addition to continued screening for those with identifiable risk factors, exposures, or elevated ALT.[23] It is important to note that individual laboratory values for normal ALT vary; the standardized normal range for ALT should be used instead: less than 30 for men and less than 19 for women.[24]

Hepatitis C Virus Treatment

Current treatment for HCV with novel DAA is well tolerated and highly effective across all genotypes, unlike previous interferon-based regimens. Treatment is no longer limited by viral genotype, fibrosis stage, or active substance use. Combination therapy is still recommended, but the development of all-oral once-daily combination tablets has substantially reduced pill burden and risk of poor adherence. AASLD updated its guidelines for the management of HCV in 2019: "Antiviral treatment is recommended for all adults with acute or chronic HCV infection except those with a short life expectancy that cannot be remediated by HCV therapy, liver transplantation, or another directed therapy".[25]

Medications approved for chronic HCV include the following:

- Combination glecaprevir 300 mg/pibrentasvir 120 mg (Mavyret) po once daily for 8 wk
- Combination sofosbuvir 400 mg/velpatasvir 100 mg (Epclusa) po once daily for 12 wk
- Combination ledipasvir 90 mg/sofosbuvir 400 mg (Harvoni) po once daily for 12 wk (only in genotype 1, 4, 5, or 6)

As with chronic HBV, patients with chronic HCV infection should be referred to a gastroenterologist, hepatologist, and/or ID specialist to ensure appropriate monitoring and risk assessment for complications, including cirrhosis, esophageal varices, and HCC.

Patient Education and Follow-Up

Immune-competent adults who recover from acute HAV or HBV develop antibodies that confer lifelong protection from reinfection. Up to 10% of adults with acute HBV will develop chronic HBV; thus, serologies should be followed for 6 months to confirm loss of HBsAg and appearance of hepatitis B surface antibody (HBsAb), indicating recovery. In contrast, up to 80% of patients with acute HCV develop chronic infection. Those who do clear HCV, whether spontaneously or with medical treatment, are not immune from reinfection, leaving patients with continued risk factors (including SUD) vulnerable.

Highlights for Clinicians

Health care providers should direct patients to credible sources of information, such as Web sites for the CDC, World Health Organization, and National Institutes of Health–National Institute for Diabetes Digestive and Kidney Disease. The American Liver Foundation (https://liverfoundation.org/for-patients/about-the-liver/health-wellness/), Hepatitis B Foundation (https://www.hepb.org/), and US Department of Veterans Affairs (https://www.hepatitis.va.gov/index.asp) also provide helpful patient education and resources.

Patients should be cautioned with viral hepatitis to avoid all alcohol, referring to recovery groups, such as Alcoholics Anonymous, if needed. Also, patients should be educated to avoid alternative remedies purported to "cure" hepatitis or "improve" liver function owing to potential hepatotoxicity. Patients should be advised to discuss all medications and supplements they are taking with their clinicians; more than 600 medications, including over-the-counter, supplements, and herbs, are documented hepatotoxins.[26] Cannabidiol, which many patients with SUD consider "safe," has also demonstrated hepatotoxicity in some studies.[27]

HUMAN IMMUNODEFICIENCY VIRUS AND SUBSTANCE USE DISORDER

HIV incidence in the United States in 2019 was estimated to be 36,337,[28] and prevalence was estimated to be close to 1.2 million.[29] Linkage to care in 2019 was estimated to be 790,800 (65.9%), and viral suppression of all persons living with HIV was estimated at 681,600 (56.8%). The HIV Care Continuum includes diagnosis of HIV infection, linkage to care, receipt of care, retention in the care, and achievement and maintenance of HIV suppression.[29] In the United States in 2019, only 7% of new HIV infections were in people who inject drugs.[29] However, substance use has a significant role in the transmission of HIV primarily owing to risky sexual behaviors by persons living with HIV who are not virologically suppressed. Although 75% of newly diagnosed patients with HIV are linked to HIV medical care, only 58% of all persons living with HIV in the United States are virologically suppressed.[28] Viral suppression is a key strategy in the Ending the HIV Epidemic Initiative, which aims to reduce new HIV infections by 75% by 2025 and by 90% by 2030.[29]

Barriers to achieving viral suppression in people living with HIV are multifactorial; however, substance use continues to play a large role in failure to achieve viral suppression and failure to remain virologically suppressed. A study by Shiau and colleagues[30] published in 2017 reviewed data from the National Survey on Drug Use and Health looking at drug use characteristics in HIV-infected patients (n = 548). Of respondents, 46.1% reported illegal drug use in the past year, and 36% reported illegal drug use in the past month. An analysis of hazardous alcohol use in persons living with HIV (n = 8567) by Crane and colleagues[31] showed 27% of persons living with HIV reported hazardous alcohol use and 34% reported binge drinking. When examining the correlation between substance use and disruption in the HIV Care Continuum, there are several key factors to consider. Persons living with HIV who use substances are less likely to obtain HIV testing, seek care, remain in care, initiate antiretroviral therapy (ART), and remain adherent to ART. It is well known that substance use interferes with judgment, decreases inhibition, and can increase risky behaviors. These may include condomless intercourse and needle or other equipment sharing. Concern over continuing ART while using substances also exists. Many substance users living with HIV fear neg. consequences, owing to possible interactions between the substance and ART regimen and choose not to take ART while using. Mental health disorders often coincide with SUD and HIV. The HIV Care Continuum can also be disrupted if the person living with HIV does not have the correct diagnosis and appropriate treatment of an underlying mental health disorder.

Human Immunodeficiency Virus Treatment

Caring for persons living with HIV who use substances or have SUD should include careful consideration of all factors. Screening for substance use and discussing sexual practices and mental health should occur with every visit. Questions should be phrased in an open and nonjudgmental manner, which improves the provider-patient relationship, as well as maintains patient trust in their ability to answer honestly. When active substance use has been identified, clinicians should aim to select an ART regimen with a high genetic barrier to resistance owing to greater possibility of poor adherence and improper follow-up. Adverse effect profile, food requirements, and ease of taking medication should also be considered in patients with substance use. A regimen with a low risk of hepatotoxicity in patients with alcohol use disorder or methamphetamine use disorder should be chosen. This is especially important in patients coinfected with HIV/HCV, which is more commonly seen in people who inject drugs. In addition, other standard factors, including resistance testing, other comorbidities, HLA-B*5701 status, and drug-drug interactions, should be reviewed before ART initiation. The Panel on Antiretroviral Guidelines for Adults and Adolescents (The Panel), updated in January 2022,[32] recommends boosted protease inhibitor (PI) regimens or a second integrase strand transfer inhibitor (INSTI) regimen with either bictegravir or dolutegravir for patients with concern about poor adherence.[33] Both bictegravir- and dolutegravir-containing regimens are included in The Panel's recommended regimens for most people with HIV.[33] Bictegravir and dolutegravir are both INSTIs and are combined with a one- or 2-drug nucleoside reverse transcriptase inhibitor (NRTI) backbone to constitute the ART regimen. Boosted PI regimens containing darunavir/cobicistat or darunavir/ritonavir combined with a 2-drug NRTI backbone are included in The Panel's recommended initial regimens for certain clinical situations.[33] PI regimens have been well known for their high genetic barrier to resistance; however, the FLAMINGO[34] and ARIA[35] trials both compared dolutegravir and boosted PI regimens with no INSTI or PI treatment-emergent resistance observed. INSTI regimens are generally well tolerated and have no food or gastric acidity requirement. Food intake is required with PI regimens. The toxicity profile of INSTIs is also low, and there are fewer drug-drug interactions than with PI regimens. Choosing a simplified regimen that is well tolerated and lacks additional requirements will improve adherence rates and allow the best opportunity for virologic suppression.

Obtaining an accurate and thorough patient history of substance use will assist in selecting the appropriate regimen to ensure there are no potential drug-drug interactions. Certain benzodiazepines and opioids, for example, are boosted by PIs. One PI, ritonavir, has been shown to increase methamphetamine effects. There are no known interactions between illicit drugs and integrase inhibitor regimens. Once an ART regimen has been selected, thorough patient education should follow. Medication adherence should certainly be addressed; however, patients with substance use should also be educated that it is acceptable and preferred to continue ART even when actively using. For patients with injection or intravenous drug use, it is essential to advise against sharing needles or other equipment. Ensuring follow-up is made before patient discharge and involving case management and nursing staff in medication and appointment adherence can also improve patient retention in care and ability to achieve and maintain virologic suppression.

Long-acting antiretroviral therapy (LA-ART) is currently being used and at the forefront of future HIV treatment modalities. Cabotegravir-rilpivirine is a LA-ART approved for the use in patients who are virologically suppressed and have no history of treatment failure. Cabotegravir-rilpivirine is a long-acting injectable administered once monthly or once every other month. Lack of adherence by missing injection appointments and drug resistance occurring as a result are concerns with the use of LA-ART in patients with active SUD. The LATITUDE Study: Long-Acting Therapy to Improve Treatment Success in Daily Life[36] is an open-label phase III study to evaluate long-acting ART in nonadherent HIV-infected individuals with an estimated completion date of October 2025. Results from this study could show effective treatment and increased adherence, thus leading to virologic suppression long term in persons living with HIV and concurrent SUD.

Despite adherence to ART and long-term virologic suppression, research shows that HIV causes a chronic, systemic inflammatory response. Substance use amplifies this response, specifically in the brain, and can lead to a more rapid disease progression as well as neurocognitive effects, such as seen in NeuroHIV.[37]

Highlights for Clinicians

Health care providers should review credible sources of information, such as CDC resources for clinicians (https://www.cdc.gov/hiv/clinicians/index.html). Mental health disorders are also quite common in persons living with HIV and SUD. Efforts should be focused on effectively treating HIV, SUD, as well as mental health disorders if present. An integrated and comprehensive care model centered on HIV testing in persons with SUD and subsequent extension into the HIV Care Continuum for persons diagnosed with HIV could reduce barriers, aid in slowing disease progression, and reduce the likelihood of neurocognitive effects. Effective treatment of SUD has also been proven to increase virologic suppression and retention in care, thereby reducing HIV transmission[37] and moving us closer to Ending the HIV Epidemic.

Clinicians should have continuing dialogue with their patients regarding their substance use, high-risk sexual behavior, social support, mental illness, comorbidities, and economic factors.[38] All health care team members, including HIV specialists, primary care providers, pharmacists, social workers, behavioral health workforce, and all other medical and support professionals, should team up and manage patients with HIV.[39] When managing these patients, having a multidisciplinary approach, evidence-based practices, and patient-centered care will lead to favorable outcomes.[38]

Figs. 7 and **8** reveal some helpful information to clinicians and other health care workers. According to current trends, white people (see **Fig. 8**) and gay and bisexual categories have the highest risk of contracting HIV through injecting drugs in the United States. **Fig. 9** demonstrates that ages between 25 and 34 years are the highest risk for contracting HIV through drug use. All these statistics are helpful when developing plans to alleviate HIV infections through drug use.

The evidence is clear that increased SUD will lead to more IDs, including HIV. At the same time, the development of ART has allowed HIV to be a chronic and manageable condition. Collectively, it is anticipated that HIV infections will stay in the United States for many years to come. However, there are not enough clinicians to manage patients with HIV, and so the challenge continues. Wijesinghe and Alexander[39] concluded that encouraging more primary care clinicians to get involved with HIV medicine may be the solution to this problem. Therefore, it is important to find novel approaches to motivate more PAs, NPs, and physicians to treat and manage patients with HIV.

Other Highlights for Clinicians

According to **Fig. 9**, it is reasonable to state that despite the allocated federal funds to prevent SUDs, the prevalence of SUDs has increased: this outcome warrants an analysis, explanation, and inquiry into whether the funds were used sagaciously. Most important of all will be to figure out the best strategy to alleviate this problem in the future.

Thirty-nine percent of physicians and 9% of pharmacists were responsible for the opioid crisis. It is critical to have an urgent intervention on this. The solution is not to

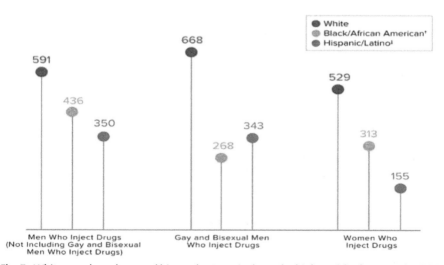

Fig. 7. White people and gay and bisexual categories have the highest risk of contracting HIV through injecting drugs in the United States. †, Black refers to people having origins in any of the Black racial groups of Africa. African American is a term often used for people of African descent with ancestry in North America. ‡, Hispanic/Latino people can be of any race. HIV and People Who Inject Drugs. https://www.cdc.gov/hiv/group/hiv-idu.html. Accessed 5/20/2022.

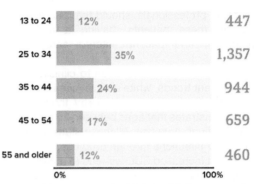

Fig. 8. Ages between 25 and 34 years are the highest risk for contracting HIV through drug use. HIV and People Who Inject Drugs. https://www.cdc.gov/hiv/group/hiv-idu.html. Accessed 5/20/2022.

avoid prescribing any opioids even for patients who are experiencing excruciating pain after surgery. However, additional training for clinicians on how to assess benefits and risks regarding treatment plans is important. The consequences of overprescribing substances should be considered and implemented in policies.

ID clinicians treat and manage patients with infectious consequences of SUD. Although ID clinicians are capable of handling the ID, a multidisciplinary team approach is the best way to successfully manage these patients as they require collaboration with other specialties, such as addtion medicine. However, ID clinicians may need to initiate managing some SUDs and maintain care until they consult an

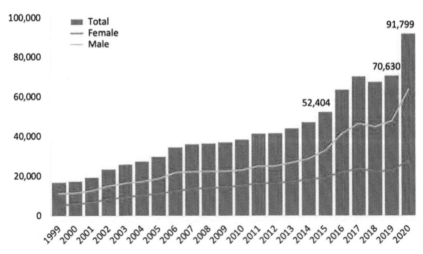

*Includes deaths with underlying causes of unintentional drug poisoning (X40–X44), suicide drug poisoning (X60–X64), homicide drug poisoning (X85), or drug poisoning of undetermined intent (Y10–Y14), as coded in the International Classification of Diseases, 10th Revision. Source: Centers for Disease Control and Prevention, National Center for Health Statistics. Multiple Cause of Death 1999-2020 on CDC WONDER Online Database, released 12/2021.

Fig. 9. National drug-involved overdose death: number among all ages, by gender, United States 1999 to 2020. *, Based on sex assigned at birth and includes transgender people. Drug Overdose Death Rates - Trends & Statistics. https://nida.nih.gov/research-topics/trends-statistics/overdose-death-rates. Accessed 5/20/2023.

addiction medicine specialist. Therefore, having additional training on SUD to ID specialist is recommended.

While the current number if HIV infections is approx. A 36,000, up until a few years ago, infection rates were as high as 50,000 annually. We have come a long way since. However, it remains vital to not only plan for but fight HIV infections as a continued threat to humankind. Hepatitis is no different. When fighting these infections, preventing SUD-led HIV and hepatitis should be a priority. A deliberate plan may help to reduce many HIV and hepatis infections.

SUMMARY

SUDs increase a user's odds of contracting IDs. The viral infections of highest concern related to substance use include HIV and hepatitis. Individuals may contract or transmit a viral infection when they inject drugs and share needles or other drug equipment. Substances also impair judgment and may cause users to make risky decisions, including having unprotected sex. Women who become infected with a virus may pass it to their baby during pregnancy or while breastfeeding. Individuals can reduce their risk of contracting or transmitting a viral infection by avoiding drugs, taking PrEP if they are at high risk for infection, screening for HIV and hepatis, consistently practicing safer sex, receiving the HBV/HAV vaccine, and seeking treatment for substance use. Every clinician treating and managing ID should have a fundamental knowledge about SUD as well as strategies to help pts before referring them to addiction specialists. It appears that despite recent efforts, that SUD-related cases of HIV and hepatitis have been increasing. Therefore, we must re-evaluate and appropriately update the current approach.

CLINICS CARE POINTS

- Review the highlights for clinicians on all sections: substance use disorders, hepatitis, and human immunodeficiency virus.

- Understand the correlation between substance use disorder and HIV/hepatitis.

- Both competent care and compassionate care are equally important when managing patients with infectious diseases and substance use disorders.

- When treating a patient for an infectious disease, investigate if there is an underlying substance use disorder and help him/her as appropriate.

- When prescribing opioids to patients, weigh both risks and benefits and prescribe only if appropriate.

- Educate patients about screening, prevention (vaccine, preexposure prophylaxis), and treatments of these viral infections.

- Despite largely allocated funds and efforts, the number of infectious diseases linked with substance use disorders has been increasing. Therefore, it is time to reassess the current system and restructure it as appropriate; the authors believe every clinician can a play a role to lessen the problem.

ACKNOWLEDGMENTS

N.K. Wijesinghe, BSc and Ariana O'Malley, PA-S supported us with proofreading and by making sure all the references are accurate. The authors appreciate their support.

DISCLOSURE

The authors have nothing to disclose.

REFERENCES

1. Centers for Disease Control and Prevention. National Hospital Ambulatory Medical Care Survey: 2018 Emergency Department Summary Tables. Available at: https://www.cdc.gov/nchs/data/nhamcs/web_tables/2018-ed-web-tables-508.pdf. Accessed July 17, 2022.

2. Centers for Disease Control and Prevention. Death rates Maps and Graphs: Drug Overdose Deaths Remains High. Updated June 2, 2022. Available at: https://www.cdc.gov/drugoverdose/deaths/. Accessed July 10, 2022.

3. Hedegaard H, Miniño AM, Spencer MR, et al. Drug Overdose Deaths in the United States, 1999–2020. National Center for Health Statistics. 2021. Available at: https://www.cdc.gov/nchs/products/databriefs/db428.htm. Accessed July 10, 2022.

4. Centers for Disease Control and Prevention. Diagnoses of HIV infection in the United States and dependent areas, 2019. HIV Surveillance Report 2021;32, 2021. Available at: https://www.cdc.gov/hiv/pdf/library/reports/surveillance/cdc-hiv-surveillance-report-2018-updated-vol-32.pdf. Accessed July 12, 2022.

5. Centers for Disease Control and Prevention. Viral hepatitis surveillance—United States, 2017. 2019. Available at: https://www.cdc.gov/hepatitis/statistics/2017 surveillance/index.htm. Accessed July 10, 2022.

6. Centers for Disease Control and Prevention. Viral Hepatitis Surveillance—United States, 2019. Updated May 19, 2021. Available at: https://www.cdc.gov/hepatitis/statistics/2019surveillance/index.htm. Accessed July 5, 2022.

7. Patel EU, Thio CL, Boon D, et al. Prevalence of Hepatitis B and Hepatitis D virus infections in the United States, 2011–2016. Clin Infect Dis 2019;69(4):709–12.

8. Tohme RA, Drobeniuc J, Sanchez R, et al. Acute hepatitis associated with autochthonous hepatitis E virus infection–San Antonio, Texas, 2009. Clin Infect Dis 2011; 53(8):793–6.

9. American Psychiatric Association. Diagnostic and statistical manual of mental disorders DSM-5. 5th edition. DSM-5: American Psychiatric Publishing; 2013. https://doi.org/10.1176/appi.books.9780890425596.

10. U.S. Department of Health and Human Services. Key substance use and mental health indicators in the United States: Results from the 2020 National Survey on Drug Use and Health. 2021;PEP21-07-01-003. Available at: https://www.samhsa.gov/data/sites/default/files/reports/rpt35325/NSDUHFFRPDFWHTMLFiles2020/2020NSDUHFFR1PDFW102121.pdf. Accessed June 30, 2022.

11. Kolla BP, Oesterle T, Gold M, et al. Infectious diseases occurring in the context of substance use disorders: A concise review. J Neurosci 2020;411:116719.

12. Gossop M, Griffiths P, Powis B, et al. Severity of dependence and route of administration of heroin, cocaine, and amphetamines. Br J Addic 1992;87(11):1527–36.

13. Zibbell JE, Asher AK, Patel RC, et al. Increases in Acute Hepatitis C Virus Infection Related to a Growing Opioid Epidemic and Associated Injection Drug Use, United States, 2004 to 2014. Am J Pub Health 2018;108(2):175–81.

14. US Department of Health & Human Services. Viral Hepatitis National Strategic Plan Overview. Updated January 7, 2021. Available at: https://www.hhs.gov/hepatitis/viral-hepatitis-national-strategic-plan/national-viral-hepatitis-action-plan-overview/index.html. Accessed June 15, 2022.

15. Pramoolsinsap C, Poovorawan Y, Hirsch P, et al. Acute, hepatitis-A super-infection in HBV carriers, or chronic liver disease related to HBV or HCV. Ann Trop Med Parasitol 1999;93(7):745–51.

16. Consumer Health Ratings. How much does an Organ Transplant cost? Available at: https://consumerhealthratings.com/?healthcare_entry=how-much-does-an-organ-transplant-cost. Accessed July 5, 2022.

17. Latt NL, Niazi M, Pyrsopoulos NT. Liver transplant allocation policies and outcomes in United States: A comprehensive review. World J Methodol 2022; 12(1):32–42.

18. Nelson NP, Weng MK, Hofmeister MG, et al. Prevention of Hepatitis A Virus Infection in the United States: Recommendations of the Advisory Committee on Immunization Practices. MMWR Recomm Rep (Morb Mortal Wkly Rep) 2020;69(No. RR-5):1–38.

19. Hepatitis B Foundation. Pregnancy and Hepatitis B. Updated September 2020. Available at: https://www.hepb.org/treatment-and-management/pregnancy-and-hbv/. Accessed June 30, 2022.

20. American Association for the Study of Liver Diseases. American Association for the Study of Liver Diseases Hepatitis C Guidance 2019 Update: American Association for the Study of Liver Diseases–Infectious Diseases Society of America Recommendations for Testing, Managing, and Treating Hepatitis C Virus Infection. Hepatology 2020;71(2). Available at: https://aasldpubs.onlinelibrary.wiley.com/doi/pdf/10.1002/hep.31060. Accessed June 10, 2022.

21. Boucher CM, Walsh A, Forest CP. Healing livers, saving lives: Hepatitis C screening in an era of cure. JAAPA 2016;29(5):20–8.

22. US Preventive Services Task Force. Hepatitis C Virus Infection in Adolescents and Adults: Screening. Updated March 2, 2020. Available at: https://www.uspreventiveservicestaskforce.org/uspstf/recommendation/hepatitis-c-screening. Accessed July 5, 2022.

23. Schillie S, Wester C, Osborne M, et al. CDC Recommendations for Hepatitis C Screening Among Adults — United States, 2020. MMWR Morb Mortal Wkly Rep 2020;69(2):1–17. Available at: https://www.cdc.gov/mmwr/volumes/69/rr/rr6902a1.htm. Accessed June 10, 2022.

24. Neuschwander-Tetri BA, Ünalp A, Creer MH. The upper limits of normal for serum ALT levels reported by clinical laboratories depend on local reference populations. Arch Intern Med 2004;168(6):663–6.

25. Björnsson ES. Hepatotoxicity by drugs: the most common implicated agents. Int J Mol Sci 2016;17(2):224.

26. Ewing LE, Skinner CM, Quick CM, et al. Hepatotoxicity of a Cannabidiol-rich cannabis extract in the mouse model. Molecules 2019;24(9):1694.

27. National Center for HIV, Viral Hepatitis, STD, and TB Prevention. HIV Hepatitis STD TB Social Determinants of Health Data. 2021. Available at: https://www.cdc.gov/nchhstp/atlas/index.htm. Accessed May 14, 2022.

28. HIV.Org. New HIV Infections (HIV Incidence). 2021. Available at: https://www.hiv.gov/hiv-basics/overview/data-and-trends/statistics. Accessed May 14, 2022.

29. HIV.Org. What Is Ending the HIV Epidemic in the U.S.? Updated July 1, 2022. Available at: https://www.hiv.gov/federal-response/ending-the-hiv-epidemic/overview. Accessed July 6, 2022.

30. Shiau S, Arpadi SM, Yin MT, et al. Patterns of drug use and HIV infection among adults in a nationally represented sample. Addict Behav 2017;39–44.

31. Crane H, McCaul ME, Chandler J, et al. Prevalence and factors associated with hazardous alcohol use among persons living with HIV across the US in the current era of antiretroviral treatment. AIDS Behav 2017;1914–25.

32. HIV.Org. Guidelines for the Use of Antiretroviral Agents in Adults and Adolescents Living with HIV. Updated June 3, 2021. Available at: https://clinicalinfo.hiv.gov/en/guidelines/adult-and-adolescent-arv/substance-use-disorders-and-hiv?view=full. Accessed May 14, 2022.

33. Molina JM, Colet B, Van Lunez J, et al. Once-daily dolutegravir versus darunavir plus ritonavir for treatment-naive adults with HIV-1 infection (FLAMINGO): 96 week results from a randomised, open-label, phase 3b study. Lancet HIV 2015;127–36.

34. Orrell C, Hagins DP, Belonosova E, et al. Fixed-dose combination dolutegravir, abacavir, and lamivudine versus ritonavir-boosted atazanavir plus tenofovir disoproxil fumarate and emtricitabine in previously untreated women with HIV-1 infection (ARIA): week 48 results from a randomised, open-label. Lancet HIV 2017;536–46.

35. ClinicalTrials.gov. The LATITUDE Study: Long-Acting Therapy to Improve Treatment SUccess in Daily LifE, 2021. Available at: https://clinicaltrials.gov/ct2/show/NCT03635788. Accessed May 14, 2022.

36. National Library of Medicine. Common Comorbidities with Substance Use Disorders Research Report. 2021. Available at: https://www.ncbi.nlm.nih.gov/books/NBK571451/. Accessed May 25, 2022.

37. Van Rhee J, Bruce C, Neary S. *Clinical Medicine for Physician Assistants*. In: Wijesinghe S, Van Rhee J, editors. Infectious diseases. 1st ed. Springer Publishing; 2022.

38. Mathematica Policy Research. Gap in supply of HIV clinicians expected to increase. Available at: https://www.mathematica-mpr.com/news/hiv-specialist. Accessed May 25, 2022.

39. Wijesinghe S, Alexander JL. Management and treatment of HIV: are primary care clinicians prepared for their new role? BMC Fam Pract 2020;21(1):130.

Moving?

Make sure your subscription moves with you!

To notify us of your new address, find your **Clinics Account Number** (located on your mailing label above your name), and contact customer service at:

Email: **journalscustomerservice-usa@elsevier.com**

800-654-2452 (subscribers in the U.S. & Canada)
314-447-8871 (subscribers outside of the U.S. & Canada)

Fax number: 314-447-8029

Elsevier Health Sciences Division
Subscription Customer Service
3251 Riverport Lane
Maryland Heights, MO 63043

*To ensure uninterrupted delivery of your subscription, please notify us at least 4 weeks in advance of move.

Printed and bound by CPI Group (UK) Ltd, Croydon, CR0 4YY

03/10/2024

01040475-0001